# Laser Procedures

# A Practical Guide to

# Laser Procedures

**Series Editor**

## Rebecca Small, MD, FAAFP

Associate Clinical Professor
Department of Family and Community Medicine
University of California, San Francisco
Director, Medical Aesthetics Training
Natividad Medical Center
Family Medicine Residency Program – UCSF Affiliate
Salinas, CA

## Dalano Hoang, DC

Clinic Director
Monterey Bay Laser Aesthetics
Capitola, CA

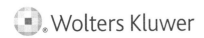

Philadelphia • Baltimore • New York • London
Buenos Aires • Hong Kong • Sydney • Tokyo

*Executive Editor:* Rebecca Gaertner
*Senior Product Development Editor:* Kristina Oberle
*Production Project Manager:* Kim Cox
*Manufacturing Manager:* Beth Welsh
*Marketing Manager:* Stephanie Kindlick
*Illustrator:* Liana Bauman
*Design Coordinator:* Doug Smock
*Production Service:* Aptara, Inc.

9  8  7  6

Printed in the United States of America

**Library of Congress Cataloging-in-Publication Data**

Small, Rebecca, author.
 A practical guide to laser procedures / Rebecca Small, Dalano Hoang.
   p. ; cm.
 Includes bibliographical references and index.
  ISBN 978-1-60913-150-0 (hardback)
 I. Hoang, Dalano, author. II. Title.
 [DNLM:   1.  Dermatologic Surgical Procedures–Handbooks.   2.  Laser Therapy–
methods–Handbooks.   3.  Cosmetic Techniques–Handbooks.  WR 39]
 RL120.L37
 617.4′770598–dc23

                                              2015017645

LWW.com

As a lecturer, editor, author, and medical reviewer, I have had ample opportunity to evaluate many speakers as well as extensive medical literature. After reviewing this series of books on cosmetic procedures by Rebecca Small, MD, I have concluded that it has to be one of the best and most detailed, yet practical presentation of the topics that I have ever encountered. As a physician whose practice is limited solely to providing office procedures, I see great value in these texts for clinicians and the patients they serve.

The goal of medical care is to make patients feel better and to help them experience an improved quality of life that extends for an optimal, productive period. Interventions may be directed at the emotional/psychiatric, medical/physical, or self-image areas.

For many physicians, performing medical procedures provides excitement in the practice of medicine. The ability to see what has been accomplished in a concrete way provides the positive feedback we all seek in providing care. Sometimes it involves removing a tumor. At other times it may be performing a screening procedure to be sure no disease is present. Maybe it's making patients feel better about their appearance. For whatever reason, the "hands on" practice of medicine is more rewarding for some practitioners.

In the late 80s and early 90s, there was resurgence in the interest of performing procedures in primary care. It did not involve hospital procedures, but rather, those that could be performed in the office. Coincidentally, patients also became interested in less invasive procedures such as laparoscopic cholecystectomy, endometrial ablation, and more. The desire for plastic surgery "extreme makeovers" waned as technology was developed to provide a gentle, more kind approach to "rejuvenation." Baby boomers were increasing in numbers and wanted to maintain their youthful appearance. This not only improved self-image, but it also helped when competing with a younger generation both socially and in the workplace.

These forces then of technological advances, provider interest, and patient desires have led to a huge increase in and demand for "minimally invasive procedures" that has extended to all of medicine. Plastic surgery and aesthetic procedures have indeed been affected by this movement. There have been many new procedures developed in just the last 10--15 years along with constant updates and improvements. As patient demand has soared for these new treatments, physicians have found that there is a whole new world of procedures they need to incorporate into their practice if they are going to provide the latest in aesthetic services.

Rebecca Small, MD, the editor and author of this series of books on cosmetic procedures, has been at the forefront of the aesthetic procedures movement. She has written extensively and conducted numerous workshops to help others learn the latest techniques. She has the practical experience to know just what the physician needs to develop a practice and provides "the latest and the best" in these books. Using her knowledge of the field, she has selected the topics wisely to include:

- A Practical Guide to: Botulinum Toxin Procedures
- A Practical Guide to: Dermal Filler Procedures
- A Practical Guide to: Chemical Peels, Microdermabrasion, and Topical Products
- A Practical Guide to: Laser Procedures

Dr. Small does not just provide a cursory, quick review of these subjects. Rather, they are an in-depth practical guide to performing these procedures. The emphasis here should be on "practical" and "in-depth." There is no extra esoteric waste of words, yet every procedure is explained in a clear, concise, useful format that allows practitioners of all levels of experience to learn and gain from reading these texts.

The basic outline of these books consists of the pertinent anatomy, the specific indications and contraindications, specific how-to diagrams and explanations on performing the procedures, complications and how to deal with them, tables with comparisons and amounts of materials needed, before and after patient instructions as well as consent forms (an immense time-saving feature), sample procedure notes, and a list of supply sources. An extensive updated bibliography is provided in each text for further reading. Photos are abundant depicting the performance of the procedures as well as before and after results. These comprehensive texts are clearly written for the practitioner who wants to "learn everything" about the topics covered. Patients definitely desire these procedures and Dr. Small has provided the information to meet the physician demand to learn them.

For those interested in aesthetic procedures, these books will be a godsend. Even for those not so interested in performing the procedures described, the reading is easy and interesting and will update the reader on what is currently available so they might better advise their patients.

Dr. Small has truly written a one-of-a-kind series of books on Cosmetic Procedures. It is my prediction that it will be received very well and be most appreciated by all who make use of it.

*John L. Pfenninger, MD, FAAFP*
*Founder and President, The Medical Procedures Center*
*PC Founder and Senior Consultant, The National Procedures Institute*
*Clinical Professor of Family Medicine, Michigan State College of Human Medicine*

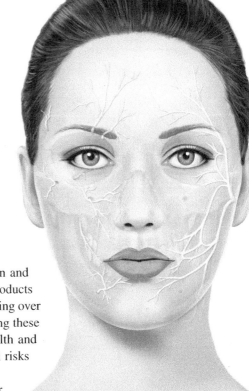

# Preface

Office-based cosmetic procedures such as botulinum toxin and dermal filler injections, chemical peels, lasers, and topical products have become the primary treatment modalities for facial aging over the last decade, and continue to be in high demand. Utilizing these procedures in an ongoing capacity can improve skin health and enhance appearance in a subtle, natural way with minimal risks relative to invasive surgical procedures.

The Practical Guide series, including this current laser book, was created to assist providers with acquiring the necessary knowledge and skill to perform minimally invasive, office-based cosmetic procedures. The books are not intended to be comprehensive, but rather focus on treatments that address the most commonly encountered aesthetic complaints. In addition, procedures were chosen that consistently achieve good outcomes and have a low incidence of side effects. While treatments can be performed independently, most procedures discussed complement and work synergistically with other aesthetic procedures to enhance results. Instruction on how to safely and effectively perform each procedure is provided using a concise step-by-step format.

The goal of this book is to bridge the gap between the operating information provided by laser manufacturers that may be too basic, and other available learning materials that may be too advanced as they assume prior knowledge of lasers. A summary of key concepts and treatment principles is provided at the beginning for convenient referencing. The introduction discusses how to perform an aesthetic consultation, assess patients' aesthetic complaints, and other fundamentals essential for successfully performing laser treatments. Each chapter is dedicated to a particular laser indication and includes sections on patient selection, contraindications, procedure preparation, treatment techniques with practical tips, desirable clinical endpoints to look for, and typical results with representative before and after treatment photographs. There are accompanying instructional videos to demonstrate procedures. Management of possible complications as well as the most commonly encountered issues seen in follow-up visits are reviewed. Up-to-date discussions of the latest technology developments and suggestions for combining lasers with other aesthetic procedures are also included for providers once they are familiarized with the basics.

The information presented in this Practical Guide series incorporates standard methods and techniques with practical suggestions and pearls from clinical experience gained from feedback teaching residents and fellow aesthetic providers. Hopefully, they will serve as clear and concise resources that assist providers to quickly and confidently gain proficiency with aesthetic procedures, and offer new treatment techniques for more seasoned providers. Books are of course not a replacement for experience and a formal training program, as well as precepting with an experienced provider, is recommended when learning aesthetic procedures.

# Acknowledgments

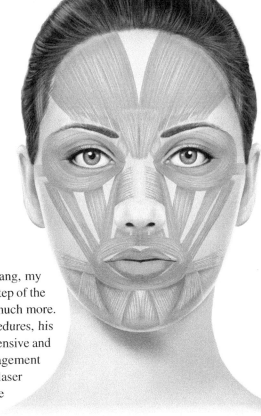

I have profound gratitude and respect for Dr. Dalano Hoang, my associate editor and husband. He has been with me every step of the way as the Clinic Director of our aesthetic practice and much more. Although he personally does not perform aesthetic procedures, his knowledge of the many facets of aesthetic medicine is extensive and invaluable. His clear, concise writing style and encouragement have been instrumental in yielding this straightforward laser procedure book as well as the other procedure books in the Practical Guide series on botulinum toxin, dermal fillers, and chemical peels and topical products.

A special thanks to Dr. John L. Pfenninger, who has inspired me, supported me and taught me much about educating and writing.

The University of California, San Francisco and the Natividad Medical Center family medicine residents deserve special recognition. Their interest and enthusiasm for aesthetic procedures led me to develop the first family medicine aesthetics training curriculum in 2008, and motivated me to write articles and editorials about aesthetics for the American Family Physician.

I'd also like to acknowledge the expert team at Wolters Kluwer Health who made these books possible, in particular, Kristina Oberle, Rebecca Gaertner, Doug Smock, and Freddie Patane. I've thoroughly enjoyed working with Liana Bauman, the gifted artist who created all of the illustrations for these books.

I am grateful to the experienced laser physicians and the specialists from Alma, Cutera, Cynosure, Lumenis, Lutronics, Sciton, and Solta for sharing their photographs and their expertise on laser technologies.

As with all my other works, I am dedicating this latest book in the series to my amazing son, Kaidan Hoang. I hope he's learning as much from me as I'm learning from him.

# Contents

*Procedure videos can be found on the book's website*

# Key References

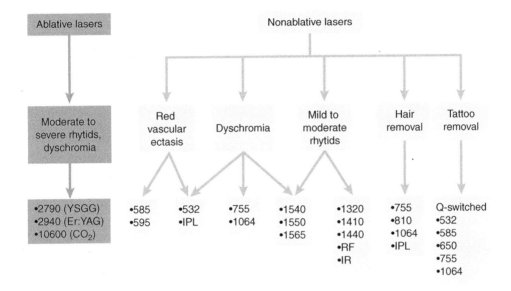

All wavelengths in nanometers

IPL = Intense pulsed light
IR = Infrared broadband light
RF = Radiofrequency

FIGURE 1 ● Lasers used for aesthetic conditions.

1

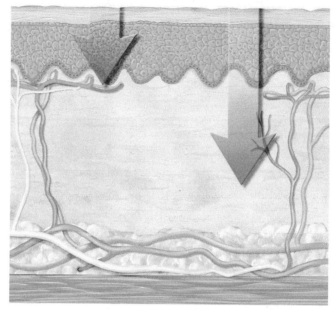

Short wavelength          Long wavelength
Short pulse width         Long pulse width
Small spot size           Large spot size
Low fluence               High fluence

*FIGURE 2* ● Factors affecting laser depth of penetration.

| Patient Characteristics | Lesion Characteristics | Laser Parameters | | |
|---|---|---|---|---|
| Dark Fitzpatrick skin type (IV–VI)<br><br>Nonfacial area | High density<br><br>Intense color | Conservative | Long wavelength<br>Long pulse width<br>Large spot size<br>Low fluence |
| Light Fitzpatrick skin type (I–III)<br><br>Face | Low density<br><br>Faint color | Aggressive | Short wavelength<br>Short pulse width<br>Small spot size<br>High fluence |

*FIGURE 3* ● Laser treatment parameters used for different patient and lesion characteristics.

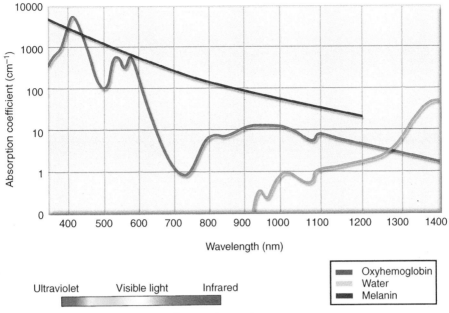

FIGURE 4 ● Absorption spectra of tissue chromophores.

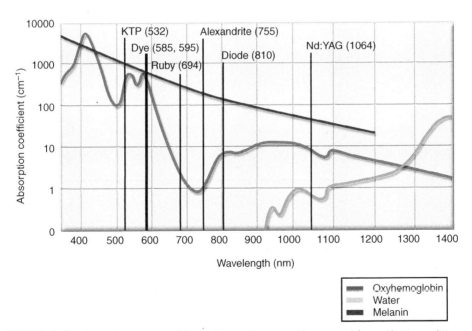

FIGURE 5 ● Absorption spectra of tissue chromophores and lasers used for aesthetic conditions.

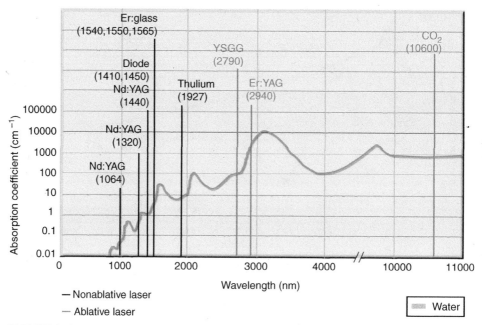

FIGURE 6 ● Water absorption spectrum and lasers used for skin resurfacing.

# Introduction and Foundation Concepts

Rebecca Small, M.D.

This Practical Guide focuses on laser and light-based technologies used to treat photoaged skin and other commonly encountered aesthetic conditions. The goals for rejuvenation of photoaged skin are to improve skin health and appearance through decreasing dyspigmentation, telangiectasias, erythema, and rhytids. A wide variety of laser and light-based technologies are available that target specific aspects of photoaging, enabling patient's individual rejuvenation needs to be met. This introduction presents the basic principles and concepts necessary to safely and effectively perform laser and light-based cosmetic treatments.

## Skin Aging

Over time skin naturally thins and loses elasticity. These intrinsic aging changes are accelerated and compounded by sun exposure. Photoaging is the term used to describe cutaneous damage caused by overexposure to UV light and is also referred to as extrinsic aging, dermatoheliosis, actinic damage, and photodamage. To appreciate the contribution of photoaging to the appearance of aged skin, photoprotected skin such as the inside of the upper forearm or under the chin can be compared to the appearance of photo-aged skin on face and back of the hands. Photoaged skin typically exhibits: **textural changes** such as rhytids (wrinkles) and roughness, **pigmentary changes** such as solar lentigines (sun spots), darkened ephelides (freckles) and actinic bronzing (background yellow-brown discoloration), **vascular changes** such as telangiectasias and erythema (redness), **sagging/laxity, fragility,** and **degenerative changes** such as actinic keratoses and neoplasia (skin cancers). Pigmentary changes, also referred to as **dyschromia,** can be darkened skin color referred to as **hyperpigmentation,** or lightened skin color referred to as **hypopigmentation**. Vascular changes are also referred to as **vascular ectasias.** Clinical findings seen in photoaged skin are reviewed in Figure 1 and Table 1.

## What Aspects of Photoaging Can Be Treated with Lasers?

Laser and light-based technologies can reduce wrinkles and rough texture of photoaged skin, treat dyschromia and vascular ectasias. Treatment of photoaged skin using laser and light-based technologies is referred to as **photorejuvenation**. These treatments can also be readily combined with other minimally invasive aesthetic procedures such as dermal fillers, botulinum toxin, and topical products to enhance results (see Combining Aesthetic Procedures section below).

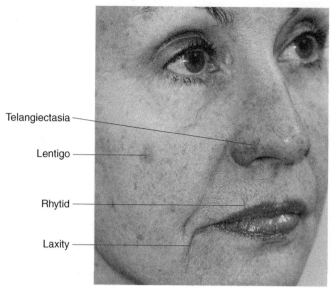

Telangiectasia —

Lentigo —

Rhytid —

Laxity —

*FIGURE 1* ● Photoaging changes. (Courtesy of R. Small, MD.)

## TABLE 1

### Clinical Findings in Photoaged Skin

**Pigmentary changes**
- Hyperpigmentation: lentigines, darkened ephelides, mottled pigmentation
- Poikiloderma of Civatte
- Hypopigmentation
- Sallow discoloration

**Vascular changes**
- Telangiectasias
- Erythema

**Textural changes**
- Rhytids
- Dilated pores
- Dry and rough skin
- Elastosis

**Sagging and laxity**

**Degenerative changes**
- Benign (e.g., seborrheic keratoses, sebaceous hyperplasia, cherry angiomas)
- Preneoplastic (e.g., actinic keratoses)
- Neoplastic (e.g., basal and squamous cell cancers and melanomas)

Laser

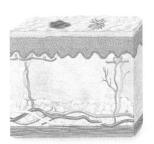
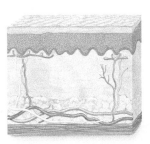

| Pretreatment | During treatment | Posttreatment |

*FIGURE 2* ● Selective photothermolysis.

## Laser Principles

The term LASER originated as an acronym for Light Amplification by Stimulated Emission of Radiation. Laser devices produce light of a single wavelength with parallel rays that minimally disperse, thus forming a monochromatic, collimated, highly focused beam. Intense pulsed light (IPL) devices emit light that has a broad spectrum of wavelengths with rays that disperse, forming polychromatic, divergent beams. Both lasers and IPL devices, collectively referred to as lasers[*] in this book, operate under the principle of **selective photothermolysis**. According to this principle, light of a specific wavelength is selectively absorbed by an undesired skin lesion such as a solar lentigo or telangiectasia; the lesion is heated, damaged and eliminated while the surrounding skin is left unaffected (Fig. 2). Unlike tracing a blood vessel with electrocautery to remove the vessel, lasers are not aimed at their target, rather they are directed at the skin and once the beam encounters its target, laser energy is selectively absorbed by the desired target.

When laser energy impacts skin, the beam may be **absorbed,** reflected, transmitted, or scattered (Fig. 3). All four interactions occur to some degree, but absorption is the most important clinically. Upon absorption, heat from the laser can elicit a spectrum of tissue responses that range from synthesis of dermal collagen which reduces wrinkles, to damaging growth structures of hair follicles and endothelial cells of blood vessels which eliminate undesired hair and vascular lesions, respectively. Absorption of laser energy depends on the presence of chromophores, light absorbing compounds. Laser treatment parameters are selected to have greater absorption by the target chromophore in the undesired lesion than chromophores in the surrounding skin.

The primary **chromophores** in skin are melanin, oxyhemoglobin, and water, and each has a unique absorption spectrum (Fig. 4, Key References). The chromophore in red vascular lesions is **oxyhemoglobin,** which shows strong absorption at 400–600 nm with peaks at 418, 542, and 577 nm and has some absorption at 750–1100 nm. The chromophore in pigmented lesions and dark hair is **melanin**. Melanin absorbs light across a wide spectrum of wavelengths with greater absorption at short wavelengths and less absorption at longer wavelengths. Wavelengths between 600 and 1100 nm are preferentially absorbed by melanin over hemoglobin. Melanin is also present in the epidermis surrounding lesions. Epidermal melanin is an important consideration in patients with dark skin as it serves as a competing chromophore with target lesions (see Laser Treatments in Patients with Dark Background Skin section). The chromophore used for

---

*Laser refers to both lasers and intense pulsed light devices, unless otherwise specified.

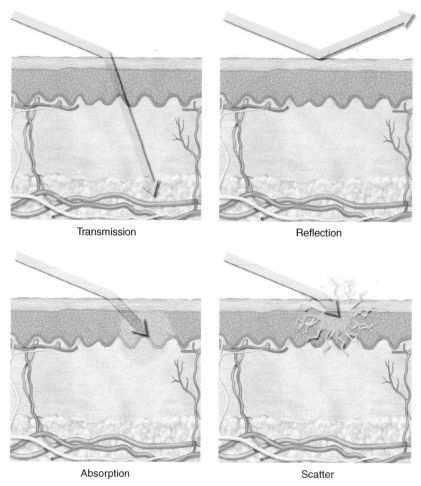

Transmission

Reflection

Absorption

Scatter

*FIGURE 3* ● Laser-tissue interactions.

treatment of wrinkles and collagen remodeling effects is **water**. Water absorption starts to become significant around 950 nm and continues up to 11000 nm, with absorption peaks between 1000–1600 nm and at 3000 nm (Fig. 6, Key References). Chromophores found in cutaneous lesions treated with lasers are summarized in Table 2.

## TABLE 2

### Chromophores in Cutaneous Lesions Targeted with Laser Treatments

| Skin Lesion | Chromophore |
| --- | --- |
| Hair | Melanin |
| Pigmented lesion | Melanin |
| Red vascular lesion | Oxyhemoglobin |
| Tattoo | Tattoo ink |
| Wrinkle | Water |

# What Are the Components of a Laser?

The key component of a laser is the lasing medium. The lasing medium is a substance, which, when stimulated by an external energy source, emits a particular wavelength of light. In other words, the lasing medium has properties that allow it to amplify light through an internal process of stimulated emission. A lasing medium can be a solid (e.g., alexandrite, ruby, neodymium-doped yttrium aluminum garnet), liquid (e.g., dyes) or gas (e.g., carbon dioxide). Lasers are often referred to by their lasing medium and the wavelength they produce. For example, a laser containing an alexandrite rod lasing medium will be referred to as a 755 nm alexandrite laser. In addition to the lasing medium, all lasers have an optical cavity surrounding the lasing medium that contains the amplification process, a power supply or "pump" that supplies energy to the lasing medium, and a delivery system such as a fiber optic cable or articulated arm with mirrors that precisely delivers laser energy to the skin. Figures 5 and 6 in Key References list lasers used for treatment of photoaged skin including their lasing medium and wavelength.

## Laser Parameters

Laser parameters are device settings that can be adjusted at the time of treatment. By appropriately selecting laser parameters of wavelength, fluence, pulse width, and spot size, specific lesions can be targeted with maximal efficacy and safety.

- **Wavelength (nm)** is selected such that it is preferentially absorbed by the chromophore in the lesion being treated. Wavelength also affects the depth of laser penetration in the skin. Short wavelengths penetrate superficially due to greater scattering of the laser beam and longer wavelengths penetrate deeper.
- **Fluence (J/cm$^2$),** also referred to as the energy density, is the energy (measured in joules) delivered per unit area (measured in cm$^2$) and is the intensity of the laser beam. Fluence is selected such that it is high enough to destroy the targeted lesion. Very high fluences can be associated with undesirable thermal injury to tissue surrounding the targeted lesion while very low fluences may not be effective for lesion removal.
- **Pulse width (range from picoseconds to seconds),** also referred to as pulse duration, is the length of time the laser beam is in contact with the skin. Short pulse widths penetrate superficially and longer pulse widths penetrate deeper. Additionally, short pulse widths are used for small lesions and long pulse widths are used for larger lesions.
- **Spot size (mm)** is the diameter of the laser beam on the skin surface. Small spot sizes penetrate superficially due to greater scattering of the laser beam and larger spot sizes penetrate deeper. Spot sizes used with fractional devices, also referred to as pixels, are very small (measured in μm) and are not adjustable. Pixels can penetrate very deeply and the principle of larger spot sizes having increased depth of penetration does not hold true when considering the tiny spot sizes used with fractional lasers.
- **Repetition rate (Hz)** is the rate at which the laser pulses. One hertz (HZ) is one pulse per second. Fast repetition rates allow for more rapid coverage of large, flat treatment areas and can shorten treatment times. Slower repetition rates aid in precise placement of laser pulses and are useful for treatment of single, discrete lesions or contoured treatment areas.
- **Power (W)** is the rate at which energy is emitted from the laser. One watt (W) is 1 joule per second. The power delivered per unit area is the **power density (W/cm$^2$),**

also referred to as irradiance. These variables are not adjusted during treatments but rather are discussed when comparing different laser devices.

- **Cooling** affects treatment efficacy and protects the epidermis from thermal injury, however, is not usually adjusted during treatments. Some lasers utilize cooling methods such as cryogen sprays and contact cooling to protect the epidermis during treatment; external forced refrigerated air is also used. Too much cooling can reduce the efficacy of the treatment and even cause epidermal injury.
- **Scanners.** Some devices, particularly for ablative resurfacing, utilize scanners and computer software to "randomly" deliver pulses within a set pattern so that the pulses are not adjacent to one another. Using nonadjacent pulses allows for high energies to be delivered to the skin without the effects of bulk heating and associated risk of thermal injury.
- **Spot density.** Fractional devices also have a density setting which determines the percentage of skin that is treated with a pulse. High-density settings are associated with more intense treatments, have longer healing times, and potentially greater improvements.
- **Variable pulse sequencing.** Some IPL devices have variable pulse sequencing where one output pulse is delivered as single, double, or triple pulses. Multipulse modes (e.g., triple pulsed mode) have delays between pulses and are safer on the skin as they allow thermal energy to dissipate between pulses. In addition, the overall pulse width is lengthened in multipulse modes and they are used to treat deeper lesions.

Laser parameters are typically selected using a computerized touch screen (Fig. 10). Other laser components used for treatments are also shown in Figure 10 including the laser arm, handpiece, and distance guide that aids in maintaining a constant distance between the laser tip and skin.

## Thermal Relaxation Time

To understand how pulse width contributes to selectively targeting lesions, one must first understand the concept of thermal relaxation time. **Thermal relaxation** time is the time it takes a lesion to dissipate ~50% of its energy into the surrounding tissue. The most selective heating of a target lesion is achieved when laser energy is delivered to the target at a rate faster than the rate of heat dissipation away from the target. In other words, laser energy is confined to the target when the laser pulse width is shorter than the thermal relaxation time of the target. The ideal pulse width is long enough to heat the desired target, while short enough to limit transfer of damaging heat to surrounding tissues. A target's thermal relaxation time is proportional to the square of the target diameter. Small targets, such as fine telangiectasias, have short thermal relaxation times and require short pulse widths for treatment; larger caliber vessels have longer thermal relaxation times and require longer pulse widths for treatment. By choosing a wavelength that is selectively absorbed by the chromophore in the lesion, using adequate fluence to damage the lesion, and choosing a pulse width that allows for heating of the lesion rather than adjacent tissue, lasers selectively destroy lesions with minimal nonspecific thermal damage to surrounding skin. This is the principle of **selective photothermolysis** as it relates to laser parameters. Liquid nitrogen treatments provide a good analogy. If a wart is treated with liquid nitrogen for example, the freeze time (i.e., pulse width) needs to be long enough to freeze the wart but not so long that the cold extends beyond the wart and damages the tissue surrounding the wart.

## Depth of Penetration

Deep penetration of laser energy is safer for the epidermis as it reduces superficial absorption of heat and the likelihood of epidermal thermal injury. In addition, understanding how laser parameters affect the depth of penetration allows providers to better target lesions at different depths in the skin. Superficial penetration is associated with short wavelengths, short pulse widths, low fluences, and small spot sizes. Deeper penetration is associated with long wavelengths, long pulse widths, high fluences, and large spot sizes. These laser concepts, summarized in Figure 2, Key References apply to nonfractional devices. The depth of penetration with fractional lasers is primarily a function of fluence and wavelength. High fluences and wavelengths poorly absorbed by the water chromophore, have deep cutaneous penetration (see Wrinkles—Nonablative Resurfacing, Chapter 5 for further discussion).

## Skin Anatomy

The skin is divided into three layers: the epidermis, dermis, and subcutaneous layer. The **epidermis** is the top layer of the skin and is composed of the outermost nonliving layer, the stratum corneum, and the living cellular layers of the stratum granulosum, stratum spinosum, and stratum basale (Fig. 4). The stratum corneum is composed of

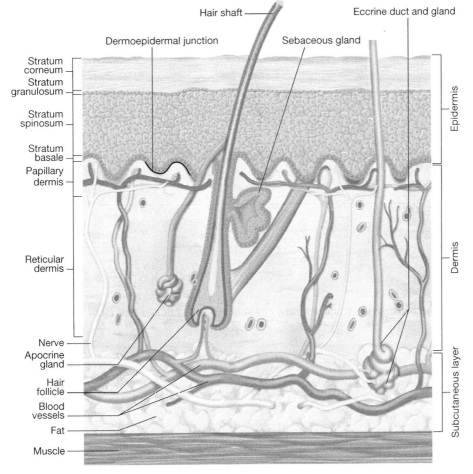

**FIGURE 4** ● Skin anatomy.

corneocytes (nonliving keratinocytes) and lipids and is often referred to as the epidermal barrier. It functions as an evaporative barrier to maintain skin hydration and suppleness, and as a protective physical barrier against microbes, trauma, irritants, and UV light. Constant renewal is necessary for the epidermis to maintain its integrity and function effectively. In healthy young skin, it takes approximately 1 month for keratinocytes to migrate from the living basal layer of the epidermis to the stratum corneum surface and desquamate during the process of epidermal renewal.

**Melanin** pigment, which determines skin color and dyschromias, is primarily concentrated within the epidermis, and in some conditions is found in the dermis (e.g., some forms of melasma). There are two types of melanin pigment: pheomelanin and eumelanin. Pheomelanin is yellow to red in color and is the predominant type in light skin. Eumelanin is brown to black in color and is predominant in dark skin. The number of melanocytes is similar for both light and dark skin; however, the type and distribution of melanin within the epidermis differ. In light skin, melanosomes are small and contain few melanin granules, which are closely aggregated. In darker skin, melanosomes are large, and contain many melanin granules that are distributed singly. The key regulatory step in melanin synthesis (melanogenesis) is the enzymatic conversion of tyrosine to melanin by tyrosinase. This occurs within melanocytes that reside in the basal layer of the epidermis. Once synthesized, melanin is packaged into intracellular organelles called melanosomes that are distributed within the melanocyte and to surrounding epidermal keratinocytes. One melanocyte can contact 30–40 keratinocytes; referred to as an epidermal-melanin unit.

The **dermis** lies beneath the epidermis and is divided into the more superficial papillary dermis and deeper reticular dermis. The main cell type in the dermis is the fibroblast, which is more abundant in the papillary dermis and sparse in the reticular dermis. Fibroblasts synthesize most components of the dermal extracellular matrix, which include, structural proteins (such as collagen and elastin), glycosaminoglycans (such as hyaluronic acid) and adhesive proteins (such as fibronectin and laminins). Hyaluronic acid binds water and augments skin thickness by increasing skin hydration. Appendageal structures, also referred to as adnexa, such as hair follicles and sebaceous glands also reside in the dermis. These structures contain regenerative precursor cells that are integral in wound healing.

The **subcutaneous layer** or superficial fascia, lies below the dermis and above the muscle. This layer is composed of both fatty and fibrous components.

## Histology of Photoaging

In the **epidermis,** UV exposure results in disorganized keratinocyte maturation and abnormal retention of cells. This creates a rough and thickened stratum corneum with poor light reflectance evident as skin dullness (also referred to as sallow discoloration). The disrupted epidermal barrier allows water to escape more freely from the skin, measured as increased transepidermal water loss, which causes dehydration. Impaired barrier function also allows for increased irritant penetration that can be associated with skin sensitivity. Pigmentary changes in photoaged skin are due to dysregulation of melanin synthesis and deposition in the epidermis. The number of melanocytes in the skin decreases naturally over time, however, chronic UV exposure results in an increased number of overactive melanocytes and disorganized melanin deposition in the epidermis. Regions with excess melanin are evident as hyperpigmentation such as freckles and lentigines, and regions with melanin deficiency are evident as hypopigmentation.

In the **dermis,** UV exposure has many damaging effects on the extracellular matrix. Hyaluronic acid diminishes and structural proteins such as collagen and elastin are

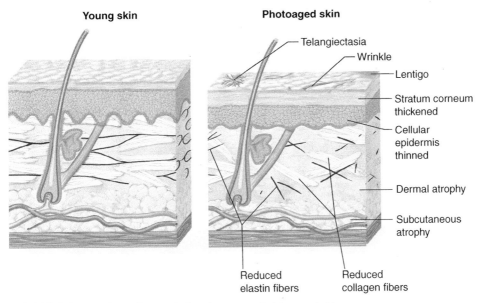

**FIGURE 5** ● Histologic characteristics of young and photoaged skin.

degraded due to upregulation of enzymes (e.g., matrix metalloproteases) and weakened due to crosslinkage. Overall collagen content decreases by approximately 1% per year in adults. The resultant dermal atrophy contributes to formation of fine lines and wrinkles. Advanced photoaged skin also has solar elastosis, which is disorganized clumping of damaged elastin fibers seen clinically as coarse wrinkling, sallow discoloration, and skin thickening. Abnormal dilation and proliferation of dermal blood vessels is visible as telangiectasias and erythema.

Histologic changes seen in photoaged skin are illustrated in Figure 5. Relative locations of epidermal pigmented lesions such as lentigines, and dermal vascular lesions such as telangiectasias are shown in Figure 6.

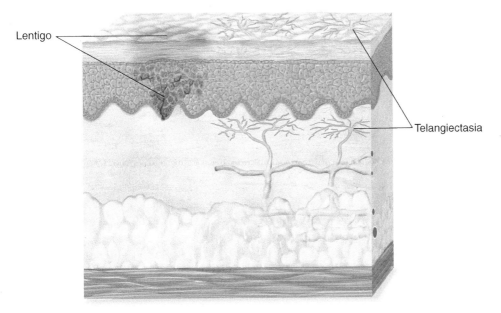

**FIGURE 6** ● Lentigo and telangiectasia cutaneous locations.

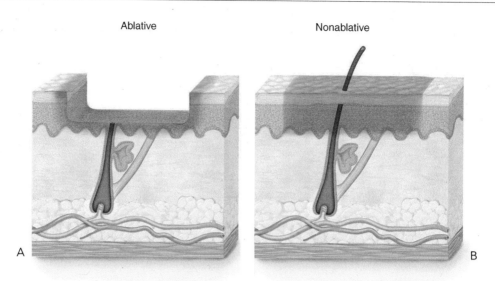

Ablative                                    Nonablative

A                                                                                          B

*FIGURE 7* ● Ablative **(A)** and nonablative **(B)** laser-tissue interactions.

## Laser Devices Overview by Type of Technology

Lasers can be broadly categorized into **ablative devices** (Fig. 7A) that heat and vaporize skin, and **nonablative devices** (Fig. 7B) that heat skin without vaporizing or removing tissue. Ablative devices target water as the chromophore and are primarily used for skin resurfacing to reduce wrinkles and pigmented lesions. Nonablative devices can target a broad range of chromophores. Some nonablative devices target water such as those used for nonablative skin resurfacing to reduce wrinkles. Other nonablative devices target melanin, oxyhemoglobin or tattoo ink, and have broad applications that include hair removal, tattoo removal, and treatment of vascular and pigmented lesions. Figure 1 in Key References gives an overview of lasers used for aesthetic conditions associated with photoaging including pigmented lesions, vascular lesions, wrinkles, and common aesthetic complaints such as hair removal and tattoo removal. A list of laser companies that manufacture devices used for treatments discussed in this book are provided in Appendix 6.

### Fractional Lasers

Fractional refers to a method of delivering laser energy to the skin, whereby a portion or "fraction" of the skin is heated in microscopic columns, called microthermal zones (MTZs). MTZs are typically 100 μm wide and distributed in a grid-like pattern that appears as tiny dots, or pixels, on the skin surface (Fig. 8B). The penetration depth of fractional (also referred to as fractionated) lasers ranges from 300 μm–1.5 mm. Untreated tissue between MTZs serves as a reservoir of regenerative cells that migrate into the treated areas and facilitate rapid healing. The wound healing process stimulates collagen synthesis and dermal remodeling. Treating skin with fractional lasers is referred to as **fractional photothermolysis**. Fractional lasers are most commonly used for skin resurfacing and can be ablative or nonablative. Ablative fractional lasers vaporize tissue in the MTZs, leaving an open wound. Nonablative fractional lasers coagulate tissue in the MTZs, leaving the stratum corneum intact.

Fractional lasers deliver the fractionated beam to the skin using different methods. Some devices use a disposable roller on the tip that is continuously moved across the

Nonfractional                                    Fractional

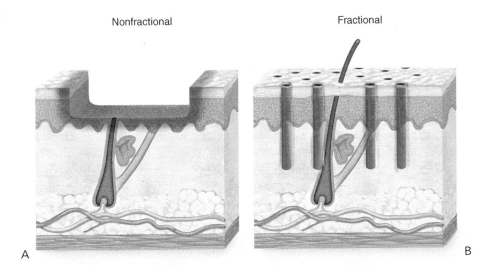

A                                                                                                          B

*FIGURE 8* ● Nonfractional **(A)** and fractional **(B)** laser-tissue interaction.

skin during treatment. Other devices use a stamping technique, where a lens inside the handpiece fractionates the beam each time the laser pulses and all pixels are created at once. Other devices use scanners to fractionate the beam placing pixels sequentially on the skin during the pulse in a fixed or randomly distributed pattern. Fractional lasers are discussed further in Skin Resurfacing.

## Intense Pulsed Light

Intense pulsed light (IPL) devices emit a **broad spectrum of wavelengths** ranging from 500–1200 nm. IPL emissions are generated from flashlamps and transmitted to the skin via a sapphire or quartz tip. Output is refined using filters to select for certain desirable wavelengths and remove undesirable wavelengths. Although the light emitted by IPLs is polychromatic and noncoherent (nonlaser), they still operate under the principle of selective photothermolysis. Emitting a range rather than a single wavelength allows IPLs to target multiple chromophores (melanin, oxyhemoglobin, and to a lesser extent water) and lesions at different depths simultaneously. Consequently, IPLs have a wide variety of applications including treatment of photoaged skin for vascular and pigmented lesions, hair removal, and to a lesser extent, skin texture and rhytids. Short wavelengths (515–550 nm) are used to treat superficial lesions and patients with light Fitzpatrick skin types; long wavelengths (greater than 570 nm) are used for deeper lesions and dark Fitzpatrick skin types.

Various methods for **filtering wavelengths** are used in IPL devices, which vary by manufacturer. Lumenis' IPL devices use cutoff filters to eliminate undesired short wavelengths. The filter's value indicates the shortest wavelength that is emitted to the skin. Common cutoff filters are 515, 550, 560, 570, 590, 615, 645, 690, 695 and 755 nm. These IPL devices utilize one handpiece for all treatments and have removable cutoff filters that slide into the handpiece. For example, a 515 nm cutoff filter eliminates all wavelengths shorter than 515 nm and is used to treat epidermal lesions; a 590 nm filter is used to treat deeper vascular lesions; and 695 nm is used for hair removal. Other manufacturer's such as Palomar/Cynosure use a combination of filters inside their IPL handpieces to generate emission peaks at desired wavelengths and remove short undesired wavelengths. For example, the IPL handpiece used for treatment of pigmented and vascular lesions (MaxG) has two output peaks at 500–670 nm and 870–1200 nm to target oxyhemoglobin and melanin chromophores respectively (Fig. 2, Chapter 2). The handpiece for hair removal (MaxRs) has different internal filters that create one emission peak at 600–800 nm to target melanin (Fig. 3, Chapter 1). The entire handpiece must be changed when treating different conditions. Another IPL manufacturer, Cutera, selects for certain emission wavelengths using a variable current that allows changes to be made electronically, avoiding the need for connecting different handpieces or filters.

Like lasers, IPLs have **variable fluences and pulse widths**, which aid in targeting specific lesions in the skin. For example, treatment of a patient with Fitzpatrick skin type II with large, deep telangiectasias may use a pulse width of 100 ms and fluence of 50 $J/cm^2$. Treatment of the same patient with background erythema, which represents fine vessels located superficially in the skin, may use a pulse width of 10 ms and fluence of 34 $J/cm^2$. Some IPL devices have **variable pulse sequencing**, where one output pulse is delivered as single, double, or triple pulses. Multipulse modes (e.g., triple pulses) have greater dissipation of heat, are safer for the epidermis and used in darker skin types. In addition, the overall pulse width is lengthened with multipulse modes; they penetrate deeper and are preferable for treatment of deeper dermal targets such as large caliber telangiectasias.

IPLs have **large spot sizes** (e.g., $1.6 \times 4.6$ cm) and consequently cover a larger area with each pulse. While large spot sizes typically translate into faster treatment times, this is offset by low repetition rates (e.g., 0.3–1 Hz) when high fluences are used. For precise treatment of small lesions, the spot size may be reduced by covering a portion of the treatment tip with an opaque paper (Fig. 8, Chapter 3). Some IPL devices have adaptors that can be attached to the treatment tip to reduce the spot size to 4 or 6 mm. High quality devices use **built-in cooling** for epidermal protection which also provides some anesthesia.

## Very Short Pulse Lasers (Q-switched and Mode-locking)

Lasers with Q-switching (or quality-switching) and mode-locking capabilities generate very short pulse widths, in the nanosecond and picosecond range respectively. These very short pulse lasers are used for tattoo removal and treatment of pigmented lesions. They operate under the principles of selective photothermolysis and photoacoustic vibration. **Photoacoustic vibration** results from rapid, high-energy pulses with short pulse widths that oscillate and fragment targeted lesions into smaller particles, thereby enhancing elimination. Tattoo ink particles and melanosomes are very small in size with short thermal relaxation times and therefore, respond well to extremely short pulse widths. While most short pulse lasers treat epidermal pigmented lesions, QS 1064 nm lasers have deeper penetration due to their longer wavelength and are used to treat dermal pigmentation such as melasma. Q-switched (QS) lasers commonly used include 532, 585, 650, 694, 755 and 1064 nm; picosecond lasers include 532 and 755 nm.

## Neodymium-doped Yttrium Aluminum Garnet Laser

Neodymium-doped yttrium aluminum garnet (Nd:YAG) can produce many different wavelengths. Nd:YAG is a crystal that has a small fraction of the yttrium replaced by neodymium (i.e., it is doped with neodymium), which provides the lasing activity for the crystal. Nd:YAG typically emits light with a wavelength of 1064 nm. However, based on how it is pumped from an external energy source, it can emit either 940 nm, 1320 nm, or 1440 nm. These are not interchangeable, and a given Nd:YAG laser only emits one of these wavelengths.

## Potassium Titanyl Phosphate Laser

Potassium titanyl phosphate (KTP) laser is actually a misnomer. The primary lasing medium in a KTP laser is neodymium-doped yttrium aluminum garnet (Nd:YAG) and the primary wavelength is 1064 nm. The 532 nm wavelength is produced by passing the 1064 nm wavelength through a frequency doubling potassium titanyl phosphate (KTP) crystal. So, a KTP laser is actually a frequency doubled Nd:YAG laser.

## Radiofrequency Devices

Radiofrequency (RF) devices are nonlaser, non–light-based devices. They employ **rapidly alternating current** that creates heat when applied to the skin, due to the skin's resistance to current flow (impedance). RF energy is concentrated in the dermis. Heating tissue with RF is controlled by several factors, including the type of electrodes used (e.g., monopolar, bipolar, tripolar), amount of current, duration of current, and cooling times. Newer RF devices utilize fractional methods for delivering current that create microwounds below the skin surface. RF devices are used primarily for reduction of skin laxity and have shown benefits in areas such as the periocular region, nasolabial folds, jowls, neck and abdomen, and for reduction of cellulite, which is outside the scope of this book.

## Light-Emitting Diodes

Light-emitting diodes (LEDs) are nonlaser, light-based devices that emit a narrow range of low-intensity wavelengths. Red LED devices (570–670 nm) are used for mild wrinkle reduction and blue LED devices (400–500 nm) for acne. They do not operate based on the theory of selective photothermolysis but rather are based on the principle of **photomodulation**, where cellular activity is modulated through illumination by particular wavelengths of light. While devices have similarities to lasers and other light-based technologies, their histologic effects on skin and clinical results are extremely modest. The main advantage of LEDs is their ease of use.

## Photodynamic Therapy

Photodynamic therapy (PDT) involves the use of a topical **photosensitizing medication** activated by a light source such as an LED, IPL or laser (e.g., 595 nm). Commonly used photosensitizers include 5-aminolevulanic acid (ALA) and methyl ALA. ALA (e.g., Levulan™) is selectively absorbed and concentrated in proliferating cells and pilosebaceous units where it is converted to protoporphyrin. Upon activation with a light source, protoporphyrin forms free radicals that selectively destroy the target. PDT is used off-label for photorejuvenation of pigmented lesions and photodamage, and is FDA approved for treatment of nonhyperkeratotic actinic keratoses on the face. While PDT has impressive results, there is significant postprocedural erythema and crusting, strict patient avoidance of ambient sunlight for 48 hours is necessary as exposure can lead to extended photosensitizer activation and associated complications, and treatment cost is higher than with laser alone due to the medications used.

## Laser Devices by Indication

### Skin Resurfacing

Wrinkle reduction with lasers, also referred to as laser skin resurfacing, is based on the principle of creating a controlled wound in the skin using heat and evoking a healing response. The healing process stimulates collagen remodeling with fibroblast production of new collagen, elastin, and other extracellular matrix components that thickens the dermis. In addition to wrinkle reduction, dermal remodeling also improves rough skin texture, pore size, and scars. Lasers are not the only means by which the skin can be resurfaced; other modalities include mechanical resurfacing with microdermabrasion and chemical resurfacing with chemical peels. Regardless of the method used, skin resurfacing can be performed to varying degrees of aggressiveness, based on the depth of skin penetration. Greater depths of wounding produce more dramatic results but require longer recovery times, more intensive postprocedure care, and have greater risks of complications. Figure 9

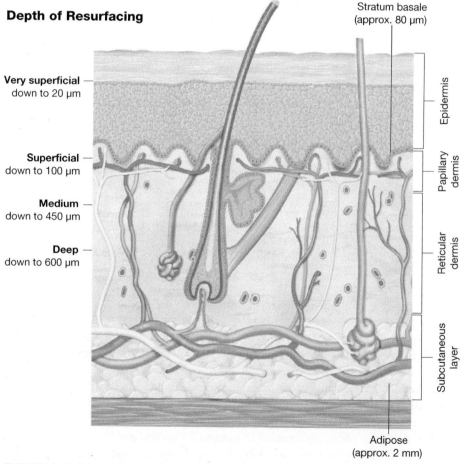

**FIGURE 9** ● Skin resurfacing terminology and cutaneous depth of penetration.

## TABLE 3

### Laser Resurfacing Treatments for Wrinkle Reduction

| Resurfacing Lasers | Patient Presentation and Treatment Characteristics | | | | |
| | Wrinkle Severity | Results | # Treatments | Recovery Time | Complication Risk |
| --- | --- | --- | --- | --- | --- |
| Nonablative | + | + | 6–8 | + | + |
| Fractional nonablative | ++ | ++ | 4–6 | ++ | ++ |
| Fractional ablative | +++ | +++ | 1 | +++ | +++ |
| Ablative | ++++ | ++++ | 1 | ++++ | ++++ |

Nonablative = 532 nm, 585 nm, 595 nm, 755 nm, 1064 nm, 1320 nm, 1450 nm, and IPL (500–1200 nm).

Fractional nonablative = 1410 nm, 1440 nm, 1540 nm, 1550 nm, 1565 nm, and 1927 nm.

Fractional ablative and ablative = 2790 nm, 2940 nm, and 10600 nm.

+ mild; ++ moderate; +++ significant; ++++ very significant.

shows the standard depths associated with very superficial, superficial, medium, and deep skin resurfacing procedures. Skin resurfacing with lasers can be achieved using ablative and nonablative lasers. Selecting the appropriate laser resurfacing procedure depends on a combination of factors including wrinkle severity, patient expectations for results, number of treatments needed to achieve results, tolerance for postprocedure downtime, and complication risks (Table 3).

**Ablative skin resurfacing lasers** vaporize and remove skin. They can achieve profound wrinkle reduction results but have longer recovery times and greater risks of complications such as pigmentary alterations, infection, and scarring compared to nonablative treatments. Ablative lasers wavelengths are highly absorbed by the water chromophore and they vaporize tissue by raising the skin temperature to over 100°C. The two wavelengths used most often for ablative resurfacing are: 2940 nm (erbium:yttrium-aluminum-garnet or Er:YAG) and 10600 nm (carbon dioxide). Treatments with ablative lasers also improve epidermal pigmented lesions such as freckles and lentigines as a result of epidermal tissue removal. Ablative skin resurfacing is most commonly performed using fractional devices as they offer more rapid recovery times and significantly decreased risks of complications compared to nonfractional ablative lasers. Ablative skin resurfacing treatments are discussed in detail in Chapter 6.

**Nonablative skin resurfacing lasers** provide milder treatments compared to ablative lasers, gently heating the skin (to approximately 60°C) without removing tissue. Results are much less significant, but recovery times are shorter, and complications are less common and less severe relative to ablative lasers. They appeal to patients who desire to continue daily activities with minimal to no disruption. Some nonablative skin resurfacing lasers target the water chromophore and others target colored chromophores (melanin and oxyhemoglobin). Out of all nonablative skin resurfacing lasers, fractional lasers that target water (1410 nm, 1440 nm, 1540 nm, 1550 nm, 1565 nm, 1927 nm) offer the most impressive wrinkle reduction results. Nonablative skin resurfacing treatments are discussed in Chapter 5.

## Pigmented Lesions

Lasers used for benign pigmented lesions such as lentigines and ephelides work by either specifically targeting melanin, or by targeting water and non-specifically removing pigmentation through skin resurfacing. Lasers used for treatment of pigmented lesions that target melanin include: 532 nm, 694 nm, 755 nm, 810 nm, and 1064 nm. These wavelengths are effective for treatment of pigmented lesions when used as long-pulse lasers and are even more effective when used as QS lasers (QS 532 nm, QS 694 nm, QS 755 nm, QS 1064 nm). Some wavelengths are well absorbed by both melanin and oxyhemoglobin such as 532 nm and IPL (500–1200 nm). They are commonly used to treat both pigmented and red vascular lesions. Skin resurfacing lasers that target water, while commonly used for wrinkle reduction, can also be used to remove pigmented lesions in a nonspecific manner. Ablative lasers remove pigmented lesions through vaporizing melanin in epidermal tissue. Nonablative fractional lasers remove pigmented lesions through extruding melanin from MTZs along with other epidermal and dermal necrotic debris. Treatment of pigmented lesions is discussed in Chapter 2.

## Hair Removal

Lasers used for hair removal target melanin, which damages follicular structures necessary for hair growth. Wavelengths that penetrate deeply into the skin and do not target red vascular chromophores are used for laser hair removal; they include: 755 nm, 810 nm, 1064 nm, and IPLs with filters that remove short wavelengths. Epidermal melanin serves as a competing chromophore for short wavelengths and use of cooling methods and short wavelength cutoff filters with IPLs is important to prevent epidermal thermal injury. The 1064 nm laser has poor epidermal melanin absorption and is safe for hair removal in dark skin types such as Fitzpatrick type VI. Laser hair removal is reviewed in Chapter 1.

## Vascular Lesions

Lasers used for red vascular lesions such as telangiectasias, erythema, and cherry angiomas target oxyhemoglobin. These lasers include: 532 nm, pulsed-dye lasers (585 nm, 590 nm, 595 nm, 600 nm), and IPL (500–1200 nm). Epidermal melanin is a competing chromophore for these wavelengths; therefore, lasers used for treatment of red vascular lesions typically employ a method for epidermal cooling to protect the epidermis from thermal injury. Blue vascular lesions such as reticular leg veins contain deoxyhemoglobin and are more effectively treated with wavelengths that are well absorbed by deoxyhemoglobin and penetrate deeply such as 755 and 1064 nm. Blue vascular lesions are not typically part of photoaging presentations and are excluded from the discussions in this book, which focus on rejuvenation of photoaged skin. Treatment of red vascular lesions is discussed in Chapter 3.

## Tattoo Removal

Lasers used for tattoo removal target exogenous ink chromophores. These treatments are performed with Q-switched (nanosecond) and mode-locking (picosecond) lasers that emit rapid, high-energy pulses with very short pulse widths. These lasers operate under the principles of selective photothermolysis and photoacoustic vibration. Wavelengths used for treatment of tattoos include: QS 1064 nm, QS 755 nm, QS 694 nm, QS 650 nm, QS 585 nm, QS 532 nm, picosecond 532 nm and picosecond 755 nm. Laser tattoo removal is discussed in the Very Short Pulse Lasers section and in Chapter 4.

## Laser Maintenance

The output of a laser may vary slightly over time and with extended use. Periodic servicing and annual maintenance can help ensure consistent performance. After servicing, it is advisable to use caution with initial treatments and pay close attention to clinical endpoints as lasers may have higher outputs than anticipated. For example, a patient's tattoo treated using a QS 1064 nm laser with a spot size of 6 mm and fluence of 3.5 J/cm$^2$ before servicing may require lower settings such as 1064 nm with a 6 mm and lower fluence of 3.0 J/cm$^2$ after servicing to achieve desireable clinical endpoints.

## Laser Safety

The **American National Standards Institute (ANSI)** laser safety requirements have established guidelines to assist with safety for both patients and providers. Specific manufacturer guidelines for safety and maintenance for the device used should also be followed. Written **laser safety policies and procedures** are established in practices using lasers, and a Laser Safety Officer designated who is responsible for ensuring proper maintenance and functioning of laser equipment and adherence to standards for laser operation. It is advisable to perform a **laser safety check list** prior to treatment, which includes covering reflective surfaces such as mirrors and windows in the treatment room, posting laser warning signs outside the treatment room, providing patients and providers with wavelength-specific eyewear to protect from ocular injury, and stowing the foot pedal out of the way when the laser is not in use. All lasers are equipped with an emergency shut-off button that may be depressed if the device needs to be rapidly turned off (Fig. 10). For example, if someone unintentionally walks into a treatment room without eye protection.

**Ocular safety** is paramount with laser treatments. Lasers produce high-intensity beams that can travel long distances and reflect off surfaces without loss of intensity, unlike IPLs, which lose intensity over distance. Due to the beam characteristics, IPLs are more ocular safe than lasers. Both lasers and IPLs can cause ocular injury and require protective eyewear for the provider operating the device, patient, and all people in the treatment room. Protective eyewear indicates the wavelengths protected against and the optical density (OD) of the lens. An OD of at least 4 for the wavelength being used is recommended for adequate eye protection. Provider goggles with clear,

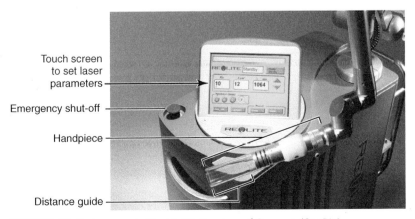

*FIGURE 10* ● Laser parts (RevLite™, Courtesy of Cynosure/ConBio).

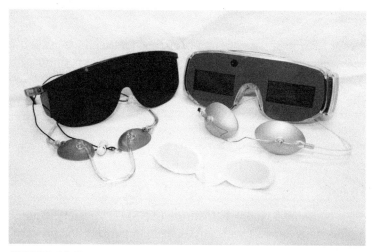

**FIGURE 11** ● Protective eye wear used for laser or IPL treatments including provider goggles, small lead goggles and adhesive lead eye shields for patients. (Courtesy of R. Small, MD.)

light-colored lenses (with appropriate OD for the wavelength used) offer the best visualization. Goggles should fit snugly to the face without big gaps, particularly if glasses are worn underneath. When working on a patient's face, extraocular lead eye shields, either goggles or adhesive pads, are used for the patient. When working on the eyelids, intraocular lead eye shields are used. Figure 11 shows a variety of protective eyewear used for laser and IPL treatments. Even with protective eyewear, the operator should never look directly into the laser tip while the laser is connected to a power source. There are reported cases of experienced laser operators doing so using 1064 nm lasers with resultant permanent visual field deficits. **Plumes** of aerosolized tissue are created with ablative lasers, and tattoo lasers may **splatter blood or tissue,** which poses risks of airborne and contact exposure to bacteria and viruses. Use of a smoke evacuator and mask is necessary with ablative lasers. Distance guide cones fitted to the tip of tattoo lasers may reduce exposure to tissue debris (Fig. 10). Lasers present a **fire hazard** and a fire extinguisher should be readily available. Use of flammable products such as alcohol is avoided immediately prior to pulsing the laser.

## Aesthetic Consultation

Aesthetic consultation is an important part of successfully performing laser treatments. In addition to identifying the patients' concerns and clarifying their specific goals, consultation provides the physician with the opportunity to establish realistic expectations for treatment results and discuss possible complications.

The patient's **medical history** is reviewed including: medications, allergies, past medical history, contraindications to treatment (see General Laser Contraindications section below), pigmentary changes (either hormonally induced or postinflammatory), and history of herpes in the treatment area. Cosmetic history is also reviewed including: previous aesthetic procedures and surgeries (modality, frequency, date of treatments, response, satisfaction with results, and complications). Identifying activities that can interfere with treatments is important such as routine sun exposure and water-related activities (e.g., surfing, swimming). An example of an aesthetic intake form that may be used is shown in Appendix 1.

A focused **physical examination** is performed and the main areas of concern determined. It is recommended that the provider and patient simultaneously examine the desired treatment areas using a handheld mirror. Lesions indicated for treatment are identified such as lentigines, freckles, erythema, and telangiectasias as well as lesions suspicious for skin cancers, and it is documented in the chart. Lesions suspicious for melanoma or other skin cancer are biopsied or referred, and benign results confirmed prior to proceeding with laser treatments. Pigmented lesions suspicious for melanoma can be screened using the "ABCDE" criteria: asymmetry, borders are irregular, color is variegated, diameter is greater than 6 mm, evolving with new characteristics such as enlargement, bleeding, or is elevated. Note that basal cell carcinomas can also be pigmented. Patients considering aesthetic treatments are advised to avoid direct sun exposure and use a broad-spectrum sunscreen with sun protection factor (SPF) 30 containing zinc oxide or titanium dioxide daily prior to and throughout the course of treatment. Baseline assessments of the patient's skin type (Fitzpatrick Skin Type) and severity of photoaging (Glogau Classification of Photoaging) are also typically performed at the time of consultation (see respective sections below).

Early on in the consultation process, it is advisable to assess whether patients will derive adequate benefit from minimally invasive treatments or require surgical intervention. Patients presenting with severe wrinkles and excessive skin laxity may not have significant improvements from minimally invasive treatments and may be better served by surgery. For patients who are candidates for minimally invasive procedures, treatment options and recommendations are reviewed including the expected degree of improvement and anticipated number of treatments. It is important to note that treatment outcomes vary from person to person and a specific percentage of improvement cannot be guaranteed for a given patient. Using terms such as "significantly improve" rather than "remove" can help set realistic expectations. Meeting or exceeding patients' expectations contributes to patient satisfaction. Patients with unrealistic expectations or body dysmorphic disorder may have a history of repeated dissatisfaction with prior aesthetic treatments and these are contraindications for aesthetic procedures. An individualized aesthetic treatment plan is created and recorded in the chart. The risks of complications, recovery time, and costs for the proposed procedures are discussed. The informed consent process is followed for each procedure with inclusion of a signed consent form in the chart (see Informed Consent section below). Photographic documentation of conditions and lesions indicated for treatment and results are recommended (see Photodocumentation section below).

## Fitzpatrick Skin Type

Fitzpatrick skin type classification is used to describe background skin coloration and the skin's response to sun exposure (Table 4). In general, individuals with more melanin in their skin have a darker baseline skin color, are more resistant to sunburn, and are classified as a high Fitzpatrick skin type. Skin types I–III are Caucasian, IV–V have olive or light brown skin tones such as people of Mediterranean, Asian, and Latin descent, and VI are black, typically of African-American descent. Fitzpatrick skin type may grossly predict complication risks with treatments and can be used as a guide to selecting the type of aesthetic treatment most appropriate for a patient and the aggressiveness of that treatment. For example, patients with light Fitzpatrick skin types (I–III) have low risks of pigmentary changes and can generally tolerate aggressive treatments. Patients with dark Fitzpatrick skin types (IV–VI) have greater risks of pigmentary changes, such as

## TABLE 4

Fitzpatrick Skin Types

| Fitzpatrick Skin Type | Skin Color | Reaction to Sun | |
|---|---|---|---|
| I | Very white or freckled | Always burns | |
| II | White | Usually burns | |
| III | White to olive | Sometimes burns | |
| IV | Brown | Rarely burns | |
| V | Dark brown | Very rarely burns | |
| VI | Black | Never burns | |

hyperpigmentation and hypopigmentation, and require more conservative treatments to minimize the likelihood of these complications. An example of a form that may be used to determine Fitzpatrick skin type is provided in Appendix 2.

## Glogau Classification of Photoaging

Glogau classification is used to assess the severity of photoaging (Table 5), especially with regard to wrinkles. It is a baseline measure performed at the time of aesthetic consultation and may also be used to grossly guide treatment selection and the aggressiveness of treatment. Glogau types I–III have less severe wrinkling and tend to show the most noticeable improvements with aesthetic treatments such as botulinum toxin and dermal filler injections, nonablative lasers, superficial and fractional ablative lasers, and superficial skin resurfacing procedures such as light chemical peels and microdermabrasion. Glogau type IV patients have severe photoaging and often require deep ablative laser treatments and/or surgery for significant skin rejuvenation.

## TABLE 5

### Glogau Classification of Photoaging

| Glogau Type | Photoaging | Typical Age | Skin Characteristics | |
|---|---|---|---|---|
| I | Mild | 20s to 30s | Minimal wrinkles<br>No lentigines<br>No keratoses | |
| II | Moderate | 30s to 40s | Wrinkles in motion<br>Rare, faint lentigines<br>Skin pores more prominent<br>Keratosis palpable but not visible | |
| III | Advanced | 50s to 60s | Wrinkles at rest<br>Prominent lentigines<br>Telangiectasias<br>Visible keratosis | |
| IV | Severe | 60s and older | Wrinkles throughout<br>Numerous lentigines<br>Elastosis, coarse pores<br>Yellowish skin color<br>Skin malignancies and premalignant lesions | |

## Informed Consent

Patients seeking elective aesthetic treatments typically have high expectations for results and low tolerance for side effects. All aspects of the informed consent process are covered prior to performing procedures, and this consist of: (i) discussing the risks, benefits (with emphasis on realistic expectations), alternatives, and complications of the procedure; (ii) providing adequate opportunity for all questions to be asked and answered; (iii) educating the patient about the nature of their aesthetic issue and procedure details; (iv) signing the consent form; and (v) documenting the informed consent process in the chart. Examples of consent forms for the laser procedures in this book are shown in Appendix 4.

## Photodocumentation

Photographs that are used to document clinical findings and incorporated into the medical record are referred to as photodocumentation. Taking photographs is recommended prior to treatment, midway through a series of treatments, and posttreatment. Consent for photographs is typically included in the procedure consent form and obtained prior to taking photographs. Consistent lighting and positioning is important, particularly with wrinkle reduction treatments as results can be subtle and challenging to capture photographically. Patients are usually positioned for photographs fully upright looking straight ahead. Photographs are taken of the full face and zoomed in to specific treatment areas from the front, 45 and 90 degrees.

## Selecting the Appropriate Laser Procedure for Photoaged Skin

Skin rejuvenation involves optimizing treatment efficacy while minimizing recovery time and procedural risks. There is no right or wrong approach to treatment of photoaged skin, and the approach taken largely depends on the devices available to the provider and balancing the patient's expectations for results with tolerance for downtime and risks. As a general rule, it is prudent to use the least aggressive and least painful laser initially such as nonablative lasers, and progress to more aggressive laser treatments such as ablative lasers when less invasive modalities will not achieve desired results.

Treatment of photoaged skin usually requires addressing multiple issues including dyschromia, vascular ectasias, skin texture and wrinkles. Providers can approach treatment of multiple issues sequentially by addressing dyschromia and vascular ectasias first and then addressing texture and wrinkles afterward. Treating in this order is advisable as improvements in texture are more apparent once dyschromia and vascularities are improved. For example, a patient presenting with photoaging might initially receive IPL treatments to address lentigines and telangiectasias and then receive nonablative skin resurfacing treatments (e.g., fractional 1550 nm) for wrinkle reduction. Another approach is to use a more aggressive laser that addresses multiple aspects of photoaging at once such as fractional ablative skin resurfacing. These lasers can treat pigmented lesions and wrinkles simultaneously but require more downtime and have more risks than nonablative lasers. Assuming a variety of laser devices are on-hand for treatment, the approach used is often determined by patient preference. Some patients prefer a less aggressive approach with a greater number of treatments, others, particularly those with advanced photoaging changes, desire the more aggressive approach.

## Laser Treatments in Patients with Dark Background Skin

Dark background skin color is associated with increased epidermal melanin concentration. Dark Fitzpatrick skin types (IV–VI) have dark background skin color as they inherently have higher epidermal melanin content. Light skin types (I–III) have lower epidermal melanin. However, light skin types can develop darkened background skin color as a result of UV exposure and formation of diffuse dyschromia (i.e. tanned skin, actinic bronzing, extensive lentigines). Epidermal melanin serves as a competing chromophore with cutaneous lesions for laser absorption during treatment, and can reduce treatment efficacy and increase risks of epidermal thermal injury. Complications such as postinflammatory hyperpigmentation, hypopigmentation, and burns are more likely to occur in patients with dark background skin color. Treatments in patients with dark background skin are performed using conservative laser parameters: long wavelengths (the safest of which is 1064 nm), long pulse widths, large spot sizes, and low fluences. These parameters allow for deep cutaneous penetration that decreases absorption by epidermal melanin, reducing the risk of complications.

## Alternative Therapies

Other aesthetic procedures that treat facial lines and wrinkles include: botulinum toxin for dynamic wrinkles, nonlaser skin resurfacing procedures such as microdermabrasion and dermabrasion (rarely used today due to risks of pigmentary changes and scarring), and chemical peels for treatment of static wrinkles. Dermal fillers are also used for static wrinkles and to improve facial contours. For severe wrinkling with redundant lax skin, surgery is an option. Pigmented lesions can be treated with liquid nitrogen and topical skin care products. Red vascularities can be treated with electrocautery (though not recommended due to scarring risks). Hair can be permanently removed with electrolysis, and tattoos can be minimized with topical caustic agents (also not recommended due to risks of scarring). Further discussion of alternative therapies to particular laser treatments are discussed in each chapter.

## Advantages of Laser Treatment

- Lesion specificity
- Short treatment times
- High efficacy when appropriate device is selected

## Disadvantages of Laser Treatment

- Expensive relative to most other procedures (except surgery)
- Risks of cutaneous thermal injury
- Risks of ocular injury
- Typically require multiple treatments, and if not, then singular aggressive treatments are associated with procedural discomfort, have longer recovery times and higher risks of complications

## General Laser Contraindications

- Active infection in the treatment area (e.g., herpes simplex, pustular acne, cellulitis)
- Dermatoses in the treatment area (e.g., vitiligo, psoriasis, atopic dermatitis)
- Melanoma, or lesions suspected for melanoma in the treatment area
- Deep chemical peel, dermabrasion or radiation therapy in the treatment area within the preceding 6 months
- Keloidal scarring[*]
- Impaired healing (e.g., immunosuppressive medications, collagen vascular diseases such as scleroderma, poorly controlled diabetes mellitus)
- Peripheral vascular disease
- Bleeding abnormality (e.g., thrombocytopenia, anticoagulant use)
- Seizure disorder

---

*Caution should be used in patients with hypertrophic scarring.*

- Uncontrolled systemic condition
- Cardiac pacemaker
- Skin atrophy (e.g., chronic oral steroid use, genetic syndromes such as Ehlers–Danlos syndrome)
- Livedo reticularis, a vascular disease associated with mottled skin discoloration of the arms or legs exacerbated by heat exposure
- Erythema ab igne, a rare acquired reticular erythematous or pigmented rash exacerbated by heat exposure
- Direct sun exposure or tanning bed use within the preceding 2 weeks resulting in reddened or sunburned skin
- Tanned skin
- Self-tanning product within the preceding 2 weeks
- Topical prescription retinoid within the preceding week
- Isotretinoin (Accutane™) within the preceding 6 months
- Gold therapy (e.g., used for treatment of arthritis)
- Photosensitizing medications (e.g., tetracyclines, St. John's wort, thiazides)
- Photosensitive disorder (e.g., systemic lupus erythematosus, polymorphous light eruption)
- Pregnant or nursing
- Unrealistic patient expectations
- Body dysmorphic disorder
- Treatment inside the eye orbit (i.e., without intraocular eye shields)

Certain dermatoses such as **vitiligo, psoriasis,** and **atopic dermatitis** can erupt at sites of trauma (referred to as koebnerization) and occurrence in the treatment area is a contraindication; the risk is greatest with lasers that cause the most trauma such as ablative skin resurfacing and tattoo removal lasers. **Oral retinoids** (isotretinoin) within the prior 6–12 months are associated with increased risks of scarring and poor healing due to impaired sebaceous gland function. Although these risks are clearly associated with ablative laser treatments, some recent studies show no adverse effects in patients undergoing nonablative laser treatments while using oral retinoids. Other conditions may also impair healing such as **collagen vascular diseases, poorly controlled diabetes mellitus,** and use of **immunosuppressive drugs** as well as prior procedures that reduce adnexal structures in the treatment area such as **deep chemical peels, dermabrasion, radiation therapy,** and **extensive electrolysis.** Patients with poorly controlled diabetes and those using immunosuppressive medications are also at increased risk of infection. **Tanned skin** has increased risks of hyperpigmentation, hypopigmentation, and burns. Laser treatment (particularly with QS lasers) is contraindicated in patients with a history of taking **gold therapy** due to the risk of inducing permanent dark blue dyspigmentation known as chrysiasis. Additional treatment-specific contraindications are listed in individual chapters.

## Indications

The chapters in this book are organized by treatment indication: hair removal, pigmented lesions, vascular lesions, tattoo removal, nonablative skin resurfacing for wrinkle reduction, and ablative skin resurfacing for wrinkle reduction. Individual lasers typically have multiple applications. Each chapter has a section on Devices Currently Available where the devices used for the chapter's indication and other common applications for those devices are discussed.

# Preprocedure Checklist

- Aesthetic consultation
- Fitzpatrick skin type
- Examination of treatment area
- Informed consent
- Pretreatment photographs
- Sun protection
- Antiviral and other pretreatment medications

A preprocedure checklist is performed prior to treatment to help ensure safety and maximize results, and each chapter includes a checklist specific to that procedure. Ablative laser treatments require more advanced preprocedure planning and the preprocedure checklist is usually started 4–6 weeks prior to treatment. The checklist for laser hair removal treatments is begun 4 weeks prior to treatment to ensure patients discontinue certain methods of hair removal. The checklist for other laser treatments can be performed on the day of treatment.

Prophylactic antiviral medications may be given for a history of herpes in or near the treatment area 2 days prior to the procedure and continued for 3 days postprocedure (e.g., valacyclovir/famciclovir 500 mg 1 tablet twice daily). If there is a remote history and the patient is low risk, an antiviral medication may instead be started on the day of treatment and continued for 5 days. Some patients require other oral or topical medications such as analgesics prior to treatment and pretreatment medications commonly used for specific procedures are discussed in each chapter.

## Preprocedure Skin Care Products for Laser Treatments

- **Sunscreen.** All patients are started on a daily broad-spectrum sunscreen with an SPF of at least 30 containing zinc oxide or titanium dioxide at the time of consultation. SPF values greater than 30 do not correlate with significantly increased protection from the sun. Broad-spectrum sunscreens protect from both UVA and UVB rays.
- **Skin lightening product.** Patients prone to hyperpigmentation and dark Fitzpatrick skin types (IV–VI) can use a topical lightening agent such as hydroquinone cream 2–8%, as it may reduce the risk of postinflammatory hyperpigmentation (PIH) with laser procedures. Cosmeceutical hydroquinone alternatives include kojic acid, arbutin, niacinamide, and azelaic acid. Ideally, a lightening product is begun 1 month prior to procedure.
- **Discontinuation of active products.** If patients are using active products such as retinoids (e.g., tretinoin) and hydroxy acids (e.g., glycolic acid), it is advisable to discontinue use 1–2 weeks prior to laser procedures to ensure the epidermis is intact at the time of treatment and reduce skin sensitivity.

Preprocedure patient instructions for each procedure are provided in Appendix 3.

## Anesthesia for Laser Procedures

Providing adequate anesthesia for laser procedures reduces anxiety, offers the patient a more tolerable experience and can facilitate greater treatment precision and optimal technique to improve outcomes. The most common anesthetic modalities used with cosmetic laser procedures are epidermal cooling and topical anesthetics. The anesthetic

## TABLE 6

### Anesthesia for Laser Treatments

| Laser Treatment | Topical Anesthetics | Contact Cooling | Forced Air Cooling | Anxiolytic and Analgesic Medications | Injectable Anesthetics |
|---|---|---|---|---|---|
| Hair removal | X | X | | X | |
| Pigmented lesions | X | X | | | |
| Vascular lesions | | | | X | |
| Tattoo removal | X | | | X | Local |
| Fractional nonablative resurfacing | X | | X | X | |
| Ablative resurfacing | X | | X | X | Regional |

modality chosen is dependent on the discomfort level associated with the procedure, procedure duration, and patient tolerance for pain. Anesthesia for less painful procedures, such as laser hair removal, can usually be accomplished with contact cooling using ice and/or topical anesthetic. More painful procedures such as ablative laser resurfacing often require a combination of modalities such as topical anesthetic, oral analgesic, and forced air cooling (Table 6).

### Epidermal Cooling

Epidermal cooling is a commonly used method for achieving anesthesia with laser treatments. In addition to reducing discomfort, it also improves safety by protecting the epidermis from thermal injury. Epidermal cooling can be achieved by directly applying ice, a chilled roller, or a cool laser tip to the skin, referred to as contact cooling (Fig. 12). Many lasers have built-in **contact cooling** mechanisms that maintain the laser tip at a constant safe temperature during pulsing. Built-in cooling methods can be

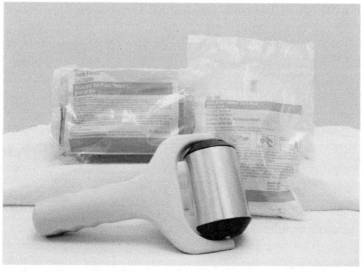

*FIGURE 12* ● Ice packs and chilled roller.

synchronized with the laser pulse or released a few milliseconds before or after the pulse. IPLs, for example, have integrated contact cooling typically consisting of a chilled sapphire window in the treatment tip that provides epidermal cooling through continuous contact with the skin during treatment. Other cooling methods include cryogen spray and forced air cooling. **Cryogen sprays** are released immediately before and/or after laser pulses and are an integrated component of the laser handpiece. Sprays are a consumable requiring replacement fairly often. **Forced air cooling** involves directing air through a hose that is aimed at the treatment area. Forced air cooling is provided by stand-alone devices (e.g., ArTek Air™ and Zimmer Cryo 6™). This noncontact method of cooling is particularly useful with ablative laser treatments.

Adequate epidermal cooling with any method is indicated by skin erythema or brief blanching. Excessive cooling is indicated by prolonged blanching of the skin and can reduce treatment efficacy and cause epidermal injury. Dark skin types (IV–VI) have a greater risk of pigmentary changes such as hyperpigmentation and hypopigmentation due to cold injury. Cooling may be used alone or adjunctively with most other anesthetic modalities for laser treatments.

## Topical Anesthetics

Topical anesthetics are often used for laser procedures due to their effectiveness and ease of application. Commonly used topical anesthetic products include: L.M.X. (lidocaine 4–5%) available over the counter, EMLA (lidocaine 2.5%:prilocaine 2.5%) available by prescription, and lidocaine 30% and BLT (benzocaine 20%:lidocaine 6%:tetracaine 4%), which require compounding by a pharmacy.

The skin is degreased with alcohol prior to application, the product rubbed gently onto the treatment area, and then occluded with plastic wrap. The degree of anesthesia achieved with a topical anesthetic is related to the strength of the product and the duration and method of application. For less painful procedures, such as laser hair removal, an application of BLT for 15 minutes is adequate for most patients. More painful procedures, such as tattoo removal and ablative resurfacing, require an application of BLT for 45 minutes under occlusion. Due to the time required for topical anesthetics to take effect, procedure times are significantly increased.

Toxicity of topical anesthetics is related to systemic absorption of the product. Several factors affect systemic absorption including surface area covered, duration of application, and the presence of an intact skin barrier. Most topical anesthetics are safe with proper use as the systemic blood levels reached are usually only a small fraction of the toxicity level. For example, 60 gm of EMLA cream placed on a 400 $cm^2$ area (equivalent to half a back) for 4 hours produces peak blood levels of lidocaine that are 1/20th the systemic toxic level of lidocaine and 1/36th the toxic level of prilocaine. Cases where topical anesthetic use has resulted in toxicity are associated with patient self-application of large quantities to large surface areas (e.g., full legs) or with procedures that disrupt the skin barrier such as fractional laser resurfacing. Signs and symptoms of systemic lidocaine toxicity range from mild dizziness to respiratory depression, hypotension, seizure, and death. To minimize the risk of systemic toxicity application to areas no greater than 400 $cm^2$ for most topical anesthetics is recommended at each treatment. It is also advisable to apply higher strength topical anesthetics such as BLT in the office under supervision.

Methemoglobinemia has been reported with anesthetics, primarily topical prilocaine and benzocaine. Metabolites of these medications can increase methemoglobin in the blood, which creates a functional anemia resulting in impaired oxygen carrying capacity of blood. Patients present with shortness of breath, cyanosis, mental status changes, headache, fatigue, dizziness, loss of consciousness, and with severe methemoglobinemia may exhibit seizures, coma, and death. They usually have low oxygen saturation as measured by pulse oximetry, and normal oxygen saturation calculated from arterial blood gas analysis. Blood with methemoglobinemia appears chocolate-brown in color and does not change color with the addition of oxygen. Methemoglobinemia is treated with supplemental oxygen and methylene blue 1% solution (10 mg/mL) 1–2 mg/kg administered intravenously slowly over 5 minutes. Methylene blue converts iron in hemoglobin to its normal state and restores the blood's oxygen carrying capacity.

## Injectable Anesthetics

Injectable anesthetics are rarely used for aesthetic laser treatments. Local infiltration may be used with laser tattoo removal treatments for patients intolerant of treatment using topical anesthetics and oral analgesics. Occasionally, a perioral regional nerve block may be necessary for ablative laser treatments. The most commonly used injectable anesthetic preparation for laser procedures is 1–2% lidocaine (10 mg/mL) with 1:100000 of epinephrine. This has a rapid onset of anesthesia within a few minutes and wears off within a few hours. Epinephrine is associated with vasoconstriction, which keeps the lidocaine in the area where it was injected, thereby decreasing systemic absorption and toxicity. Lidocaine may be buffered with sodium bicarbonate in a 1:8 or 1:10 ratio to reduce the burning sensation upon injection. When performing local infiltration, care should be taken to inject the smallest possible anesthetic volumes necessary to minimize the risk of lidocaine toxicity.

Maximal safe doses of 2% lidocaine with and without epinephrine are listed below. Above these doses there is an increased risk of neurotoxicity and seizures.

| Lidocaine Solution | Maximum Adult Dose by Body Weight (mg/kg) | Maximum Injection Volume for 140 lb Adult (mL) |
| --- | --- | --- |
| 2% lidocaine without epinephrine | 4 | 13 |
| 2% lidocaine with epinephrine | 7 | 22 |

## Anxiolytic and Analgesic Medications

Anxiolytic and analgesic medications may be required by a small number of patients who are intolerant of laser procedures using other anesthetic modalities. These medications are typically administered in-office 1 hour prior to the procedure. Patients taking anxiolytics or opioids such as hydrocodone require a driver to take them home after their procedure. Common in-office anxiolytic and analgesic medications include the following:

## Anxiolytic

- Diazepam (Valium®) 5–10 mg orally

## Analgesics

- Tramadol (Ultram®) 50–100 mg orally
- Ketorolac (Toradol®)10–20 mg orally or 30–60 mg IM
- Hydrocodone with acetaminophen (Vicodin® 5/500) 1–2 tablets orally

### Pneumatic Skin Flattening

Pneumatic skin flattening devices utilize negative pressure to elevate and flatten skin against the laser window, which reduces pain. The mechanism of action of these devices is based on the gate theory of pain, whereby the pressure generated by pneumatic flattening inhibits pain sensation by overwhelming and blocking the pain pathways. Pneumatic skin flattening has been used to provide anesthesia with hair removal, and it may also increase treatment efficacy by bringing the hair bulb closer to the skin surface. Some laser devices have pneumatic skin flattening incorporated into the laser and others have a separate external device that attaches to the treatment tip.

# Laser Procedure

Procedural recommendations are provided in each chapter and include: guidelines for selecting initial laser parameters, technique recommendations, desirable and undesirable clinical endpoints, aftercare, treatment intervals, parameter modifications for subsequent treatments, follow-up issues, and complications and their management. While the general principles discussed apply to most lasers used for a particular indication, it is advisable to follow manufacturer recommendations for the specific device used at the time of treatment.

## Aggressive Versus Conservative Laser Parameters

Laser parameters used for treatments are often described as aggressive or conservative. **Aggressive** laser parameters refer to the use of short wavelengths, short pulse widths, small spot sizes, and high fluences. **Conservative** laser parameters refer to the use of long wavelengths, long pulse widths, large spot sizes, and low fluences (Fig. 3, Key References).

## Selecting Initial Laser Parameters for Treatment

Laser parameters of wavelength, fluence, pulse width, spot size, and repetition rate can be selected at the time of treatment. **Patient characteristics** and **lesion characteristics** are both considered when selecting laser parameters for treatment and each chapter discusses how these factors are taken into consideration.

### Patient Characteristics

- **Fitzpatrick skin type.** Patients with dark Fitzpatrick skin types (IV–VI) have high epidermal melanin. These patients have greater risks of epidermal injury and associated complications of hyperpigmentation, hypopigmentation, and burns. It is advisable to use conservative laser parameters of long wavelengths, long pulse widths, large spot sizes, and low fluences when treating these patients (Fig. 3, Key References). Patients with light Fitzpatrick skin types (I–III) can tolerate more aggressive parameters of short wavelengths, short pulse widths, small spot sizes, and high fluences.
- **Anatomic location.** Nonfacial areas such as the neck, chest, and extremities have decreased healing capacity and delayed healing, due to fewer adnexal structures. Relative to the face, these areas have a greater risk of complications such as scarring and it is advisable to use more conservative parameters when treating nonfacial areas (Fig. 3, Key References). Slow repetition rates are also used for treatment of discrete lesions to aid in precise laser pulsing; fast repetition rates are used for confluent treatment of large areas.

- **Treatment area contour.** The contour of the treatment area often determines the repetition rate selected. Flat areas such as the chest and back can be treated with fast repetition rates, which shorten treatment times. Contoured areas such as the face usually require slow rates to help ensure careful placement and complete contact between the skin and laser tip.

## Lesion Characteristics

- **Target lesion chromophore.** Treatment areas that contain a lot of target chromophore such as high density of lesions (e.g., numerous lentigines) or intensely colored lesions (e.g., dark brown lentigines) require conservative parameters. Treatment areas that contain less target chromophore such as low density of lesions (e.g., sparse lentigines) or faintly colored lesions (e.g., light brown lentigines) require more aggressive parameters (Fig. 3, Key References).
- **Other chromophores.** In addition to the lesions targeted, the treatment area is assessed for the presence of other chromophores that are targets for the wavelength being used. Photodamaged skin often has both vascular and pigmented lesions, particularly on the face and chest. Treatment areas may also have dark hair present, which is a chromophore for many wavelengths used to treat photoaging. These lesions often overlie one another and lasers cannot discriminate between desirable targets or otherwise. Therefore, conservative treatment parameters are used when multiple chromophore targets are present. For example, if a patient presents for treatment of sparse, faintly colored lentigines but these lesions overlie intense erythema, then based on having a lot of target, conservative laser parameters are used. Similarly, if a patient presents for treatment of lentigines that overlie dark hair, conservative parameters are used.

## General Treatment Technique

- The provider is comfortably positioned (usually seated) at the head of the treatment table (Fig. 13). It is helpful to tuck elbows into the body at 90 degrees to alleviate upper back strain and repetitive motion injury.
- Snugly fitted laser-safe eye protection that corresponds to the wavelengths used (with an OD greater than or equal to 4) is worn by the provider, patient, and all people in the treatment room. When working on the face, patient contact lenses are removed and extraocular lead eyeshields worn.
  **TIP: Patients will still see a flash of light with most lasers during the procedure even when proper eye protection is used. Reassuring patients that they are adequately protected puts them at ease.**
- Laser treatments on the face are typically performed outside of the ocular region: above the supraorbital ridge (roughly where the eyebrows sit) and below the inferior orbital rim (Fig. 14). Treatment of the eyelids (e.g., with ablative lasers) or lips (e.g., with lasers for vascular or pigmented lesions) are advanced techniques and outside the scope of this book.
- The face can be broken down in to regions that are treated sequentially, and this provides a systematic approach for complete coverage of the face. Figure 14 shows facial regions and one possible treatment sequence starting with region 1 and progressing to region 6.
- The laser tip is held perpendicular to the skin at all times.
  **TIP: In the periocular area, the laser tip is directed away from the eyes to reduce the risk of ocular injury and laser reflection off the patient's lead goggles.**

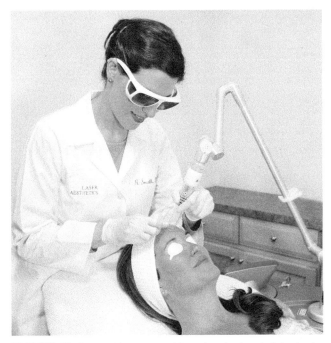

FIGURE 13 ● Providers are positioned at the head of the bed when treating the face. (Courtesy of R. Small, MD.)

- The laser handpiece is moved across the skin in a vertical (Fig. 15A) or horizontal (Fig. 15B) direction toward the provider to allow for good visualization of laser pulses on the skin.

  **TIP: It is advisable to start on the lateral face as it is less sensitive, and progress medially.**

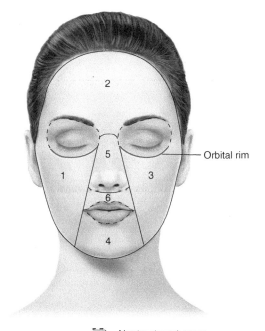

● = Nontreatment areas

FIGURE 14 ● Laser treatment areas on the face.

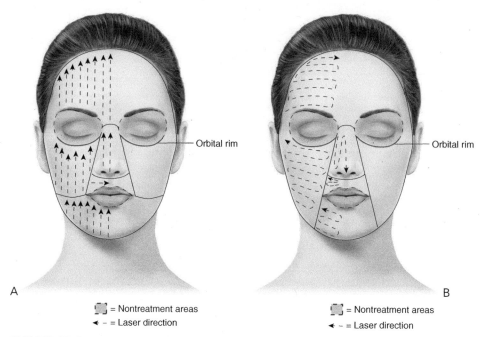

Orbital rim

Orbital rim

A

B

= Nontreatment areas
◄ – = Laser direction

= Nontreatment areas
◄ – = Laser direction

**FIGURE 15** ● Laser handpiece directions: **(A)** vertical and **(B)** horizontal.

- Bulky handpieces such as IPLs (Fig. 16A) can obscure the providers view, and moving the handpiece vertically usually gives the best visualization. Laser handpieces (Fig. 16B) are typically smaller, which makes it easier to visualize the treatment area; vertical or horizontal motion can be used based on provider preference.
- The degree of overlap between laser pulses varies for different technologies. In general, nonablative lasers have greater pulse overlap than ablative lasers.
- Confluent coverage of the treatment area with laser pulses is referred to as one pass.
- Test spots may be performed for patients with higher risk Fitzpatrick skin types (IV–VI) prior to the initial treatment. Test spot parameters are selected based on the patient's Fitzpatrick skin type and lesion characteristics following the manufacturer's guidelines for wavelength, pulse width, spot size, and fluence. It is advisable to place test spots discretely near the intended treatment area (such as under the chin, behind or inferior to the ear) and overlap pulses to simulate the technique used with treatment. Test spots are viewed 3–5 days after placement for evidence of erythema, blister, crust, or other adverse effect. It is important to inform patients that lack of an adverse reaction with test spots does not ensure that a side effect or complication will not occur with a treatment.

## Desirable Clinical Endpoints

Desirable clinical endpoints are the intended tissue response seen on the skin after pulsing the laser. Although clinical endpoints discussed in each chapter are in regard to the specific technology used to demonstrate the procedure, clinical endpoints are generalizable for most technologies used for that indication. For example, when treating a telangiectasia, most laser technologies (e.g., 532 nm, 585 nm, 590 nm, 595 nm, 600 nm, IPL) will yield clinical endpoints of increased erythema, vessel clearance, or darkening and may have purpura.

Clinical endpoints are clearly visible in light skin types (I–III) and are typically seen immediately after or within a few minutes of the laser pulsing. Patients with dark skin types (IV–VI) tend to be treated with less aggressive settings; endpoints

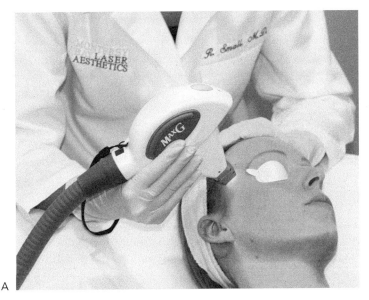

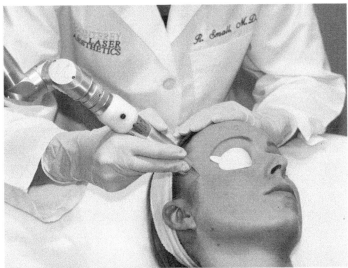

FIGURE 16 ● Intense pulsed light (A) and laser (B) handpieces. (Courtesy of R. Small, MD.)

develop more slowly and are less obvious. For example, clinical endpoints for laser treatment of lentigines in a light Fitzpatrick skin type usually consist of lesion darkening, enhanced lesion demarcation against background skin, and perilesional erythema almost immediately after laser pulsing. In dark skin types, clinical endpoints may only consist of enhanced lesion demarcation without erythema and may appear 10 minutes after pulsing the laser.

Having a clear understanding of the desired endpoints obtained during treatment is essential to successfully performing laser treatments. By continuously monitoring the treatment area, the provider can detect whether desirable endpoints are achieved and whether parameters are adequate. In addition, the provider can immediately detect whether undesirable tissue responses occur and modify treatment parameters accordingly to provide a safe, effective treatment.

## Undesirable Clinical Endpoints

Undesirable clinical endpoints are unintended tissue responses seen on the skin after pulsing the laser. They indicate potential thermal injury to the epidermis and are usually due to overly aggressive laser parameters for a given Fitzpatrick skin type. Undesirable clinical endpoints include: graying, severe whitening, blistering, and bleeding. If any of these occur, it is advisable to discontinue treatment and cool the skin using wrapped ice packs for 15 minutes and compression for bleeding. Patients are monitored over the next few weeks for formation of enlarged blisters (bullae), intense erythema and induration (firmness), which may precede scarring.

## Performing Laser Treatments

Guidelines for laser treatments using one device are provided in each chapter for the indication discussed. While the principles apply to most lasers used for that chapter's indication, manufacturer recommendations for the specific device used at the time of treatment should be followed.

- Inquires about sun exposure and sunscreen use are made prior to treatment. If the patient is recently sun exposed or has tanned skin in the treatment area, it is advisable to wait 1 month before treating to reduce the risk of complications.
- The patient is positioned supine on a flat treatment table.
- The skin is cleansed with a nonalcohol wipe.
- If the treatment is not intended for removal of tattoos or permanent makeup, then those areas are avoided and may be covered with gauze. It is advisable to keep the laser tip approximately 1 inch away from tattoos during treatment.
  **TIP: Full thickness burns may result from treating over tattoos using devices that are not indicated for tattoo removal (e.g., IPL).**
- Wavelength-specific protective eyewear is provided to everyone in the treatment room.
- The laser is operated in accordance with the clinic's laser safety policies and procedures using manufacturer guidelines and recommended settings.
- Selection of wavelength, pulse width, spot size, and fluence is based on the indication, Fitzpatrick skin type, facial or nonfacial anatomic location, and lesion characteristics in the treatment area including lesion density, lesion color intensity, and the presence of other chromophores that are targets for the wavelength used (see Selecting Initial Laser Parameters for Treatment section).
- Selection of repetition rate is based on the size and contour of the treatment area (see Selecting Initial Laser Parameters for Treatment section).
  **TIP: Care must be taken to keep pulses adjacent when fast repetition rates are used to avoid skipping areas.**
- Some lasers, particularly IPLs, require application of a layer of clear colorless gel to the skin.
- The treatment tip is either placed on the skin as with most IPLs (Fig. 16A), or maintained at a constant distance from the skin determined by a distance guide (Fig. 16B).
- A single pulse is performed at the lateral margin of the treatment area (e.g., anterior to the ear if treating the face) to assess for patient tolerance and observe the skin for clinical endpoints (see Desirable Clinical Endpoints section). In general, there should be subtle endpoints with initial treatments and pain should be less than or equal to 5 on a scale of 1–10. Allow a few minutes for endpoints to evolve for light skin types (I–III) and up to 10 minutes for darker skin types (IV–VI). If no endpoints

are observed, gradually increase the fluence in small increments as tolerated by the patient until desirable clinical endpoints are achieved.

- The whole region is treated confluently with laser pulses or discrete lesions are treated individually, depending on the indication.
- Laser–tissue interactions and clinical endpoints are continually assessed throughout the treatment and settings adjusted accordingly to ensure adequate treatment but not overtreatment.
- Ice may be applied immediately after treatment for 15 minutes to soothe skin in the treatment area and reduce erythema and edema.
- When not in use, the foot pedal is properly stored and the key removed from the laser.

## Postprocedure Skin Care for Laser Treatments

Selection of postprocedure skin care products is determined by whether or not the skin is intact after treatment. The goal with all postprocedure products is to soothe, protect and hydrate the skin to promote healing and hasten resolution of erythema. Prolonged postprocedure erythema can be associated with PIH and therefore, rapid resolution of erythema is desirable. Postprocedure patient instructions for each procedure are provided in Appendix 3.

### Intact Skin

Skin is intact after nonablative laser treatments for pigmented lesions, vascular lesions, hair removal, nonablative skin resurfacing, and for most tattoo removal treatments. However, if bleeding or blistering occurs with a laser treatment, such as tattoo removal, the skin is not intact and should be treated as such.

- **Erythema.** Postprocedure erythema is managed with a topical corticosteroid cream applied twice daily, and the potency is based on the severity of erythema: low potency steroids (e.g., hydrocortisone 1% or 2.5%) are used for mild erythema, medium potency steroids (e.g., triamcinolone acetonide 0.1%) for moderate erythema, and high potency steroids (e.g., triamcinolone acetonide 0.5%) for severe erythema. If erythema is not present, a topical corticosteroid is not necessary.
- **Soothe, protect and hydrate.** A gentle cleanser, broad-spectrum sunscreen of SPF 30 containing zinc oxide or titanium dioxide, and a nonocclusive moisturizer are used for 2 weeks postprocedure. Nonocclusive moisturizers used postprocedure usually contain ingredients to soothe skin (such as borage and evening primrose seed oils) and promote healing (such as beta glucan and peptides). Examples include Biafine® (OrthoNeutrogena), Epidermal Repair® (SkinCeuticals), Bio-Cream® (Neocutis) and TNS Ceramide Treatment Cream® (SkinMedica).
- **Routine skincare products.** Patients' routine skincare regimens are typically resumed 2 weeks postprocedure.

### Nonintact Skin

Laser treatments that create a wound, such as ablative skin resurfacing and some tattoo removal treatments, are managed differently from intact skin.

- **Occlusive moisturizers** are used immediately postprocedure to facilitate moist wound healing. These products are usually ointments and examples include Aquaphor® (Beiersdorf), Hydra Balm® (SkinCeuticals), Protective Recovery Balm® (biO2

Cosmeceuticals), and Puralube® (Nycomed). Puralube® is an ophthalmologic grade petrolatum product that may be used in the periocular area. Occlusive moisturizers are continued until re-epithelialization occurs, usually for 4–7 days after fractional ablative lasers, and up to 2 weeks or more after nonfractional ablative lasers. Prolonged use of occlusive products can lead to acne and milia formation.

- **Cleansing.** Cleansing nonintact skin after ablative laser treatment is discussed in the Aftercare section of Chapter 6.
- **Sunscreen.** It is not possible to layer other products such as sunscreen on top of ointments. Therefore, sun protective measures such as hats and sun avoidance during this period of healing are very important to prevent pigmentary complications in the treatment area.
- **Intact skin.** Once the skin has fully re-epithelialized and is intact, a nonocclusive moisturizer is used and skin care is followed as outlined above.
- **Skin lightening product.** If PIH is a concern, skin lightening products such as hydroquinone may be started 1 month postprocedure (see Preprocedure Skin Care Products for Laser Treatments section).

## Treatment Intervals

In general, nonablative laser procedures are performed as a series of treatments with consistent intervals between treatments for optimal results, while more aggressive procedures such as ablative laser treatments are performed less frequently, or singly. **Nonablative laser** treatments are usually performed every month or every 2 months, depending on the procedure and the treatment area. For example, laser hair removal treatments on the face are performed every month for 6 months. Laser treatments for telangiectasias are usually performed monthly for 3 months. **Ablative laser** treatments for wrinkle reduction by comparison, are typically performed once every year or every few years. Specific recommendations for treatment intervals are discussed in each chapter.

## Subsequent Treatments

**Nonablative laser** procedures are usually progressive, whereby treatment intensity is increased at each subsequent visit to enhance results. Target lesions usually lighten and have less chromophore over the course of treatments. Fluence is usually increased and pulse width decreased to appropriately match the changing lesion characteristics. It is advisable to intensify treatments by changing only one parameter at any given visit. Typically, the fluence is initially increased for a few treatments and pulse width is decreased in later treatments. **Ablative laser** treatments are not progressive and, if a subsequent treatment is performed the following year, parameters may not change.

## Common Follow-Ups

Patients may seek posttreatment follow-up for mild issues that are not necessarily complications and each chapter has a section on Common Follow-ups that discusses commonly encountered follow-up issues and provides recommendations for management. While **nonablative laser** treatments do not typically require scheduled follow-up visits, **ablative laser** treatments do require postprocedure visits to evaluate for wound healing, manage postprocedure skin care products, and assess for complications. Recommendations for ablative laser follow-up visits are provided in the Follow-up Visit section of Chapter 6.

## Results

Photographs taken before and after laser procedures showing representative results are included in each chapter.

## Complications

- Pain
- Erythema
- Edema
- Hyperpigmentation
- Hypopigmentation
- Burn
- Scar
- Infection
- Contact dermatitis
- Milia
- Failure to reduce or improve the intended lesion
- Reduction of hair in or adjacent to the treatment area
- Ocular injury
- Urticaria
- Petechiae and purpura

This list is representative of some of the complications encountered with laser treatments. Complications specific to each procedure are reviewed in the respective chapters of this book along with strategies for management.

Complications associated with laser treatments range from mild to severe. Fortunately, most complications encountered are mild and spontaneously resolve without permanent sequelae. Mild complications from laser treatments include prolonged erythema and edema, acne eruptions, milia formation, and contact dermatitis. Moderate complications include local infections and postinflammatory hyperpigmentation. Severe complications include hypertrophic scarring, delayed onset hypopigmentation, ectropion, disseminated infection, and ocular injury. Nonablative lasers usually leave the skin intact and have milder complications compared to ablative lasers that create an open wound, which increases the frequency and severity of complications.

Some of the most common and problematic adverse effects with lasers are associated with cutaneous thermal injury. Thermal injury can result in burns, scarring, and pigmentary changes (hyperpigmentation and hypopigmentation) and can occur with any laser. In a recent study by Zelickson looking at nearly 500 cosmetic laser adverse events reported to the FDA, the most common complications for all lasers were burns (36%), scarring (20%), and pigmentary changes (9%). Thermal injury occurs most often in patients with dark Fitzpatrick skin types (IV–VI) and patients with dyschromia such as actinic bronzing, recently tanned, and severely sun damaged skin. These patients have abundant epidermal melanin, which serves as a competing chromophore for lasers, increasing laser energy absorption and the risk of thermal injury. Use of aggressive laser parameters including short wavelengths, short pulse widths, small spot sizes, high fluences, and inadequate epidermal cooling are also associated with increased risk of thermal injury (Table 7).

Provider error and device malfunction are the most common causes of laser complications. Use of checklists, such as the Preprocedure Checklists in each chapter of this

## TABLE 7

Risk Factors for Severe Laser Complications of
Hyperpigmentation, Hypopigmentation, and Burns

Patient characteristics (dark background skin)
- Dark Fitzpatrick skin types (IV–VI)
- Tanned skin
- Actinic bronzing
- Severe photodamage

Laser treatment parameters (aggressive settings)
- Short wavelength
- Short pulse width
- Small spot size
- High fluence
- Inadequate cooling

book, is recommended to reduce the likelihood of laser complications from provider error. However, it should be noted that lasers are complex devices, laser–tissue interactions can vary with individual patients and even in the best of hands with the best technique, complications can occur.

**Hyperpigmentation and hypopigmentation** are pigmentary complications resulting from alteration to background skin color. **Hyperpigmentation,** darkened skin coloration relative to surrounding skin, is a very common complication and has been reported with virtually every laser device. Hyperpigmentation associated with laser treatments is primarily due to upregulation of melanin synthesis and deposition in the epidermis as a result of inflammation, referred to as PIH. Prolonged erythema posttreatment combined with direct sun exposure is associated with PIH, particularly in dark skin types. Excessive cooling can also injure the epidermis, inducing PIH or hypopigmentation. Hyperpigmentation usually resolves spontaneously over several months, although in rare instances it may be permanent. **Hypopigmentation,** lightened skin coloration relative to surrounding skin, is a less common but more significant complication than hyperpigmentation. It is most often seen with short pulse widths (e.g., Q-switched lasers) and short wavelengths (e.g., 532 nm). Hypopigmentation is also almost always transient but rarely can be permanent.

**Burns** are defined by the degree of tissue damage resulting from thermal injury. First degree burns involve the epidermis and are visible as erythema and edema. Second degree burns extend into the dermis and are visible as erythema, edema and blisters that may rupture and form crusts or erosions. Third-degree burns, also called full-thickness burns, extend to the subcutaneous fat. First- and second-degree burns rarely scar, but third-degree burns usually form scars. Third-degree burns have been reported with treatment over tattoos using devices not intended for tattoo removal, such as IPL pulsing over decorative tattoos.

**Scarring** is an uncommon but serious complication with laser treatments. A **keloid** is defined as an abnormal scar that grows beyond the boundaries of the original site of skin injury. A **hypertrophic scar** is defined as a widened or raised scar that does not extend beyond the boundaries of the site of injury. Unlike keloids, hypertrophic scars typically reach a certain size and then stabilize or regress. An **atrophic scar** is a depressed well defined area, most commonly resulting from collagen destruction associated with inflammatory conditions such as cystic acne, or as a result of tension on a surgical wound. A subtle **textural change**, detected as a palpable unevenness in the skin, is also a form of scarring. Signs of impending scar formation include focal, persistent areas of erythema and induration. Interventions to prevent scarring are most effective at this stage and are reviewed in the Scarring section, Chapter 6. Scarring is a rare complication with the use of appropriate settings, but can result with any laser at sites that have been overtreated or burned, especially if healing has been complicated by infection or repetitive abrasion. Hypertrophic scarring is more common with laser treatments that create an open wound such as ablative lasers. Subtle textural changes commonly occur with Q-switched tattoo laser treatments due to epidermal injury from high absorption of laser energy by darkly pigmented targets. Recent use of isotretinoin, previous radiation therapy in the treatment area, and a history of keloid formation are also risk factors for hypertrophic and keloidal scarring. Certain areas of the body such as the lower eyelids, mandible, anterior neck and chest are more susceptible to scarring. Additionally, patients of Asian and African decent may have a greater predisposition to hypertrophic and keloidal scarring.

**Ocular injury** is the most severe complication associated with laser use, and both patients and providers are at risk. IPL devices have fewer ocular risks than lasers due to their less intense, divergent beams. Wavelengths less than 1100 nm (e.g., 1064 nm) are strongly absorbed by melanin in the pigmented cells of the choroid and retina. Unprotected eye exposure to these wavelengths can lead to retinal burns and blindness. These wavelengths can also be absorbed by the vitreous humor, forming 'floaters' that drift across the visual field. Retinal detachment due to floaters is rare, but reported with lasers. Wavelengths greater than 1100 nm are strongly absorbed by water in the cornea and can lead to corneal burns and cataract formation. Protective eye wear appropriate for the wavelengths used is essential for providers, patients, and personnel in the treatment room and is reviewed in Laser Safety.

**Pain** is common with laser treatments. Most patients experience discomfort only when the laser pulses the skin, and this rapidly resolves once the pulse ceases. The goal for patient discomfort is no more than moderate pain, 5 on a standard pain scale of 1–10. Structures in the midline of the face such as the lips, nose, and chin are more sensitive than the periphery of the face. Ablative laser treatments are more painful than nonablative lasers. Certain nonablative laser treatments such as tattoo removal with Q-switched lasers, fractional resurfacing, and RF are relatively more painful than other nonablative lasers.

**Erythema and edema** are expected after most laser treatments. While this is not usually problematic for women as makeup can be worn, erythema can be more of a concern for men. Erythema and edema are considered abnormal if they persist longer than or are more intense than routinely observed. Nonablative lasers generally have a shorter duration of postprocedure erythema usually lasting 3–4 days, ablative lasers have a longer duration of erythema, which can persist up to a few weeks or even months with deep nonfractional ablative resurfacing. Worsening erythema and edema can be associated with contact dermatitis or infection. Contact dermatitis is typically associated with pruritus (itchiness) and infection with tenderness. Treated skin is vulnerable to irritation from various substances found in topical products such as preservatives and fragrances. Over-the-counter herbal and vitamin remedies such as vitamin E and aloe products are common causes of contact dermatitis.

**Infection** postprocedure can be viral, bacterial, or fungal. **Reactivation of herpes simplex virus** is the most common and can occur following any laser treatment. Herpes simplex eruptions are usually preceded by tingling and burning and appear as small vesicles on the lip (i.e., cold sores) or less commonly the nose and rarely in the eye area. Reactivation of herpes zoster is infrequent but can also occur. Prophylactic antiviral medications are given to reduce the occurrence in patients with a known history of viral infections in the treatment area. **Bacterial** infections are rare (apart from acne), and if they occur usually result from *Streptococcus* or *Staphylococcus*. **Acne vulgaris** infection due to Propionibacterium acnes is visible as erythematous papules and pustules and can occur following any laser treatment. Acne may be due to the laser treatment itself or postprocedure skin care, particularly with prolonged use of occlusive moisturizers. **Impetigo** is a superficial bacterial infection that can occur following treatments on the face and extremities; lesions progress from papules to vesicles, pustules, and crusts. The main pathogens are *Staphylococcus aureus* (methicillin-resistant *Staphylococcus aureus* is uncommon) and group A *Streptococcus*. Impetigo often occurs in patients who are known carriers. **Folliculitis** is a superficial infection of hair follicles visible as small, erythematous papules and pustules that are less than 5 mm in diameter. Folliculitis most often occurs after vigorous exercise or shaving immediately following treatments and is due to S. *aureus* and *Candida;* folliculitis associated with swimming and hot tub use is most often due to *Pseudomonas aeruginosa*. Ablative laser treatments have the greatest risk of any infection as the skin is not intact posttreatment, and they have a greater risk of rapidly spreading. Furthermore, the appearance of infections in nonintact resurfaced skin does not always have the characteristic signs seen with intact skin.

    **Tattoos and permanent makeup** have concentrated ink pigments and treating over them with lasers that are not intended for tattoo removal can result in severe epidermal injury such as a full thickness skin burn (i.e., third-degree burn).

    **Unintended hair reduction** can occur with laser treatments. Hair growth structures are susceptible to thermal injury and reduction of hair growth can occur with most lasers, especially those that are absorbed by the melanin chromophore. In addition, when performing hair removal treatments, it is possible to reduce hair adjacent to the intended treatment area as hair follicles grow at angles to the skin. This is of particular concern when treating near the eyebrows.

    **Milia** are tiny 1–2 mm white papules that result from occlusion of sebaceous glands. Ointments used to hydrate skin can occlude sebaceous glands and contribute to milia formation.

    **Urticaria** (hives) may occur with nonablative laser treatments. Urticaria is seen most often in patients prone to developing hives. Urticaria appears as erythematous welts in the treatment area.

    **Petechiae and purpura** (bruise) represent bleeding underneath the skin and usually appear a few minutes after treatment. They are defined based on size where petechiae are pinpoint dots less than 3 mm, purpura is 3–10 mm, and ecchymoses are greater than 10 mm. These commonly occur with lasers using short pulse widths such as Q-switched lasers and short wavelengths that are highly absorbed by oxyhemoglobin such as 532 nm and pulsed-dye lasers. While they are not a serious complication, purpura in particular, is an unsightly inconvenience due to the 2–3 week duration necessary for clearance.

## Learning Techniques

When getting started with lasers or incorporating a new laser procedure into practice, it is advisable to treat friends, family and staff prior to treating patients. Selecting light Fitzpatrick skin types (I–III) is also advisable as they have relatively low risks of complications. Striving for subtle endpoints by using conservative settings also reduces the risk of complications.

## Current Developments

New technologies under development are discussed at the end of each chapter. **Home-use laser devices** are a new area of laser medicine that's expanding rapidly and are discussed below.

The US FDA has approved home devices for hair removal and wrinkle reduction (Table 8). The evidence behind these devices is limited and there is wide variation in effectiveness, safety, and quality. Home-use devices use lower parameters than office devices to reduce patient risks, and when compared to in-office devices, more treatments are required at frequent intervals to achieve effects. Lasers used for treatment of vascularities require relatively high energy and as yet there are no home devices for this indication. Although physicians may not use home laser devices directly, patients will likely seek guidance from healthcare professionals about these devices.

There are currently two main types of home devices used for wrinkle reduction: fractional lasers and LEDs. Home fractional lasers create MTZs of coagulated tissue like office devices but uses lower energies (15 mJ vs. up to 70 mJ for office devices) and have lower MTZ density (2% vs. up to 50% for in-office devices). LEDs have marginal efficacy; their main advantage is their lack of side effects.

Home devices used for hair removal include diode, IPL, and thermal devices, of which the diode and IPL have demonstrated efficacy. Some of these devices have restricted areas for use. For example, the Tria, which is one of the most popular and effective home devices for hair removal, is not indicated for use on the face, neck, or genital area. Tria is indicated for Fitzpatrick skin types I–IV and, like all FDA approved home laser devices, it has an optical sensor that measures skin color and disables the laser output if the melanin content of the skin is too high. The Tria has a built-in diffuser that reduces risks to the retina from laser exposure. Use of goggles is not required with home laser devices.

## TABLE 8

### Home-use Laser Devices

| Indication | Laser (Wavelength) | Brand Name | Manufacturer | Parameters |
|---|---|---|---|---|
| Hair removal | Diode (810 nm) | Tria Laser™ | Tria Beauty | Fluence 13–22 J/cm$^2$ Pulse width 300–600 ms |
| | IPL (475–1200 nm) | Silk'n SensEpil™ | Home Skinovations | Fluence 3–7 J/cm$^2$ Pulse width 5 ms |
| | Thermal | No!no! Hair™ | Radiancy | Hot wire razor |
| Periocular wrinkles | Fractional nonablative (1410 nm) | PaloVia™ | Palomar | Fluence 15 mJ Pulse width 10 ms 200–250 μm depth, 1–2% MTZ density |
| | LED red (660 nm) | Tanda Luxe™ | Syneron | |
| | LED red (645 nm) and IR | Silk'n FaceFx™ | Home Skinovations | |

# Combining Aesthetic Procedures

Facial aging is a multifaceted process associated with changes on the skin surface, such as formation of wrinkles, textural changes, pigmented lesions, and vascular lesions. In addition, diminishment and redistribution of fat, hyperdynamic muscle contraction, volume loss and bone resorption also contribute to facial aging changes. To help improve the signs of photoaging and enhance overall aesthetic appearance, an array of minimally invasive cosmetic procedures are currently available including injectable botulinum toxin and dermal fillers, nonablative and ablative lasers, chemical peels and topical prescription, and cosmeceutical products. Many of these aesthetic procedures can be safely combined to enhance facial rejuvenation outcomes. Some are performed together on the same day during one visit, others are incorporated into a multiple visit treatment plan. Common combination treatments using the procedures discussed in this book are reviewed below.

## Pigmented Lesions

- **Nonablative lasers with exfoliation treatments.** Nonablative lasers used to treat benign pigmented lesions (e.g., IPL and 755 nm lasers) may be combined with microdermabrasion to facilitate removal of pigmentation. Following laser treatment of pigmented lesions such as lentigines, lesions clinically darken due to formation of microcrusts. Microcrusts will slough off spontaneously; however, the addition of an exfoliating microdermabrasion treatment expedites exfoliation and enhances overall skin appearance. Microdermabrasion is typically performed 2 weeks after nonablative laser treatment on the face and 3 weeks after treatment on nonfacial areas. This combination may be alternated every 2 weeks for the duration of the patient's series of laser treatments.
- **Multiple nonablative lasers.** Nonablative lasers of different wavelengths may be combined at different visits to treat dyschromia and target pigmentation at different depths in the skin. Figure 17 shows a patient with dyschromia before (A) and after

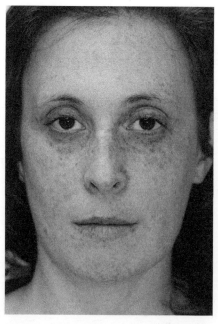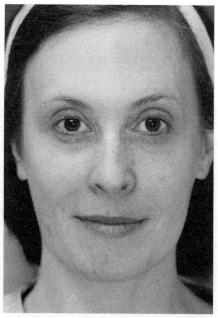

A                                                                                          B

*FIGURE 17* ● Dyschromia before **(A)** and after **(B)** combination treatment using multiple nonablative lasers. (Courtesy of R. Small, MD.)

(B) three IPL treatments (StarLux 500™ with LuxG handpiece, Cynosure/Palomar), followed by a QS 532 nm laser (RevLite™, Cynosure/ConBio) to target faintly colored, superficial pigmented lesions.

## Vascular Lesions

- **Nonablative lasers with exfoliation treatments.** Nonablative laser treatments used to treat red vascular lesions (e.g., IPL and 532 nm lasers) may be combined with microdermabrasion. Red vascular lesions such as telangiectasias and rosacea can be pretreated with microdermabrasion immediately before a laser treatment during one visit. Microdermabrasion enhances red vascular targets by temporarily increasing blood flow and intensity of erythema. This combination approach improves efficacy of the laser treatment and is particularly useful when treating faintly colored vascular lesions.

## Wrinkle Reduction

- **Nonablative lasers with exfoliation treatments.** Nonablative skin resurfacing lasers (e.g., 1320 nm, 1064 nm) may be combined with superficial resurfacing procedures such as microdermabrasion and chemical peels to enhance wrinkle reduction and other collagen remodeling effects such as reduction of coarse pores, rough texture, and to treat dyschromia. One such technique uses a nonablative skin resurfacing laser (e.g., QS 1064 nm) followed by microdermabrasion and then a chemical peel all in the same visit. This approach to skin rejuvenation targets the dermis with the laser and epidermis with exfoliation treatments. Exfoliation of the epidermis may be performed immediately after the laser treatment using microdermabrasion and then a light chemical peel. Microdermabrasion removes the stratum corneum barrier and allows for even and deeper chemical peel penetration in the skin. This combination treatment of nonablative skin resurfacing laser and exfoliation treatments can be safely performed at monthly intervals for cumulative benefits.
- **Multiple ablative lasers.** Severe wrinkles associated with advanced photoaging can be addressed by combining different ablative skin resurfacing lasers. Superficial ablative skin resurfacing addresses rough texture and fine lines and fractional ablative resurfacing penetrates deeper and addresses coarser wrinkles. Figure 18 shows a patient with severe wrinkles and rough skin texture before (A) and after (B) combination treatment with superficial ablative skin resurfacing of the full face and fractional ablative skin resurfacing of the cheeks and perioral area with an YSGG laser (Pearl Fusion™, Cutera).
- **Lasers and botulinum toxin injections.** Wrinkles typically have a dynamic and static component. By addressing both dynamic muscle contraction with botulinum toxin and static lines with skin resurfacing lasers, wrinkle reduction results can be enhanced, particularly in the periocular area. Figure 19 shows crow's feet lines and ephelides before (A) and after (B) combination treatment with botulinum toxin in the crow's feet muscles and superficial ablative skin resurfacing using an erbium laser (DermaSculpt™, Cynosure/ConBio). Botulinum toxin treatments are usually performed on a different day from laser treatments to eliminate the risk of migration of toxin in areas that are manipulated or heated. Performing botulinum toxin injection at least 1 week prior to ablative skin resurfacing treatments allows the toxin to have some effects and the skin to be smoother during the postlaser healing phase.
- **Lasers with dermal filler injections.** Dermal fillers can restore volume loss and treat static wrinkles. Wrinkle reduction results are enhanced when dermal fillers

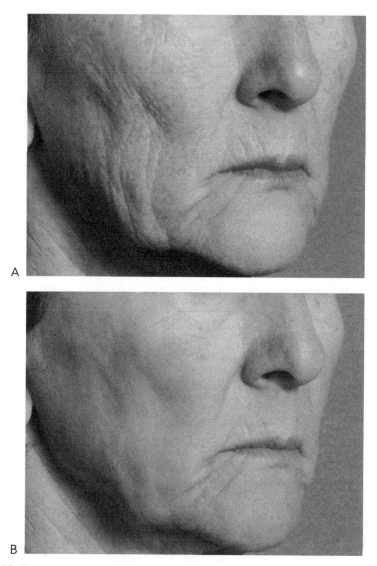

A

B

*FIGURE 18* ● Wrinkles and rough skin texture before **(A)** and after **(B)** combination treatment using multiple ablative lasers. (Courtesy of J. Turkle, MD and Cutera.)

are combined with laser skin resurfacing. However, the type of laser used and the order with which treatments are performed are important considerations that affect outcomes. Nonablative and superficial ablative lasers have been shown to have no adverse effects on fillers. These laser treatments can be performed following dermal filler injection on a different day, once bruising resolves. Deeper ablative and fractional ablative laser treatments have been found to alter dermal fillers and it is advisable to perform ablative laser treatments prior to dermal filler injection, on separate days once skin is fully healed. Static radial lip lines can be challenging to treat and often require combination treatment. Figure 20 shows radial lip lines before (A) and after (B) combination treatment with fractional ablative skin resurfacing using an erbium laser (Lux2940™, Cynosure/Palomar) combined with bolutinum toxin and dermal filler above the upper lip. Figure 21 shows full face rejuvenation before (A) and after (B) combination treatment with fractional ablative skin resurfacing using an erbium

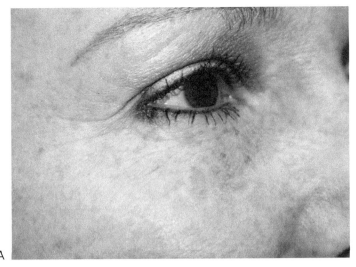

A

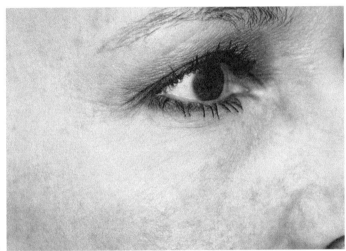

B

*FIGURE 19* ● Periocular rhytids and ephelides before **(A)** and after **(B)** combination treatment with an ablative laser and botulinum toxin. (Courtesy of R. Small, MD.)

laser (ProFractional™, Sciton) for texture combined with dermal filler in the lips, botulinum toxin in the frown, and tattooing of the eyebrows and lips.

## Wrinkle Reduction and Pigmented Lesions

- **Multiple nonablative lasers.** Nonablative lasers of different wavelengths may be combined during the same visit to treat wrinkles and pigmented lesions. Typically, nonablative lasers for wrinkles (e.g., 1320 nm, 1064 nm) are performed first on the full face, and if the treatment area is not overly warm or too erythematous, this can be followed by lasers that target discrete pigmented lesions (e.g., 755 nm, IPL). For example, a nonablative full face laser treatment for wrinkles using a QS 1064 nm laser can be immediately followed by spot treatment of discrete lentigines using a 755 nm laser. Another nonablative laser combination involves two fractional lasers; one that preferentially targets wrinkles and the other that targets epidermal pigmented lesions. For example, a full face fractional

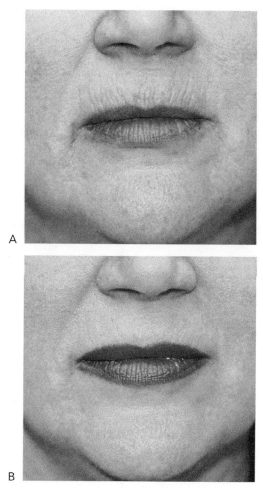

**FIGURE 20** ● Radial lip lines before **(A)** and after **(B)** combination treatment with an ablative laser, dermal filler, and botulinum toxin. (Courtesy of R. Small, MD.)

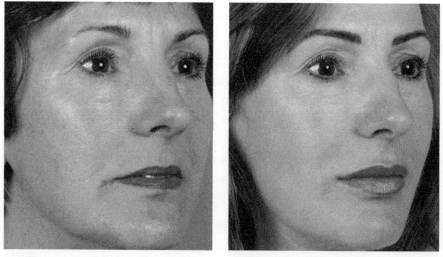

**FIGURE 21** ● Full face rejuvenation before **(A)** and after **(B)** combination treatment with an ablative laser, dermal filler, and botulinum toxin. (Courtesy of D. Holcomb, MD and Sciton.)

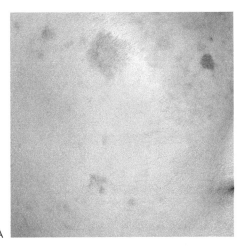
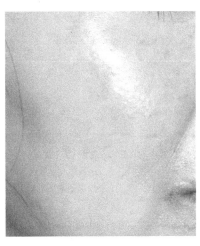

A                                                                                    B

FIGURE 22 ● Dyschromia and rough skin texture before (A) and after (B) combination treatment with a nonablative and ablative lasers. (Courtesy of W. Baugh, MD and Iridex.)

treatment using a 1550 nm laser that targets the dermis for wrinkle reduction can be performed, and immediately followed by a full face fractional treatment using a 1927 nm laser that targets epidermal pigmented lesions. Results of combination nonablative fractional lasers appear to be improved, but patients may experience greater discomfort and longer recovery times compared to use of these lasers alone.

- **Nonablative lasers with ablative lasers.** Nonablative lasers can be combined with ablative lasers to treat wrinkles and pigmented lesions. Figure 22 shows a patient with lentigines, fine lines, and rough skin texture before (A) and after (B) a 532 nm laser (Gemini™, LaserScope) for treatment of lentigines and superficial ablative skin resurfacing using an erbium laser (Venus i™, LaserScope) for textural improvement. Figure 23 shows a patient with severely photodamaged skin before (A) and after (B)

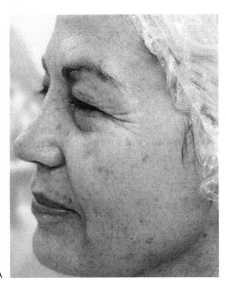
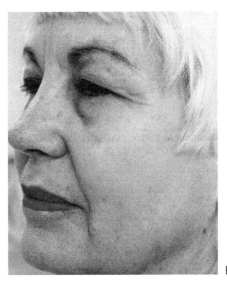

A                                                                                    B

FIGURE 23 ● Dyschromia, wrinkles, and rough skin texture before (A) and after (B) combination treatment with nonablative and ablative lasers. (Courtesy of T. Bessinger, MD and Sciton.)

IPL (BBL™ with 560 nm filter, Sciton) treatment for lentigines followed by fractional ablative skin resurfacing (ProFractional-XC, Sciton) for textural improvement.

### Wrinkle Reduction and Vascular Lesions

- **Multiple nonablative lasers.** Nonablative lasers of different wavelengths can be combined during the same visit to treat wrinkles and red vascular lesions. Typically, nonablative lasers for wrinkles (e.g., 1320 nm, 1064 nm) are performed first on the full face, and if the treatment area is not overly warm or too erythematous, this can be followed by lasers that target discrete vascularities (e.g., 532 nm, IPL). For example, a nonablative full face laser treatment for wrinkles using a 1064 nm QS laser can be immediately followed by spot treatment of discrete telangiectasias using a 532 nm laser.

## Financial Considerations

Most cosmetic laser treatments are not covered by insurance. Treatment of some conditions such as rosacea may be covered, but this benefit varies widely with different insurance carriers. Fees for laser treatments are based on the type of treatment performed and the size of the treatment area, and vary according to community pricing and geographic region. Some laser procedures, such as hair removal and tattoo removal, require several treatments to achieve optimal results and a series of treatments may be offered to patients.

# Treatments

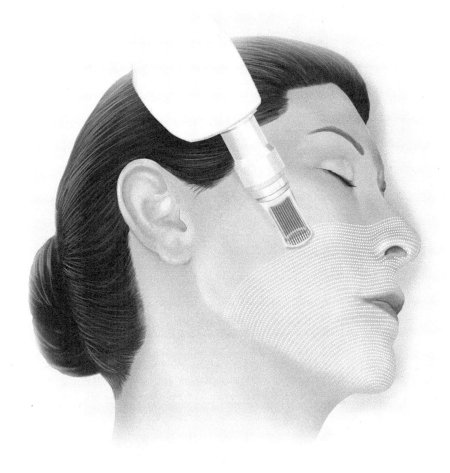

## Chapter 1

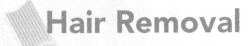

# Hair Removal

### Rebecca Small, M.D.

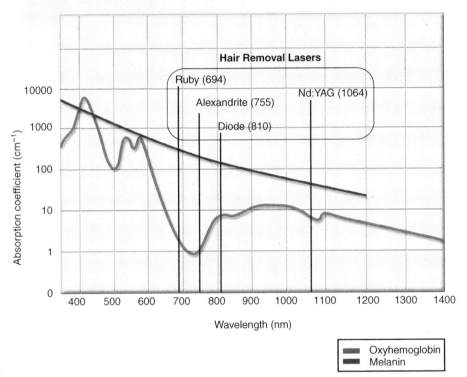

*FIGURE 1* ● Absorption spectra of tissue chromophores and lasers commonly used for hair removal.

Undesired hair growth is a common aesthetic problem affecting both men and women. For women, body areas typically affected include the face, axilla, groin, and legs and for men, the chest, back, shoulders, neck, and ears are common areas of concern. Since its approval by the U.S. Federal Drug Administration in 1995, laser hair removal (LHR) has become one of the most popular cosmetic procedures. While some seek hair removal for cosmetic reasons; others may have underlying medical causes for hirsutism such as polycystic ovarian syndrome (PCOS) and hypothyroidism. In either case, unwanted hair growth, if left untreated, can lead to significant distress for affected individuals and negatively impact self-image and self-esteem. This chapter reviews laser[*] principles as they relate to hair removal and provides a practical approach to the treatment of unwanted hair.

## Anatomy

**Hair follicles** are composed of the bulb (matrix and dermal papilla), outer root sheath, bulge, and hair shaft (Fig. 2). The hair matrix depth in the skin ranges from 2 to 7 mm, depending on the body location, and the hair bulge is approximately 1.5 mm. Hair growth occurs in three phases with distinct changes below the skin in the hair bulb: (1) **anagen,** the active growth phase during which the hair bulb is most darkly pigmented; (2) **catagen,** the regression phase when cell division ceases and the follicle begins to involute; and (3) **telogen,** the resting phase during which the hair bulb is minimally pigmented (Fig. 3). Hair growth is initiated by epithelial stem cells located in the bulge, a protrusion near the attachment of the arrector pili muscle. During anagen, the rapidly dividing matrix cells of the hair bulb cause the hair to elongate and transfer melanin to the hair shaft giving it pigmentation. The hair shaft, visible above the skin surface looks unchanged during the three phases of hair growth.

　　**Two types of hairs** are present in adults: **vellus and terminal. Vellus** hairs are fine (i.e., thin) usually with a diameter of 20–50 μm and are lightly colored. Vellus hairs are often referred to as "peach fuzz." **Terminal** hairs are coarse (i.e., thick) usually with a diameter of 150–300 μm and are darkly colored. The type of hair produced

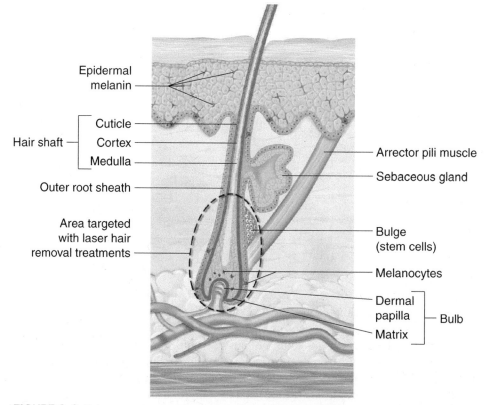

Epidermal melanin

Cuticle

Hair shaft — Cortex

Medulla

Outer root sheath

Area targeted with laser hair removal treatments

Arrector pili muscle

Sebaceous gland

Bulge (stem cells)

Melanocytes

Dermal papilla

Matrix

Bulb

*FIGURE 2* ● Hair anatomy.

*Laser refers to both lasers and intense pulsed light devices, unless otherwise specified.*

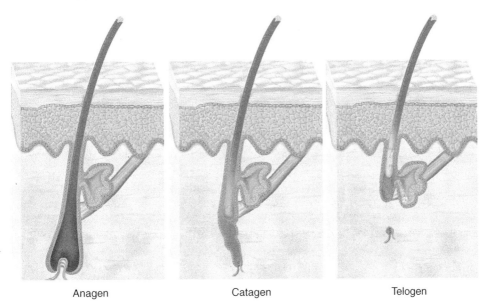

| Anagen | Catagen | Telogen |

**FIGURE 3** ● Phases of hair growth.

by an individual follicle can change over time. For example, during puberty increased androgenic hormone levels cause vellus hair to be replaced with terminal hair in certain parts of the body. In androgenic alopecia, terminal hair can be replaced with vellus hair.

**Melanin** pigment gives hair and skin its color. Melanin is located in several areas of the hair follicle including the hair shaft, bulb, and outer root sheath. Two types of melanin pigment are synthesized by melanocytes: eumelanin and pheomelanin. Eumelanin is brown to black in color; it is the predominant type in dark Fitzpatrick skin types (IV–VI) and is found in darkly pigmented hair. Pheomelanin is yellow to red in color; it is the predominant type in light Fitzpatrick skin types (I–III) and is found in red and blonde hair. White and gray hairs have no melanin.

**Hairs in the early anagen phase** are most susceptible to laser treatment as the matrix has the greatest melanin content and the hair bulb is darkest. The percentage of hairs in anagen varies for different parts of the body (Table 1). Those areas with the greatest percentage in anagen, such as the scalp, respond most rapidly to laser treatments. The

## TABLE 1

Percentage of Hairs in Anagen Phase at Any Given Time and Duration of Telogen Phase for Different Body Areas

| Body Area | Anagen Hair (%) | Telogen Duration (Months) |
| --- | --- | --- |
| Scalp | 85 | 3–4 |
| Beard | 70 | 2.5 |
| Upper lip | 65 | 1.5 |
| Axillae | 30 | 3 |
| Pubic area | 30 | 3 |
| Arms | 20 | 4.5 |
| Lower legs | 20 | 6 |

duration of telogen serves as a rough guideline for the interval between treatments. For example, the upper lip has a short telogen phase and requires intervals of approximately 1 month between treatments, whereas the lower legs have a longer telogen phase and require 2 months or more between treatments.

## Laser Principles

Laser hair removal is based on the principle of selective photothermolysis, the conversion of laser energy to heat, which selectively destroys hair follicles. To achieve hair reduction, laser energy is applied to the skin and absorbed by **melanin,** the target chromophore in hair. Melanin, specifically eumelanin, preferentially absorbs laser energy between 600 and 1200 nm (Fig. 4, Key References). Pheomelanin found in red and blonde hair is poorly absorbed by these wavelengths. Laser energy is converted to heat in the hair which selectively destroys the hair, growth structures. The surrounding skin minimally absorbs energy and remains unaffected.

## Laser Parameters for Hair Removal Treatments

By adjusting laser parameters of wavelength, fluence, pulse width, and spot size, maximal efficacy and safety can be achieved with LHR treatments (see also Introduction and Foundation Concepts, Laser Parameters section).

- **Wavelength.** Wavelength is selected to target melanin. Lasers targeting melanin that are used for hair removal are shown in Figure 1 and include: **ruby (694 nm), alexandrite (755 nm), diode (810 nm), and Nd:YAG (1064 nm). Intense pulsed light (IPL)** devices used for hair removal emit wavelengths that also target melanin and Figure 4 shows an emission spectrum from an IPL handpiece (MaxRS, Palomar/Cynosure) used for hair removal with a peak at 600–800 nm. Longer wavelengths have deeper cutaneous

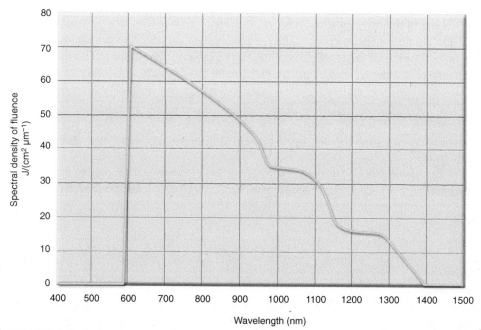

**FIGURE 4** ● Emission spectrum for an intense pulsed light handpiece used for hair removal.

penetration that makes them safer for the epidermis and are preferable for treating darker Fitzpatrick skin types (IV–VI).

- **Fluence.** High fluences are used when less target chromophore is present either due to fine, light-colored hairs or areas with sparse hair. Lower fluences are used when more target chromophore is present either due to coarse, dark hairs or areas with dense hair. From an efficacy perspective, higher fluences are associated with greater permanent hair removal.
- **Pulse width.** Short pulse widths are used when less target chromophore is present either due to fine, light-colored hairs or areas with sparse hair. Longer pulse widths are used when more target chromophore is present either due to coarse, dark hairs or areas with dense hair. In addition, the deeper cutaneous penetration of longer pulse widths makes them safer for the epidermis and they are preferable for treating dark Fitzpatrick skin types (IV–VI).
- **Spot size.** Large spot sizes have greater absorption and deeper cutaneous penetration compared to small spot sizes. The larger the spot size, the more body area covered per pulse, which translates to shorter treatment times.
- **Repetition rate.** Fast repetition rates allow for more rapid coverage of large treatment areas and can shorten treatment times.
- **Pulse modes.** Some IPL devices have variable pulse modes. Multipulse modes with long delays between pulses (e.g., triple-pulsed mode) allow more thermal energy to dissipate and are safer for the epidermis than single pulse modes. Multipulse modes with long delays are typically used when more target chromophore is present and in dark skin types. Single pulse mode is more aggressive and is used for treatment when less target chromophore is present and in lighter skin types.

Laser treatment parameters are often described as **aggressive or conservative.** Aggressive treatment parameters refer to the use of short wavelengths, short pulse widths, high fluences, and small spot sizes. Conservative laser parameters refer to the use of long wavelengths, long pulse widths, low fluences, and large spot sizes (Fig. 3, Key References).

## Patient Selection

**Light Fitzpatrick skin types (I–III) with dark, coarse hair** are the best candidates for LHR treatment. Light Fitzpatrick skin types have less epidermal melanin, which, if present, can serve as a competing chromophore for laser energy. **Dark Fitzpatrick skin types (IV–VI)** have more epidermal melanin and are at greater risk of epidermal injury with LHR treatments. Patients with Fitzpatrick skin type VI pose the greatest challenge to treatment with the highest risk of complications, and recommendations for treatment are outside the scope of this chapter. White and gray hairs have no melanin and are, therefore, nonresponsive to LHR treatments. Light-colored hair (i.e., blonde and light red) and vellus hair lack significant melanin target and patients with these hair characteristics are poor candidates for LHR. It is worth noting that attempts have been made to increase target chromophore in patients with light-colored hair by applying topical dyes (consisting of carbon in mineral oil), but this has not proven to enhance permanent hair removal.

While many people seek hair removal for cosmetic reasons; others may have underlying medical causes for excess hair growth that warrant medical work-up prior to LHR. **Hirsutism** is excessive terminal hair growth typically seen in androgen-sensitive areas such as the upper lip, chin, chest, upper abdomen, back, and buttocks. It is almost always due to increased androgen production, primarily testosterone. PCOS is the most common cause of hirsutism and patients typically have menstrual irregularities along with truncal obesity as presenting signs. Other less common causes of hirsutism include congenital adrenal hyperplasia, ovarian and adrenal androgen-secreting tumors, medications (e.g., Danazol™), and other rare disorders such as Cushing disease, hyperthecosis (a non-malignant ovarian disorder), and severe insulin resistance syndromes. **Hypertrichosis** is excessive vellus hair growth diffusely on the body that is non–androgen-dependent. While typically due to genetics or idiopathic, it can be due to medications (e.g., prednisone, phenytoin, minoxidil, cyclosporine) and can be due to systemic illnesses, such as hypothyroidism, anorexia nervosa, malnutrition, porphyria, dermatomyositis, and paraneoplastic syndromes. Patients with untreated hormonal or other underlying medical conditions that stimulate hair growth will not experience permanent hair removal with LHR treatments unless the underlying pathology is treated. For example, patients with elevated androgen levels such as PCOS typically respond to estrogen-containing oral contraceptives and/or spironolactone both of which have antiandrogen effects, and once stable on medication LHR results are permanent.

## Patient Expectations

Addressing patient expectations helps ensure patient satisfaction with LHR treatments. Prior to treatment it is important to clarify the common misconception that LHR results in complete permanent hair loss. According to the U.S. Food and Drug Administration (FDA), LHR is approved for permanent hair reduction, which is defined as "the long-term, stable reduction in the number of hairs regrowing after a treatment regime." Patients may experience a range of outcomes in addition to lack of growth, such as fewer, thinner, and lighter hairs, which are clinically significant and desirable. Patients are unlikely to be permanently bald with no hair growth in the area after a series of LHR treatments.

A series of LHR treatments is required to achieve optimal results. Typically, individuals with light Fitzpatrick skin types (I–III) require a series of 6 treatments, and dark skin types (IV–V) require 8 treatments, or occasionally more. Fluences are increased more slowly and conservatively over time with darker skin types to minimize the risk of complications. On average, hair is permanently reduced by 20–30% after 1 treatment and up to 60–90% after completing a series of treatments. During the course of LHR treatments, hair becomes finer, lighter, and patchy. Once hair becomes very fine and light, the efficacy limits of the laser may be reached. Subsequent, more aggressive treatments may not be of therapeutic benefit and may be associated with greater risks of complications.

## Indications

- Permanent hair reduction
- Hirsutism
- Hypertrichosis
- Pseudofolliculitis barbae
- Pseudofolliculitis pubis

## Alternative Therapies

**Temporary hair removal methods,** such as shaving, chemical depilatory creams (e.g., Nair™), waxing, threading (use of a cotton thread to pull hair), topical eflornithine

(Vaniqa™), and tweezing are alternative treatment options to LHR. Depilatories contain calcium or potassium thioglycolate that breaks down keratin and weakens hair, facilitating hair removal so that it is easily scraped off. **Eflornithine** is FDA approved for removal of facial hair in women. This product retards the rate of hair growth by blocking ornithine decarboxylase, an enzyme necessary for follicular cell growth and maturation into hairs. Effects are typically seen after 8 weeks with topical application twice daily. While indicated for all hair types, we have found it to be most effective for vellus hair. The only other FDA approved method for permanent hair reduction is **electrolysis.** This utilizes electrical current via a fine needle electrode to destroy individual hair follicles. Electrolysis is effective for treating fine and nonpigmented hair including blonde and gray. However, electrolysis requires longer treatment times compared to LHR and is associated with more pain as the "pulse durations" are in the order of seconds as opposed to milliseconds with lasers, and the hairs are treated individually with electrolysis as opposed to treating numerous hairs simultaneously with each pulse of the laser.

## Devices Currently Available for Laser Hair Removal

| Laser | Wavelength |
| --- | --- |
| Ruby | 694 nm |
| Alexandrite laser | 755 nm |
| Diode laser | 810 nm |
| Nd:YAG laser | 1064 nm |
| Q-switched Nd:YAG laser | QS 1064 nm |
| Intense pulsed light | 500–1200 nm |
| Electro-optical synergy | IPL and RF |

Nd:YAG, neodymium-doped yttrium aluminium garnet; IPL, intense pulsed light; RF, radiofrequency.

**Ruby lasers (694 nm)** were the first devices used for LHR and while still in use today, are not very common. This wavelength is shorter than others used for LHR and consequently it targets epidermal melanin, limiting its use to light skin types (I–III).

**Alexandrite lasers (755 nm)** are commonly used for hair removal in lighter skin types (I–III). While some studies demonstrate efficacy with darker skin types (IV–VI) complications such as postinflammatory hyperpigmentation (PIH) is common. Alexandrite devices have the advantage of being easy to use with flexible fiber optic arms. These devices typically use cryogen spray as a means of cooling the epidermis.

**Diode lasers (810 nm)** have been extensively used for LHR. They are highly effective on coarse dark hair and can treat darker skin types more safely than alexandrite lasers due to their longer wavelength with deeper penetration and contact cooling of the laser tip. They are commonly used in skin types I–V. Part of their appeal and popularity are due to their relatively compact size and lack of disposable parts.

**Nd:YAG lasers (1064 nm)** can be used for LHR in all skin types, and have the greatest safety and efficacy for skin type VI. This longer wavelength that penetrates deeply protects the skin from epidermal injury; however, it has relatively poor melanin absorption making it less effective for LHR. In order to adequately damage hair growth structures, high fluences are required that must be coupled with intense cooling to protect the epidermis from thermal injury.

**Q-switched Nd:YAG lasers (1064 nm)** offer temporary hair reduction and some studies have shown permanent reduction. The short nanosecond pulse widths of these lasers damage the hair growth structures with photoacoustic vibration in addition to selective photothermolysis. These devices can be used with all Fitzpatrick skin types and are commonly used for the treatment of fine dark hairs, particularly on the face.

**IPL devices** emit noncoherent, multiwavelength light ranging from 500–1200 nm. Filters are used that allow emission peaks at certain desired wavelengths. IPLs used for hair removal typically emit a wavelength peak between 600–800 nm that selectively targets melanin. Some IPL devices have demonstrated similar clinical efficacy in hair reduction compared to diode and alexandrite lasers. While most IPLs are not used on Fitzpatrick VI skin types, some devices now combine IPL and 1064 nm to allow for treatment of all skin types.

**Electro-optical synergy (Elos) devices** combine radiofrequency and optical energy (laser or IPL) to remove hair. The electrical radiofrequency energy heats the hair bulb and bulge, and the optical energy heats the hair shaft. Electrical radiofrequency devices are typically more painful than other LHR devices.

See Supply Sources, Appendix 6 for laser manufacturers.

## Contraindications

### General Laser Contraindications

- Active infection in the treatment area (e.g., herpes simplex, pustular acne, cellulitis)
- Dermatoses in the treatment area (e.g., vitiligo, psoriasis, atopic dermatitis)
- Melanoma, or lesions suspected for melanoma in the treatment area
- Deep chemical peel, dermabrasion, or radiation therapy in the treatment area within the preceding 6 months
- Keloidal scarring[‡]
- Bleeding abnormality (e.g., thrombocytopenia, anticoagulant use)
- Impaired healing (e.g., immunosuppressive medications, poorly controlled diabetes mellitus)
- Peripheral vascular disease
- Seizure disorder
- Uncontrolled systemic condition
- Cardiac pacemaker
- Skin atrophy (e.g., chronic oral steroid use, genetic syndromes such as Ehlers–Danlos syndrome)
- Livedo reticularis, a vascular disease associated with mottled skin discoloration of the arms or legs exacerbated by heat exposure
- Erythema ab igne, a rare acquired reticular erythematous or pigmented rash exacerbated by heat exposure
- Direct sun exposure within the preceding 4 weeks resulting in reddened or tanned skin
- Self-tanning product use within the preceding 4 weeks
- Topical prescription retinoid within the preceding week

[‡]*Caution should be used in patients with hypertrophic scarring.*

- Isotretinoin (Accutane™) within the preceding 6 months
- Gold therapy (e.g., used for treatment of arthritis)
- Photosensitizing medications (e.g., tetracyclines, St. John's wort, thiazides)
- Photosensitive disorder (e.g., systemic lupus erythematosus)
- Pregnant or nursing
- Unrealistic patient expectations
- Body dysmorphic disorder
- Treatment inside the eye orbit (i.e., without intraocular eye shields)

## Contraindications Specific to Laser Hair Removal

- Hair removal by waxing, tweezing, or electrolysis during the previous month
- Use of bleaching or depilatory cream during the previous 2 weeks
- Recent, undiagnosed increase in hair growth

## Advantages of Laser Hair Removal

- Permanent hair reduction
- Mild discomfort
- Minimal risks of complications
- Useful for large body areas, such as backs and legs
- Minimal to no recovery time

## Disadvantages of Laser Hair Removal

- Risk of skin discoloration, burns, and infection
- Darker Fitzpatrick skin types (V–VI) have higher risks of thermal injury
- Not effective for reduction of white, gray, and blonde hair

## Equipment

- Laser hair removal device
- Laser-safe eyewear for the patient and provider specific to the wavelength being used
- Nonalcohol cleansing wipes
- Topical anesthetic such as EMLA or benzocaine:lidocaine:tetracaine (BLT)
- Clear colorless gel for treatment if indicated by the manufacturer
- Gauze 4 × 4 in
- Nonsterile gloves
- Ice packs
- Hydrocortisone cream 1% and 2.5%
- Sunscreen that is broad spectrum with SPF 30 containing zinc oxide or titanium dioxide
- Alcohol wipes for cleansing the laser tip
- Germicidal disposable wipes for sanitizing the device
- Soft white eyeliner pencil to mark treatment areas

## Preprocedure Checklist

- **Aesthetic consultation** is performed to review the patient's medical history including contraindications to treatment, medications that may cause hypertrichosis (such as corticosteroids and immunosuppressives), conditions that cause hirsutism such as PCOS and ovarian and adrenal tumors, history of herpes in the treatment area, as well as previous hair reduction methods and results. See also Introduction and Foundation Concepts, Aesthetic Consultation section.

- **Fitzpatrick skin type** is determined (see Introduction and Foundation Concepts, Aesthetic Consultation section).
- **Examination of the treatment area** is performed and hair color, coarseness, and density are documented. Lesions suspicious for neoplasia are biopsied or referred, if indicated, and negative biopsy results received before proceeding with laser treatments.
- **Informed consent** is obtained (see Introduction and Foundation Concepts, Aesthetic Consultation section). An example of a consent form is provided in Appendix 4a.
- **Pretreatment photographs** are taken (see Introduction and Foundation Concepts, Aesthetic Consultation section).
- **Avoidance of direct sun exposure** and daily use of a broad-spectrum **sunscreen** with SPF 30 prior to and throughout the course of treatment is advised.
- **Lightening background skin** may be considered for dark Fitzpatrick skin types (IV–VI) to reduce risks of pigmentary changes such as PIH. Topical skin-lightening products may be used once or twice daily for 1 month prior to treatment such as prescription strength hydroquinone cream 4–8% or over-the-counter cosmeceutical products containing kojic acid, arbutin, niacinamide, and azelaic acid (which are less effective).
- **Test spots** may be considered for patients with dark Fitzpatrick skin types (IV–VI) prior to the initial treatment. Test spot parameters are selected based on the patient's skin type and lesion characteristics following the manufacturer's guidelines for wavelength, spot size, fluence, and pulse width. Test spots are placed discretely near the intended treatment area (e.g., under the chin, behind or inferior to the ear) and pulses overlapped to simulate the technique used with treatment. Test spots are viewed 3–5 days after placement for evidence of erythema, blister, crust, or other adverse effect. Patients should be informed that lack of an adverse reaction with test spots does not ensure that a side effect or complication will not occur with a treatment.
- **Antiviral medication** may be given prophylactically for a history of herpes in or near the treatment area 2 days prior to the procedure and continued for 3 days postprocedure (e.g., valacyclovir 500 mg or acyclovir 400 mg 1 tablet twice daily). Patients with a remote history of HSV infection have a lower risk of reactivation and an antiviral may instead be started on the day of treatment and continued for 5 days.
- **Hair is shaved** 1–2 days prior to treatment such that the hair is just visible (approximately 1–2 mm above the skin) at the time of treatment.
- **Snacks** such as granola bars or juice can be offered on the day of treatment to help avert hypoglycemia in patients who have not eaten for a prolonged period and are treating a large area.
- **Written preprocedure instructions** are provided to patients (see Hair Removal Before and After Instructions for Laser Treatments, Appendix 3a).

## Anesthesia

Laser hair removal treatments are uncomfortable as hair follicles are innervated. Discomfort is usually likened to a rubber band snap. Anesthesia requirements vary according to the specific device used, patients' pain tolerance, and the treatment area.

Many LHR devices have built-in cooling mechanisms, such as a cooled sapphire tip or cryogen spray, which protect the epidermis from thermal injury and provide anesthesia. Application of wrapped ice or cold packs immediately prior to pulsing the laser is a very good, cost effective method of anesthesia, and can also be used posttreatment to soothe the skin. Forced air (e.g., Zimmer Cryo 6™, LaserMed), devices direct cold air at the treatment area and have similar effects to ice. Pneumatic skin flattening is a newer method of anesthesia utilizing vacuum pressure to compress the tip of the laser against the skin thereby reducing pain sensation. This epidermal contact cooling increases safety and provides some anesthesia. Some patients may require topical anesthetics to improve treatment tolerability such as EMLA (prilocaine 21/2%:lidocaine 21/2%), ELA-Max (lidocaine 4%), or BLT (benzocaine 20%:lidocaine 6%:tetracaine 4%). See Introduction and Foundation Concepts, Anesthesia for Laser Procedures section for additional information.

## Laser Hair Removal Procedure

The following procedural recommendations for hair removal, including the sections on selecting initial laser parameters for treatment, general treatment technique, desirable clinical endpoints, undesirable clinical endpoints, aftercare, treatment intervals, subsequent treatments, and common follow-ups are based on using an IPL device (Cynosure/Palomar Icon™ with the MaxRs handpiece) that is indicated for Fitzpatrick skin types I–V. Manufacturer guidelines for the specific device used should be followed at the time of treatment.

### Selecting Initial Laser Parameters for Treatment

Many clinical factors influence laser parameter selection for treatment including the following:

- **Fitzpatrick skin type.** Dark Fitzpatrick skin types (IV–V) have a greater risk of epidermal injury. Conservative parameters of long pulse widths and low fluences are used for treatment. Light skin types (I–III) can tolerate more aggressive parameters of short pulse widths and high fluences. For example, a patient with Fitzpatrick skin type V may initially be treated using a pulse width of 100 ms and fluence using 24–28 $J/cm^2$. A patient with Fitzpatrick skin type II may initially be treated using a pulse width of 20 ms and fluence of 32–38 $J/cm^2$.

   Skin color in the treatment area may vary from the patient's Fitzpatrick skin type that is determined using the Fitzpatrick skin type form (Appendix 2). The perineum and perianal areas for example, are usually darker than other body areas. If a treatment area is darker than the patient's global skin type, consider treating more conservatively, as though their Fitzpatrick score is increased by one. For example, the perineum of a patient with a Fitzpatrick Skin Type IV may be relatively darker compared to the rest of the body, and settings appropriate for Skin Type V may be used.
- **Hair characteristics.** Treatment areas containing a lot of target (i.e., hair that is coarse, dark, or dense) typically require conservative parameters of long pulse widths and low fluences. Treatment areas with less target (i.e., hair that is fine, lightly colored or sparse) require more aggressive parameters of high fluences and short pulse widths (Fig. 5). For example, an initial treatment for a patient with Fitzpatrick skin

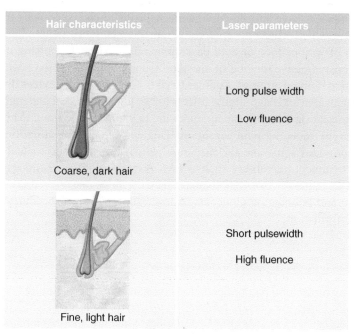

| Hair characteristics | Laser parameters |
|---|---|
| Coarse, dark hair | Long pulse width<br><br>Low fluence |
| Fine, light hair | Short pulsewidth<br><br>High fluence |

FIGURE 5 ● Hair characteristics and laser parameters.

type II having coarse, brown hair that is dense may use a pulse width of 30 ms and fluence of 32 J/cm². A patient having the same Fitzpatrick skin type with finer, brown hair that is sparse may use a pulse width of 20 ms and fluence of 38 J/cm².

- **Other chromophores in the treatment area.** When assessing the treatment area it is important to take all chromophores that are potentially targeted by the wavelength being used into account. Most hair removal lasers also target pigmented lesions. If pigmented lesions are present in the area being treated for hair, then conservative parameters of long pulse widths and low fluences are used due to the greater amount of overall target in the skin.
- **Size of treatment area.** Large flat areas such as the back and upper legs can be treated with fast repetition rates (e.g., 0.6 Hz), which shortens treatment times. Contoured areas such as the face usually require moderately slow rates (e.g., 0.4 Hz) to help ensure careful placement and complete contact between the skin and IPL tip.
- **Bony prominences.** Laser energy can reflect off the bone, increasing epidermal heat. Fluence is decreased over bony prominences such as shin bones and ankles to reduce the risk of overtreatment in these areas.

## General Treatment Technique

- IPL treatments on the face are performed outside of the orbit: above the supraorbital ridge (roughly where the eyebrows sit) and below the inferior orbital rim. Figure 14 in Introduction and Foundation Concepts shows the nontreatment areas of the face.

  **TIP: Lasers are not used for eyebrow shaping underneath the eyebrow. They can be used between the eyebrows at the glabella.**

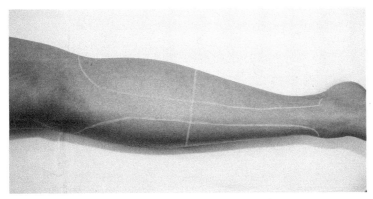

FIGURE 6 ● Grid pattern for laser hair treatments. (Courtesy of R. Small, MD.)

- When preparing to pulse the laser, the IPL tip is placed firmly on the skin surrounded by a thin layer of gel. It remains in contact with the skin throughout the treatment.
- The IPL tip is held perpendicular to the skin and is moved toward the provider, allowing for maximum visibility (Fig. 12a, Introduction and Foundation Concepts).
- A grid pattern may be drawn on the skin to divide the treatment area into sections using a soft white eyeliner pencil. This is helpful when treating large areas such as the legs and back to ensure complete coverage. (Fig. 6).
- IPL pulses are placed adjacently with approximately 20% overlap of each pulse to confluently cover the treatment area.
  **TIP: Incomplete coverage may leave noticeable stripes of hair regrowth 1–2 weeks after treatment.**

## Desirable Clinical Endpoints

When optimal parameters are used for LHR treatments, one or more of the following clinical endpoints may be observed:

- **Singed hair smell**
- **Erythema** (Figs. 7, 8 and 9)
- **Perifollicular edema (PFE)** (Fig. 8)
- **Singed hair** (Figs. 7 and 9)
- **Hair extrusion** (Fig. 9)

Singed hair smell and extrusion are evident immediately, if they occur. Erythema and PFE typically develop a few minutes after the pulse. PFE is more commonly seen with long pulse widths. Figure 9 shows the desired clinical endpoints of singed and extruded hair as well as erythema and PFE.

## Undesirable Clinical Endpoints

When overly aggressive laser parameters are used for treatment, one or more of the following undesirable clinical endpoints may be observed on the skin:

- **Graying**
- **Severe whitening**
- **Blistering**

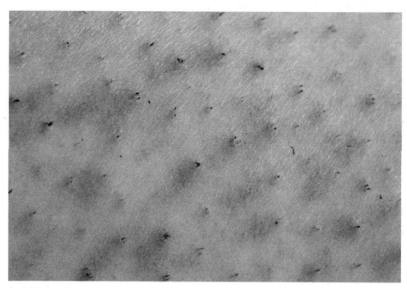

*FIGURE 7* ● Laser hair removal clinical endpoints of erythema and singed hair. (Courtesy of R. Small, MD.)

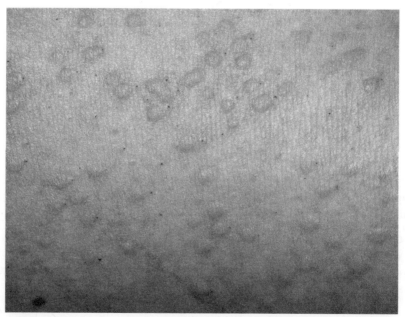

*FIGURE 8* ● Laser hair removal clinical endpoints of perifollicular edema and erythema. (Courtesy of R. Small, MD.)

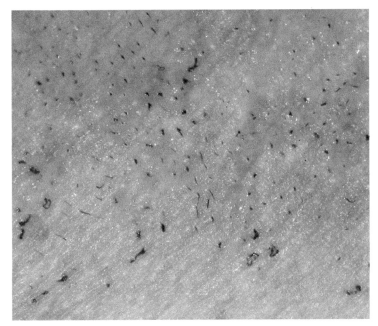

FIGURE 9 ● Laser hair removal clinical endpoints of singed and extruded hair, erythema, and perifollicular edema. (Courtesy of R. Small, MD.)

## Performing Laser Hair Removal

The following recommendations are guidelines for LHR treatments using an IPL device. These treatment steps are specific to the Cynosure/Palomar Icon™ system using the MaxRs handpiece. Providers are advised to follow manufacturer guidelines specific to the device used at the time of treatment.

1. Inquire about sun exposure and sunscreen. If the patient is recently sun exposed or has tanned skin in the treatment area, it is advisable to wait 1 month before treating to reduce the risk of complications.
2. Remove jewelry that may reflect laser light.
3. Position the patient comfortably on the treatment table, prone or supine, to allow for exposure of the treatment area.
4. Shave the treatment area if not shaved within the preceding 1 to 2 days.
5. Apply topical anesthetic (e.g., BLT) if necessary, and remove after 30-45 minutes.
6. Cleanse the skin with a nonalcohol wipe.
7. Cover tattoos and permanent makeup (e.g., with wet gauze) and keep the laser tip approximately 1 inch away from the tattoo during treatment.
   **TIP: Full-thickness burns may result from treating over tattoos.**
8. Provide wavelength-specific protective eyewear to everyone in the treatment room. If working on the face provide the patient with extraocular lead goggles and have the patient remove contact lenses.
9. Always operate the device in accordance with your clinic's policies and procedures and the manufacturer's guidelines.
10. The laser technician is comfortably positioned, usually seated, to allow for precise manipulation of the handpiece while depressing the foot pedal.
11. Select the pulse width and fluence based on the patient's Fitzpatrick skin type and hair characteristics in the treatment area taking into account hair color, coarseness, and density (see Selecting Initial Laser Parameters for Treatment section).

12. Select the repetition rate based on the size and contour of the treatment area (see Selecting Initial Laser Parameters for Treatment section).
13. Apply a clear colorless gel to the skin.
14. Hold the handpiece at a 90-degree angle to the skin and place the treatment tip firmly on the skin, ensuring the entire tip is in contact with the skin.
15. Perform a single pulse in the treatment area. Assess patient tolerance and observe the skin for clinical endpoints. Pain should be less than or equal to 6 on a scale of 1 to 10. Allow a few minutes for clinical endpoints to evolve. If no endpoints are observed, gradually increase the fluence in small increments as tolerated by the patient until desirable clinical endpoints are achieved.
    • **Clinical endpoints with short pulse widths** (e.g., 20 ms) such as singed hair and hair extrusion are visible immediately.
    • **Clinical endpoints with long pulse widths** (e.g., 100 ms) such as PFE can take 5-10 minutes to become visible.
16. Cover the entire treatment area confluently with IPL pulses, using approximately 20% overlap of pulses.
    **TIP: Care must be taken to maintain 20% overlap when fast repetition rates are used to avoid skipping areas.**
17. Continually assess laser–tissue interaction and clinical endpoints throughout the treatment and adjust settings accordingly.
    • **If undesirable endpoints occur,** discontinue treatment in the area and cool skin using wrapped ice packs for 15 minutes. Decrease fluence and/or increase pulse width to achieve desirable endpoints in the remaining treatment areas.
18. Clean the IPL tip frequently during treatment with gauze to reduce build-up of singed hair.
19. Ice packs wrapped in a towel may be applied immediately after treatment for 15 minutes to soothe the treatment area and reduce erythema and edema.
20. Hydrocortisone cream may be applied topically to erythematous areas, 1% for mild erythema and 2.5% for moderate erythema.
21. A broad-spectrum sunscreen (SPF 30 with zinc oxide or titanium dioxide) is applied to treatment areas that are sun exposed.

## Aftercare

• **Erythema and PFE** are expected and typically resolve within a few hours to a few days after LHR treatment. Instruct patients to apply a wrapped ice pack 15 minutes every 1–2 hours and 1% hydrocortisone cream 2–3 times per day for 3 to 4 days or until resolved. Patients are advised to contact their provider if erythema persists for more than 5 days as PIH can occur with prolonged erythema and may require evaluation to rule out other complications (see Complications section).
• **Singed hairs** on the skin may be evident immediately after treatment and a moist washcloth may be used to wipe these hairs off.
• **Direct sun exposure** is avoided and a broad-spectrum sunscreen of SPF 30 is applied daily for 4 weeks after treatment to help minimize the risk of pigmentary changes.
• **Written aftercare** instructions are provided to patients (see Hair Removal Before and After Instructions for Laser Treatments, Appendix 3a).

## Common Follow-Ups

• **Hair extrusion** is visible as dark hairs "growing" immediately after treatment. These are treated hairs coming out of the follicle. Extrusion can take 1–2 weeks;

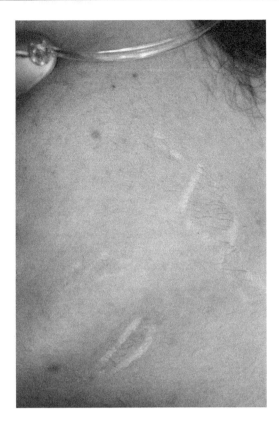

*FIGURE 10* Patchy hair growth on a patient's cheek, chin, and anterior neck outlined with a white pencil midway through an LHR treatment series. (Courtesy of R. Small, MD.)

using a washcloth when cleansing the area and wiping in the direction of the hairs can facilitate removal.

- **Prolonged delay** in hair growth can occur after the first treatment, lasting 1 to 3 months. Inform patients that this is temporary hair reduction and regrowth will occur.
- **Patchy hair growth** occurs after several LHR treatments, where hair appears in some parts of the treatment area and not others (Fig. 10). This is normal and indicates that a group of hairs in the anagen phase were effectively treated. It does not indicate poor coverage of the treatment area.

## Treatment Intervals

Laser hair removal is most effective when performed as a series of 6–8 treatments with adequately long intervals between treatments. The intervals roughly encompass the duration of the telogen phase for the treatment area (Table 2). Six months to 1 year after completion of an LHR treatment series, some patients may require a few follow-up treatments if dormant hairs have entered the hair growth cycle and become active.

**TABLE 2**

Laser Hair Removal Treatment Intervals

| Body Region | Interval Between Treatments (Weeks) |
| --- | --- |
| Face | 4–6 |
| Upper body | 8–10 |
| Lower body | 12 |

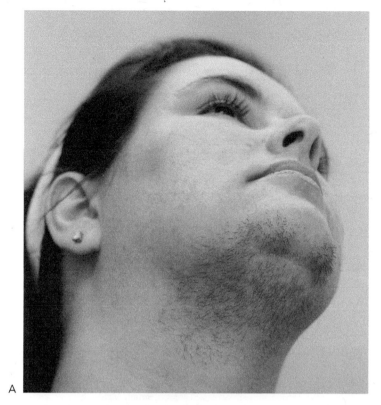

A

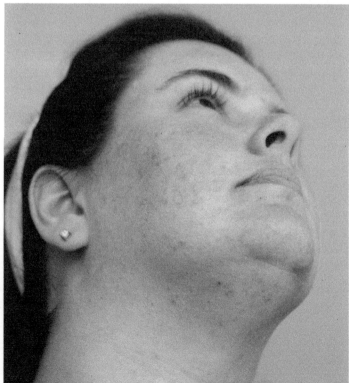

B

*FIGURE 11* ● Anterior neck and chin hair before **(A)** and after **(B)** six hair removal treatments using intense pulsed light. (Courtesy of R. Small, MD.)

## Subsequent Treatments

- **Finer and lighter hair** in the treatment area is observed as treatments progress. Fluence is increased and pulse width decreased in accordance with manufacturer's guidelines, to appropriately match the characteristics of the hair. It is recommended that only one parameter be changed to intensify treatments at any given visit. Typically, the fluence is increased initially for a few treatments and pulse width is decreased in later treatments.
- The **entire area** is treated at each LHR session.
- **Delay treatment** by 2 weeks if there is no evidence of hair growth in the treatment area.

## Results

Permanent hair removal is most effectively achieved with high fluences of at least 30 J/cm², a greater number of treatments, and adequately long intervals between treatments that encompass the telogen phase for the treatment area. Patients with light Fitzpatrick skin types (I–III) typically require 6 treatments and darker skin types (IV–VI) require 8 treatments, or occasionally more. If hairs remain after treatment, they are finer and lighter, and are usually not problematic.

- Figure 11 shows hair on the anterior neck and chin before (A) and after (B) six treatments using an IPL (StarLux™ with LuxRs handpiece, Cynosure/Palomar).
- Figure 12 shows hair on the chin before (A) and after (B) four treatments using a 755 nm laser (Elite+™, Cynosure).
- Figure 13 shows hair on the back before (A) and after (B) six treatments using an IPL (StarLux™ with LuxRs handpiece, Cynosure/Palomar).
- Figure 14 shows hair on the shoulder and upper back before (A) and after (B) a series of treatments using a 755 nm laser (Elite MPX™, Cynosure).
- Figure 15 shows hair on the axilla before (A) and after (B) four treatments using an IPL (StarLux™ with LuxRs handpiece, Cynosure/Palomar).
- Figure 16 shows fine dark upper lip hair in a dark Fitzpatrick skin type before (A) and after (B) a series of treatments using a Q-switched 1064 nm (RevLite®, Cynosure/ConBio).
- Figure 17 shows fine dark sideburn hair before (A) and after (B) a series of treatments using a 755 nm laser (Eliteplus™, Cynosure).
- Figure 18 shows pseudofolliculitis barbae in a patient with Fitzpatrick skin type VI before (A) and after (B) twelve treatments using a 1064 nm long pulse laser (ClearScan YAG™, Sciton).

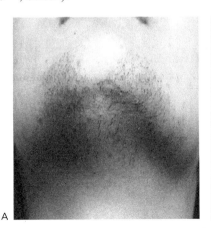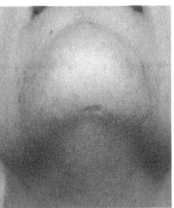

A          B

*FIGURE 12* ● Chin hair before **(A)** and after **(B)** four hair removal treatments using a 755 nm laser. (Courtesy of T. Woo, MD and Cynosure)

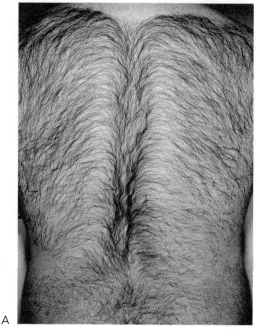

A

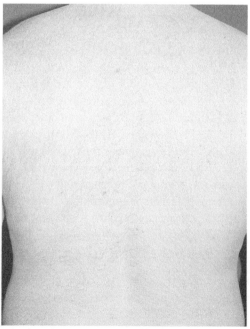

*FIGURE 13* ● Back hair before **(A)**
and after **(B)** six hair removal treatments
using intense pulsed light. (Courtesy of A.
Rockoff, MD and Cynosure)                            B

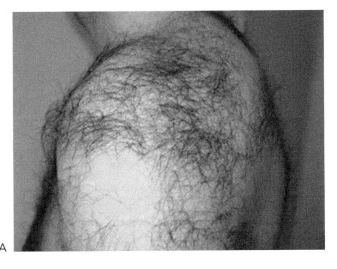

A

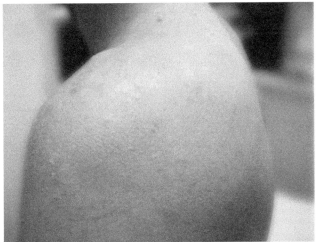

B

**FIGURE 14** ● Shoulder and upper back hair before **(A)** and after **(B)** a series of hair removal treatments using a 755 nm laser. (Courtesy of I. Aristondo, MD and Cynosure)

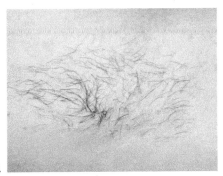

A

B

**FIGURE 15** ● Axilla hair before **(A)** and after **(B)** four hair removal treatments using intense pulsed light. (Courtesy of K. Khatri, MD and Cynosure).

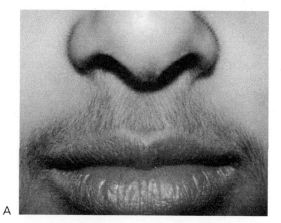

A

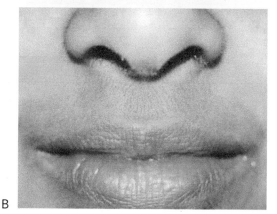

**FIGURE 16** ● Upper lip hair before
**(A)** and after **(B)** a series of hair removal
treatments using a Q-switched 1064 nm
laser. (Courtesy of J. Garden, MD and
Cynosure)

B

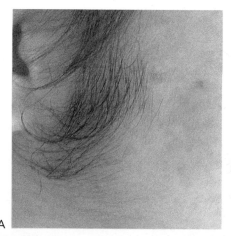

A

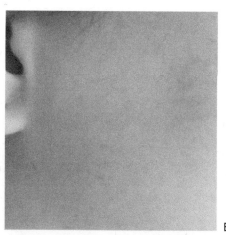

B

**FIGURE 17** ● Sideburn hair before **(A)** and after **(B)** a series of hair removal treatments using a
755 nm laser. (Courtesy of C. Arroyo, MD and Cynosure)

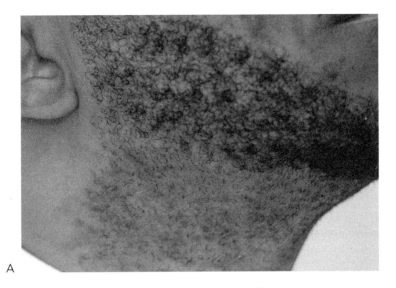

A

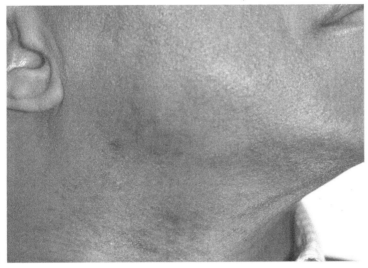

B

**FIGURE 18** ⬤ Pseudofolliculitis barbae before **(A)** and after **(B)** twelve hair removal treatments using a 1064 nm long pulse laser. (Courtesy of L. Haney, RN and Sciton)

## Complications

- Pain
- Prolonged erythema
- Prolonged edema
- Infection
- Hyperpigmentation
- Hypopigmentation
- Burn
- Tattoo alteration
- Scarring
- Failure to reduce the number of hairs or hair coarseness
- Hair reduction in or adjacent to the treatment area

- Paradoxical hair growth
- Urticaria
- Ocular injury
- Bruising
- Erythema ab igne
- Livedo reticularis

While serious complications are rare with laser hair removal, knowledge of the potential complications and their management is important to help ensure the best outcomes. Complications associated with overtreatment such as burns, hyperpigmentation, and hypopigmentation occur most often with the use of aggressive treatment parameters: short wavelengths, short pulse widths, high fluences, and inadequate epidermal cooling. Patients with dark Fitzpatrick skin types (IV–VI) and those with light skin types (I-III) that have diffuse dyschromia such as actinic bronzing, tanned skin, and severely sun-damaged skin with extensive lentigines have the highest risk of these complications.

**Temporary erythema, edema, mild pruritus, and mild sunburn-like discomfort** after treatment are common, lasting a few hours to several days, and are not considered complications.

**Pain** at the time of treatment is common with LHR as all hairs are innervated. Most patients only experience discomfort during the laser pulse, which rapidly resolves once the pulse ceases. Certain areas such as the upper lip, axillae, and genitalia are more sensitive than other areas. Epidermal cooling with application of ice pretreatment and/ or topical anesthetics can reduce discomfort (see Introduction and Foundation Concepts, Anesthesia section). Complaint of pain several days postprocedure is uncommon and evaluation is advisable, particularly to assess for thermal injury due to overtreatment and infection.

**Prolonged erythema and edema** lasting more than 5 days is unusual and may be indicators of thermal injury due to overtreatment, contact dermatitis, or infection (see below).

**Infections** postprocedure from LHR require treatment specific to the pathogen. **Herpes simplex** and varicella zoster may be reactivated in the treatment area, most commonly the lip and genital areas. Prophylactic use of an oral antiviral medication (e.g., valacyclovir/famciclovir 500 mg 1 tablet twice daily begun 2 days prior to the procedure and continued for 3 days postprocedure) in patients with a known history reduces this risk. If a herpetic outbreak occurs despite prophylaxis, consider switching to a different antiviral medication. **Acne vulgaris** is relatively common, on the face and back, particularly in patients prone to acne. It typically resolves spontaneously, but if acne persists, an oral antibiotic such as doxycycline or minocycline (e.g., 100 mg 1 tab twice daily for 2 weeks) may be used. **Folliculitis** may occur, particularly after vigorous exercise, swimming, hot tub use, and shaving immediately after treatment (Fig. 19). Folliculitis typically resolves on its own or with application of warm moist compresses. If lesions persist, topical mupirocin (Bactroban™) may be used for presumed *Staphylococcus aureus*. Pseudomonas folliculitis resulting from hot tubs or contaminated water does not usually require treatment. **Impetigo** may occur, particularly with treatments around the mouth and lower extremities, and although uncommon, is most often seen in patients who have had impetigo previously and are known carriers of *group A Streptococcus* and *S. aureus*. Topical mupirocin three times daily or retapamulin (Altabax™) twice daily for 5 days may be used for treatment of a small

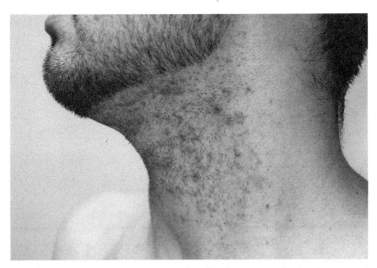

*FIGURE 19* ● Folliculitis on the neck two weeks after hair removal using intense pulsed light. (Courtesy of R. Small, MD.)

number of lesions, and for numerous lesions an oral antibiotic such as dicloxacillin (250–500 mg four times per day) or cephalexin (250–500 mg four times per day) may be used for 7 days.

**Hyperpigmentation and hypopigmentation** are pigmentary complications resulting from alteration to background skin color and are most commonly seen in patients with dark Fitzpatrick skin types (IV–VI), and light Skin types (I-III) with diffuse dyschromia such as actinic bronzing, tanned skin, severely photodamaged skin, and with aggressive treatment parameters. Hyperpigmentation from lasers is primarily in response to inflammation associated with treatment and is referred to as **PIH.** PIH is commonly seen in the setting of prolonged erythema posttreatment combined with direct sun exposure, particularly in dark skin types; it is usually transient and rarely may be permanent. Sun protection including the application of a broad-spectrum sunscreen with SPF 30 containing zinc oxide or titanium dioxide and sun avoidance are used to treat and help prevent PIH. PIH can also be treated with topical lightening agents such as hydroquinone cream 4–8% twice daily and superficial exfoliation procedures such as microdermabrasion and light chemical peels 1 month after treatment. Pretreatment of dark skin types with hydroquinone for 1 month may also aid in prevention of hyperpigmentation. **Hypopigmentation** is a more significant complication that is usually temporary but may be permanent. There are few treatment options for hypopigmentation, but it may repigment with exposure to ambient light sunlight, excimer laser (308 nm), and narrow band UVB treatment. Alternatively, skin surrounding hypopigmented areas can be lightened to reduce the demarcation between darker background skin and hypopigmented areas.

**Burns** can result from aggressive treatment parameters, particularly with short wavelengths and short pulse widths. Figure 20 shows a first-degree burn on the abdomen with prolonged erythema shortly after a hair removal treatment using an IPL that did not have built-in cooling (EsteLux™, Cynosure/Palomar) (A) and resolution at 1 month (B). Devices such as this that rely on manually spraying cryogen onto the laser tip provide less consistent cooling to the epidermis than devices with built-in cooling. While overtreatment of the epidermis is less common with devices that have built-in cooling mechanisms, it can still occur. Figure 21A shows a second-degree burn on the back

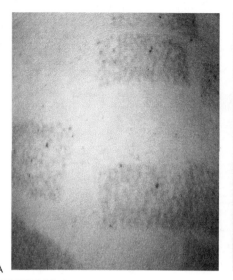

A                                                  B

*FIGURE 20* ● First-degree burn on the abdomen with excessive erythema shortly after **(A)** and one month after **(B)** hair removal using an intense pulsed light device that did not have built-in cooling. (Courtesy of Cynosure/Palomar).

1 week after a hair removal treatment using an IPL (StarLux™ with LuxRs handpiece, Cynosure/Palomar) in a patient with Fitzpatrick IV skin type who presented with a blister that crusted and prolonged erythema. This prolonged erythema in a dark Fitzpatrick skin type evolved to PIH 2 months after treatment (Fig. 21B). Prompt application of a wrapped ice pack to areas suspected of overtreatment at the time of treatment that are intensely erythematous and painful may reduce the area of injury. Blisters and crusting are managed with application of an occlusive ointment, like Aquaphor™ or bacitracin,

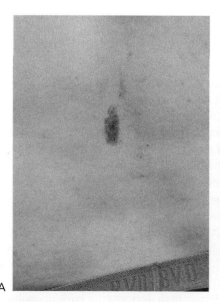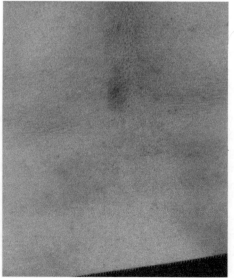

A                                                  B

*FIGURE 21* ● Second-degree burn on the back with crusting and erythema one week after **(A)** and postinflammatory hyperpigmentation two months after **(B)** hair removal using intense pulsed light in a patient with Fitzpatrick IV skin type. (Courtesy of R. Small, MD.)

and covered with a gauze dressing and tape. Patients are monitored over the next few weeks for formation of bullae, intense erythema, induration, and scarring.

**Tattoos and permanent makeup** have concentrated ink pigments and treating over them can result in severe epidermal injury such as a full-thickness skin burn (i.e., third-degree burn). It is advisable to stay 1–2 in away from tattoos and cover them with gauze during treatment.

**Scarring** is an uncommon but serious complication. It is associated with aggressive treatment, particularly in areas predisposed to scarring such as the sternum, or with treatments complicated by burns and infection. In addition, recent use of isotretinoin, previous radiation therapy in the treatment area, and a history of keloid formation are also risk factors for hypertrophic scarring. Persistent intense erythema can be an indicator of impending scar formation. Interventions for persistent intense erythema to reduce the risk of scarring and management of scarring are discussed in Chapter 6, Scarring section.

**Failure to reduce unwanted hair** can be related to undiagnosed medical conditions including hyperandrogenic conditions such as PCOS, untreated hypothyroidism, and as a result of treatments using suboptimal laser parameters with fluences below 30 J/cm$^2$. In addition, intervals that are too short between treatments do not allow adequate time for hairs to return to the anagen phase and can render laser treatments ineffective.

**Hair reduction adjacent to the treatment area** is possible as hair follicles grow at angles to the skin. It is advisable to avoid treating near the eyebrows as these hairs do grow at an angle and unwanted hair reduction can occur.

**Paradoxical hair growth** is a rare phenomenon whereby LHR increases hair. LHR may cause either conversion of vellus hair to coarse terminal hair in the treatment area, or may stimulate hair growth adjacent to the treatment area. Most cases are reported in skin types IV–V with treatment of fine hairs in the lateral face using low fluences. One study found that immediate application of ice around the treatment area and two passes of the laser in the treatment area reduced the risk of paradoxical hair growth.

**Urticaria** is extremely uncommon with LHR treatment but has been reported with nonablative lasers. It can be treated with cold compresses and an oral antihistamine (e.g., cetirizine 10 mg) taken daily until resolved. Once identified, these patients may be pretreated with an antihistamine 1 hour prior to procedure to prevent urticaria formation.

**Ocular injury** from laser light in the eye can be avoided by wearing appropriate laser-safe eyewear at all times during treatment, always directing the laser tip away from the eye and treating outside of the eye orbit. Laser light on the retina can destroy retinal melanin, resulting in blindness.

**Extremely rare and idiosyncratic complications** include bruising, erythema ab igne that is a reticular erythematous rash related to heat exposure, and livedo reticularis that is a vascular condition associated with mottled skin discoloration of the legs or arms exacerbated by heat.

## Special Populations and Additional Considerations

- **Pregnant and nursing.** Women that are pregnant or nursing typically do not undergo elective procedures such as LHR. One of the potential complications from prolonged pain during an LHR treatment might be inhibition of lactation in women who are nursing.

- **Dark Fitzpatrick skin types.** Patients with dark skin types (IV–V) are treated using conservative settings with long pulse widths and low fluences. Treatment parameters are increased gradually to reduce the risk of complications.
- **Pediatric patients.** Hirsute pediatric patients may be treated with parental consent after medical evaluation for hirsutism. Pain management is important with this population and age appropriate analgesics and dosing is necessary.
- **Polycystic ovary syndrome and other hyperandrogenic conditions.** Patients with undesired hair growth due to polycystic ovary syndrome and other conditions associated with elevated androgens will only experience temporary hair reduction from LHR treatments unless androgen excess is corrected.

## Learning Techniques for Laser Hair Removal

Consider initially performing LHR treatments on patients with light Fitzpatrick skin types (I–III) who have coarse, dark hair to minimize the risk of side effects and to better visualize clinical endpoints. Axillae are a preferred area to start with as they are flat, minimally sun exposed, and usually have coarse hair.

## Current Developments

**Pneumatic skin flattening** is being incorporated into some LHR devices to reduce discomfort associated with treatment (see Introduction and Foundation Concepts, Anesthesia for Laser Procedures section). This works by coupling a vacuum chamber to the laser tip which generates negative pressure to flatten skin against the tip thereby reducing discomfort.

**Home-use LHR devices** have recently become available. One such device, Tria™ by Tria Beauty, is a diode (810 nm) that uses a very long pulse width (400 ms) with low fluences (7–20 J/cm$^2$). There is currently no data indicating that permanent reduction can be achieved with these devices and they will likely serve as a temporary hair reduction method.

## Financial Considerations

Laser hair removal is not reimbursable by insurance. The cost for treatments are typically based on the size of the area and can vary widely based on geographic region. For example, a single LHR treatment for a small area such as underarms may be $175 and for a large area such as lower legs may be $350. LHR results are most effective with multiple treatments at appropriate intervals. A series of 6–8 treatments may be offered to help patients stay on schedule with their treatment intervals and achieve optimal results.

**Chapter 2**

# Pigmented Lesions

Rebecca Small, M.D.

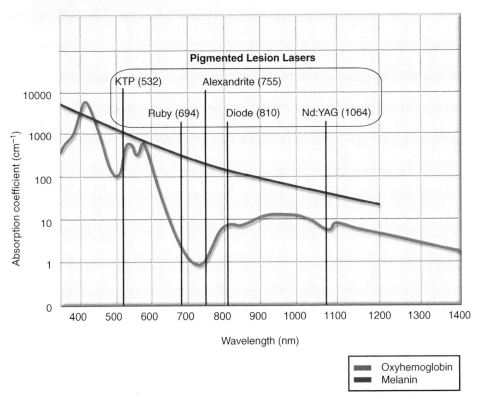

FIGURE 1 ● Absorption spectra of tissue chromophores and lasers commonly used for treatment of benign pigmented lesions.

The most common benign pigmented lesions associated with photoaging are ephelides (freckles), solar lentigines (sun spots), and mottled pigmentation. Certain dyschromic conditions are also associated with or exacerbated by exposure to ultraviolet (UV) light such as postinflammatory hyperpigmentation (PIH), melasma, and poikiloderma of Civatte. This chapter reviews laser[*] principles as they relate to treatment of benign pigmented lesions and conditions seen in photoaged skin and provides a step-by-step approach to treatment.

---

*Laser refers to both lasers and intense pulsed light devices, unless otherwise specified.

Chronic exposure to UV light also contributes to formation of neoplastic pigmented lesions such as melanomas and pigmented basal cell carcinomas. Neoplasias are not indicated for cosmetic laser treatments. When treating pigmented lesions with lasers, they must be verified as benign prior to treatment.

## Anatomy

**Solar lentigines,** also referred to as liver spots and sun spots, are one of the most common benign pigmented lesions seen in photoaged skin. These brown macules darken and increase in size and number with chronic sun exposure. They are typically located around the periphery of the face (Figs. 4a and 7a), neck, chest (Fig. 6a), and other sun-exposed areas of the body (Figs. 8a and 9a). **Ephelides (freckles)** are similar to lentigines but smaller; they darken in summer and lighten in winter (Fig. 11a). Photodamaged skin often demonstrates **mottled pigmentation,** with areas of mixed **hypopigmentation and hyperpigmentation** (Fig. 9a). Some patients with photoaging have chronically hyperpigmented skin, referred to as **actinic bronzing** (Fig. 17a).

**Pigmented conditions** exacerbated by UV exposure include PIH, melasma, and poikiloderma of Civatte. PIH is visible as brown macules or patches arising at sites of inflammation such as acne and trauma (Fig. 13a) and can be a complication from inflammation associated with laser treatments. PIH occurs most often in patients with dark Fitzpatrick skin types (IV–VI). **Melasma** presents as hyperpigmented reticular patches and brown macules on the face, typically involving the cheeks, upper lip, forehead, and chin (Figs. 14a and 15a). It is frequently observed following a change in female hormonal status such as during pregnancy (chloasma) and in response to oral contraceptives. Although much less common, melasma can also occur on the neck, chest, and forearms. **Poikiloderma of Civatte** presents as erythematous and/or brown discoloration on the chest, lateral neck and cheeks. (Figs. 3 and 4, Chapter 3).

**Melanin** pigment determines skin and pigmented lesion color. Pigmentary changes in photoaged skin are due to dysregulation of melanin synthesis and deposition in skin. Chronic UV exposure results in an increased number of overactive melanocytes and disorganized melanin deposition in the epidermis. Chronic UV exposure results in an increased number of overactive melanocytes and disorganized melanin deposition in the epidermis. This results in regions excess with melanin evident as hyperpigmentation such as freckles and lengtigines, and regions with melanin deficiency evident as hypopigmentation.

**Pigmented lesions can be classified based on depth of melanin accumulation** in the skin as epidermal, dermal, or mixed epidermal and dermal. Solar lentigines and freckles are located in the epidermis while PIH, melasma, and poikiloderma of Civatte can be located in either or both of these levels. Benign pigmented lesions and their cutaneous location are summarized in Table 1. A Wood's lamp may be used to visually determine the depth of melanin pigment in skin. When illuminated with a Wood's lamp epidermal pigmentation appears darker with more contrast against the background skin, while dermal pigmentation has less contrast.

## Laser Principles

Laser treatment of benign pigmented lesions is based on the principle of photothermolysis. There are two main categories of lasers used to treat pigmented lesions, **pigment specific lasers that target the melanin chromophore** in pigmented lesions, and **skin resurfacing lasers that target the water chromophore** in dermal tissue.

## TABLE 1

Types of Benign Pigmented Lesions in Photoaged Skin

| Cutaneous Location | Benign Pigmented Lesion |
| --- | --- |
| Epidermal | Lentigines |
| | Ephelides |
| Epidermal and/or dermal | Melasma |
| | Postinflammatory hyperpigmentation |
| | Poikiloderma of Civatte |

**Pigment specific** lasers are most commonly used for treatment of pigmented lesions. They use melanin as the target chromophore, which preferentially absorbs light between 600 and 1200 nm (Fig. 1). Melanin has greater absorption at shorter wavelengths and less absorption at longer wavelengths (Fig. 4, Key References). Lasers that produce light in this range include: KTP (532 nm), ruby (694 nm), alexandrite (755 nm), diode (810 nm), Nd:YAG (1064 nm). Many of these wavelengths are available as Q-switched (QS) lasers that generate very short pulse widths, in the nanosecond and picosecond range. Melanosomes are very small in size (approximately 1 μm) and respond well to these extremely short pulse widths. QS lasers utilize photoacoustic vibration as well as selective photothermolysis for removal of pigmented lesions. Intense pulsed light (IPL) devices emit a band of wavelengths and those used for treatment of pigmented lesions encompass the desired wavelengths for melanin absorption. When a lesion such as a lentigo is irradiated with a pigment specific laser, melanin within the melanosome absorbs energy and is heated and melanosome-containing cells (i.e., melanocytes and keratinocytes) rupture. Melanin is then eliminated through lymphatic drainage, phagocytosis, and exfoliation.

**Skin resurfacing lasers** use water as the target chromophore, which significantly absorbs light above 1200 nm (Fig. 6, Key References). These lasers are used primarily for collagen remodeling effects to treat wrinkles and scars, but can also be used to treat pigmented lesions. When skin is irradiated with a resurfacing laser, water in the dermis absorbs energy and is heated. Epidermal and dermal tissue is removed and pigmented lesions are removed nonspecifically along with this tissue. **Nonablative skin resurfacing lasers (fractional)** that treat pigmented lesions include 1410, 1440, 1540, 1550, and 1927 nm. Through a process referred to as fractional photothermolysis, these lasers heat and coagulate a portion of the skin in microscopic columns, called microthermal zones. Melanin in the treated microthermal zones is extruded from the epidermis along with other epidermal and dermal debris, thereby reducing unwanted pigmentation. The depth of penetration for these lasers is affected by their water-absorption capabilities, where wavelengths that are highly absorbed by water penetrate superficially and shorter wavelengths with lower water absorption penetrate more deeply. For example, 1927 nm has greater water absorption than 1550 nm (Fig. 6, Key References). Consequently, 1927 nm targets more superficial lesions and is effective for treatment of epidermal pigmented lesions such as lentigines and ephelides, whereas 1550 nm penetrates deeper to the dermis and is more effective for dermal pigmented lesions such as melasma. **Ablative skin resurfacing lasers (both fractional and nonfractional)** include 2790, 2940, and 10600 nm. Ablative skin resurfacing lasers are primarily used for treatment of wrinkles and scars, but ablation of epidermal and dermal tissue also removes pigmented lesions.

## Laser Parameters for Treatment of Pigmented Lesions

By adjusting laser parameters of wavelength, fluence, pulse width, and spot size, maximal efficacy and safety can be achieved when treating benign pigmented lesions (also see Introduction and Foundation Concepts, Laser Parameters section). The following discussion focuses on parameters used with **pigment specific lasers,** discussion of parameters used with skin-resurfacing lasers can be found in the chapters on nonablative and ablative lasers for wrinkle reduction (Chapters 5 and 6 respectively).

- **Wavelength.** Pigment specific lasers target melanin. Lasers used to treat pigmented lesions are shown in Figure 1 and include **KTP (532 nm), ruby (694 nm), alexandrite (755 nm), diode (810 nm), and Nd:YAG (1064 nm). IPL** devices used for treatment of pigmented lesions emit wavelengths that also target melanin. Figure 2 shows the emission spectrum for an IPL handpiece used for pigmented lesions (MaxG, Palomar/Cynosure) with peaks at 500–670 nm and 870–1200 nm. Short wavelengths penetrate superficially due to high scatter of the laser beam and longer wavelengths penetrate deeper. Shorter wavelengths are more effective for epidermal pigmented lesions and longer wavelengths are more effective for dermal pigmentation and are safer on darker skin types.
- **Fluence.** High fluences are used when less target chromophore is present either due to sparse lesions or faintly colored lesions. Lower fluences are used when more target chromophore is present either due to a high density of pigmented lesions or intensely colored lesions.
- **Pulse width.** Short pulse widths are used when less target chromophore is present either due to sparse lesions or faintly colored lesions. Longer pulse widths are used

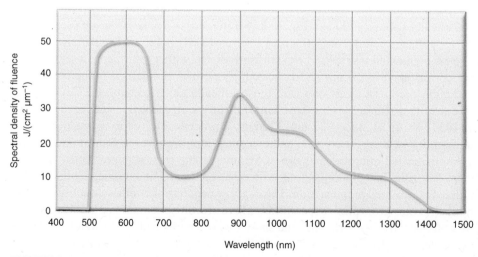

*FIGURE 2* ● Emission spectrum for an intense pulsed light handpiece used for treatment of benign pigmented lesions.

when more target chromophore is present either due to a high density of pigmented lesions or intensely colored lesions. In addition, longer pulse widths penetrate deeper into the skin, making them safer on the epidermis and preferable for treatment of dark skin types. Light skin types are treated with shorter pulse widths compared to those used with dark skin types.

- **Spot size.** Large spot sizes have deeper cutaneous penetration compared to small spot sizes. Large spot sizes are safer on the epidermis and are preferable for treatment of dark skin types. Light skin types are treated with smaller spot sizes. When treating large areas confluently, large spot sizes are used that cover more body area per pulse and have shorter treatment times. When treating discrete lesions, the spot size is chosen to match the size of the lesion. This is particularly important with QS lasers to avoid pigmentary changes to skin surrounding the lesions.
- **Repetition rate.** Fast repetition rates allow for rapid coverage of large treatment areas and shorten treatment times.
- **Pulse modes.** Some IPL devices have variable pulse modes. Multipulse modes with long delays between pulses (e.g., triple-pulsed mode) allow more thermal energy to dissipate and are safer for the epidermis than single pulse modes. Multipulse modes with long delays are typically used when more target chromophore is present and in dark skin types. Single pulse mode is more aggressive and is used for treatment when less target chromophore is present and in lighter skin types.

Laser treatment parameters are often described as **aggressive or conservative.** Aggressive treatment parameters refer to the use of short wavelengths, short pulse widths, high fluences, and small spot sizes. Conservative laser parameters refer to the use of long pulse widths, low fluences, and large spot sizes (Fig. 3, Key References).

## Patient Selection

**Light Fitzpatrick skin types (I–III)** are the best candidates for laser treatment of pigmented lesions. Treatments have high efficacy, and these patients require fewer treatments and have lower risks of complications. This is because light skin types with pigmented lesions have the greatest contrast between background skin and target lesions and aggressive treatment parameters can be used. Patients with **dark Fitzpatrick skin types (IV–VI)** also present with benign pigmented lesions; however, treatment of these patients is more challenging. Darker skin types have increased risks of complications such as hyperpigmentation, hypopigmentation, and burns due to melanin in the background skin competing with the melanin chromophore in the target lesions. Fitzpatrick skin type VI patients have the greatest risk of complications with any aesthetic procedure and treatment of this skin type is an advanced laser application, outside the scope of this book. To minimize risks, patients with dark skin types are treated using conservative parameters. Treatments are less effective and a greater number of treatments are required to achieve improvements.

## Patient Expectations

Treatment of benign pigmented may be performed on virtually any body region where photodamage is present. Treatment of the face, neck, chest, and hands are some of the most commonly treated areas. Noticeable results are evident after a single treatment in properly selected candidates, but typically a series of 3–5 treatments are required for optimal results. Patients with severe photodamage require more treatments than those with mild damage. After treatment, pigmented lesions typically darken and become more noticeable for 1–2 weeks before flaking off to reveal lightened or resolved lesions. It is important for patients to understand that treated lesions will temporarily look worse before they look better.

## Indications

- Lentigines
- Ephelides
- Mottled pigmentation
- Postinflammatory hyperpigmentation
- Poikiloderma of Civatte
- Melasma

Melasma can respond unpredictably with lasers. Nonablative lasers are preferable for melasma due to the risk of exacerbation with ablative lasers. Nonablative QS 1064 nm and fractional 1440 and 1550 nm lasers using repetitive treatments spaced well apart, and a limited number IPL treatments (e.g., 1-2) have demonstrated success with melasma. Paradoxical darkening of melasma can occur particularly with laser treatments that excessively heat the skin using aggressive parameters or short intervals between treatments.

## Alternative Therapies

Nonlaser treatment options for benign pigmented lesions include **liquid nitrogen, exfoliation treatments** such as microdermabrasion and chemical peels, and **topical skin-lightening products** such as hydroquinone and azelaic acid. Liquid nitrogen is much less costly than lasers; however, it is frequently associated with hyperpigmentation and hypopigmentation posttreatment and it is advisable to restrict use to lighter skin types. Exfoliation and topical therapies are slower to achieve improvements and results are rarely comparable to lasers.

**Photodynamic therapy (PDT)** is used off-label for treatment of pigmented lesions, and is approved by the Federal Drug Administration (FDA) for treatment of nonhyperkeratotic actinic keratoses on the face (see Introduction and Foundation Concepts, Photodynamic section). PDT has a greater cost to the patient than laser alone, more downtime with erythema and crusting and requires strict patient avoidance of ambient sunlight posttreatment for 48 hours as exposure can lead to overtreatment and associated complications.

## Devices Currently Available for Treatment of Pigmented Lesions

Lasers used for treatment of benign pigmented lesions can be broken down into 2 broad categories based on their cutaneous target: **Pigment specific lasers** target the melanin chromophore (Figs. 1 and 2), and **skin resurfacing lasers** target the water chromophore (Fig. 6 Key References).

|                   | Laser                                    | Wavelength (nm)       |
| ----------------- | ---------------------------------------- | --------------------- |
| Pigment specific  | Intense pulsed light                     | 500–1200              |
|                   | KTP                                      | 532                   |
|                   | Alexandrite                              | 755                   |
|                   | Diode                                    | 810                   |
|                   | QS: KTP, ruby, alexandrite, Nd:YAG       | 532, 694, 755, 1064   |
| Skin resurfacing  | *Nonablative fractional*                 |                       |
|                   | Diode                                    | 1410                  |
|                   | Nd:YAG                                   | 1440                  |
|                   | Er:glass                                 | 1540, 1550, 1565      |
|                   | Thulium                                  | 1927                  |
|                   | *Ablative (fractional and nonfractional)* |                      |
|                   | YSGG                                     | 2790                  |
|                   | Er:YAG                                   | 2940                  |
|                   | $CO_2$                                   | 10600                 |

KTP, potassium titanyl phosphate; Nd:YAG, neodymium-doped yttrium aluminum garnet; Er:glass, erbium glass; YSGG, Yttrium–scandium–gallium garnet; Er:YAG, erbium-doped yttrium aluminum garnet; $CO_2$, carbon dioxide.

## Pigment Specific Lasers

Short wavelength lasers that target melanin (e.g., 532 nm) are most effective for epidermal lesions as they have high melanin absorption and superficial penetration. Longer wavelength lasers (e.g., 1064 nm) are most effective for dermal pigmentation and are safer for treatment of patients with dark skin types (IV–VI).

**Intense pulsed light (IPL)** devices emit a spectrum of wavelengths and employ filters to refine the energy output selecting for wavelengths that are absorbed by the target lesions. Figure 2 shows an IPL handpiece used to treat pigmented lesions that has emission peaks at 500–670 nm and at 870–1200 nm. Both melanin and oxyhemoglobin are targeted with these wavelengths. Lesions at different depths are also targeted where shorter wavelengths target more superficial lesions and the longer wavelengths target deeper lesions. In this way, a single IPL device can be used to treat both vascular and pigmented lesions at a variety of depths in the skin. IPL devices can be used to treat large photodamaged areas confluently. Many devices also have modified treatment tips that can be used to target discrete lesions. High-quality devices use built-in cooling for epidermal protection, which provides some anesthesia as well. Due to large spot sizes, IPL devices have relatively short treatment times. Depending on the device, most IPL devices can be used for Fitzpatrick skin types I–IV and some for skin type V.

**KTP lasers (532 nm)** are highly absorbed by oxyhemoglobin as well as melanin and, while primarily used for treatment of vascular lesions, they are also used to treat discrete pigmented lesions. Due to the short wavelength and high melanin absorption, this laser targets lesions located in the epidermis such as lentigines and ephelides. The disadvantage of this superficial target depth is the formation of purpura and epidermal injury with associated hyperpigmentation and hypopigmentation, which has limited their use in the past. Newer devices have large spot sizes (e.g., 10 mm) that penetrate deeper and have improved safety with decreased risks of purpura and epidermal injury. Translucent compression spoons may be used to depress pigmented lesions, which reduce vascular target in the treatment area, thereby reducing risks of purpura and overtreatment. KTP lasers are used in light Fitzpatrick skin types (I–III).

**Ruby lasers (694 nm)** were one of the first long pulse lasers to be used for treatment of pigmented lesions, but they had a high incidence of hypopigmentation and are rarely used today. However, QS ruby lasers are still used for treatment of discrete pigmented epidermal lesions and tattoo removal. Ruby lasers are mainly used in light Fitzpatrick skin types (I–III).

**Alexandrite lasers (755 nm)** are commonly used for hair removal but are also effective for treatment of epidermal pigmented lesions. Many devices have the advantage of being easy to use with flexible fiber-optic arms. They typically use a cryogen spray for cooling; these cannisters are disposable and have an associated cost. The risk with cryogen sprays is injury to the epidermis due to overcooling. Alexandrite lasers are primarily used in light Fitzpatrick skin types (I–III).

**Diode lasers (810 nm)** are also primarily used for hair removal and, like alexandrite lasers, their high melanin absorption also makes them effective for treatment of discrete epidermal pigmented lesions. They can be used in darker skin types more safely than alexandrite lasers due to their longer wavelength with deeper penetration, and built-in cooling. Part of their appeal and popularity is due to their relatively compact size and lack of disposable parts. Diode lasers can be used in Fitzpatrick skin types I–IV.

**QS lasers** generate very short pulse widths, in the nanosecond and picosecond range. Melanosomes are very small in size (approximately 1 μm) and respond well to these extremely short pulse widths. In addition, the shorter wavelength lasers **(QS 532 nm, QS 694 nm, and QS 755 nm)** have strong absorption by melanin and are very effective for treating epidermal pigmented lesions such as freckles and lentigines in light skin types. QS lasers have clinical endpoints of crisp white spots and often induce petechiae. When treating discrete lesions with these wavelengths, spot size is chosen to match the size of the lesion to avoid pigmentary changes to the surrounding skin. In addition to treating discrete epidermal lesions, QS 532 nm and QS 755 nm lasers can be used to treat large photodamaged areas confluently in light skin types. Due to a greater depth of penetration and lower melanin absorption, the **QS 1064 nm** laser is used to treat dermal conditions such as melasma, poikiloderma of Civatte, and PIH, and is safe in all skin types (I–VI).

## Skin Resurfacing Lasers

Skin resurfacing lasers are primarily used for collagen remodeling effects to treat wrinkles and acne scars but can also reduce pigmentation. They are used to treat large areas confluently for diffuse pigmentation, rather than for discrete pigmented lesions. Water is the target chromophore for these lasers.

**Nonablative fractional lasers including diode (1410 nm), Nd:YAG (1440 nm), and erbium glass (1540 nm, 1550 nm, 1565 nm)** can treat epidermal and dermal pigmentation. While they do not generate a wound as ablative lasers do, the skin is disrupted and requires some downtime for healing. Treatments are painful and patients typically require topical anesthetic and may also require oral analgesics. Posttreatment they can be associated with acne, milia, prolonged erythema, and PIH, particularly in dark skin types. The **nonablative fractional thulium laser (1927 nm)** has greater absorption by water than the other nonablative fractional lasers, which result in more superficial penetration and more effective targeting of epidermal pigmentation. There is more downtime with 1927 nm than other nonablative fractional lasers and otherwise it has similar complication rates. See Chapter 5 for further discussion of nonablative fractional lasers used for laser resurfacing.

**Ablative lasers (2790 nm, 2940 nm, 10600 nm)** are the most aggressive lasers and are primarily used for resurfacing to reduce wrinkles and laxity but can also treat epidermal pigmented lesions. Ablative lasers create a wound and have risks of pigmentary changes such as hyperpigmentation and hypopigmentation, scarring, and infection. Ablative lasers have the longest postprocedure downtime. Treatments are painful and patients typically require oral analgesics, anxiolytics, and topical anesthetics. Fractional ablative lasers, relative to nonfractional ablative lasers, have shorter recover times and similar types of complications, but with significantly lower incidences and reduced severity. See Chapter 6 for further discussion of ablative lasers used for laser resurfacing.

See Supply Sources, Appendix 6 for laser manufacturers.

# Contraindications

## General Laser Contraindications

- Active infection in the treatment area (e.g., herpes simplex, pustular acne, cellulitis)
- Dermatoses in the treatment area (e.g., vitiligo, psoriasis, atopic dermatitis)
- Melanoma, or lesions suspected for melanoma in the treatment area
- Deep chemical peel, dermabrasion, or radiation therapy in the treatment area within the preceding 6 months
- Keloidal scarring[‡]
- Bleeding abnormality (e.g., thrombocytopenia, anticoagulant use)
- Impaired healing (e.g., immunosuppressive medications, poorly controlled diabetes mellitus)
- Peripheral vascular disease
- Seizure disorder
- Uncontrolled systemic condition
- Cardiac pacemaker
- Skin atrophy (e.g., chronic oral steroid use, genetic syndromes such as Ehlers–Danlos syndrome)
- Livedo reticularis, a vascular disease associated with mottled skin discoloration of the arms or legs exacerbated by heat exposure
- Erythema ab igne, a rare acquired reticular erythematous or pigmented rash exacerbated by heat exposure
- Direct sun exposure within the preceding 2 weeks resulting in reddened or tanned skin
- Self-tanning product within the preceding 2 weeks
- Topical prescription retinoid within the preceding week
- Isotretinoin (Accutane™) within the preceding 6 months
- Gold therapy (e.g., used for treatment of arthritis)
- Photosensitizing medications (e.g., tetracyclines, St. John's wort, thiazides)
- Photosensitive disorder (e.g., systemic lupus erythematosus)
- Pregnant or nursing
- Unrealistic patient expectations
- Body dysmorphic disorder
- Treatment inside the eye orbit (i.e., without intraocular eye shields)

---

[‡]*Caution should be used in patients with hypertrophic scarring.*

## Contraindications Specific to Laser Treatment for Pigmented Lesions

- Skin type IV with some devices
- Skin type V with most devices
- Skin type VI with all devices except 1064 nm

## Advantages of Laser Treatment for Pigmented Lesions

- Dramatic improvements in a relatively short amount of time compared to topical products such as retinoids or hydroquinone
- Minimal recovery time and minimal risks of complications such as hyperpigmentation, hypopigmentation, scarring, or infection in appropriately selected patients using nonablative lasers
- Less risk of hypopigmentation compared to liquid nitrogen

## Disadvantages of Laser Treatment for Pigmented Lesions

- Darker Fitzpatrick skin types (IV and above) have increased risks of hyperpigmentation, hypopigmentation, and scarring
- High equipment expense relative to nonlaser treatments

## Equipment

- IPL device appropriate for pigmented lesion treatment
- Laser-safe eyewear for the patient and provider specific to the wavelengths being used
- Nonalcohol facial wipes
- Clear colorless gel for treatments if necessary per the manufacturer
- Gauze $4 \times 4$ in
- Nonsterile gloves
- Ice packs
- Hydrocortisone cream 1% and 2.5%
- Sunscreen that is broad spectrum with SPF 30 containing zinc oxide or titanium dioxide
- Alcohol wipes for cleaning laser tip
- Germicidal disposable wipes for sanitizing the device

## Preprocedure Checklist

- **Aesthetic consultation** is performed to review the patient's medical history including contraindications to treatment, hormonally induced hyperpigmentation, history of PIH or abnormal scarring, medications that may worsen hyperpigmentation or erythema such as oral estrogen–containing hormones and topical steroids, as well as previous methods for treating photodamaged skin and success. See also Introduction and Foundation Concepts, Aesthetic Consultation section.
- **Fitzpatrick skin type** is determined (Introduction and Foundation Concepts, Aesthetic Consultation section).

- **Examination of the treatment area** is performed. Lesions suspicious for melanoma or neoplasia are biopsied or referred, if indicated. Lesions suspicious for melanoma may be asymmetric, have irregular borders, variegated color, diameter greater than 6 mm, changing or new characteristics such as enlargement or bleeding. Note that basal cell carcinomas can also be pigmented. Await negative biopsy results before proceeding with laser treatments.
- **Informed consent** is obtained (see Introduction and Foundation Concepts, Aesthetic Consultation section). An example of a consent form is provided in Appendix 4b.
- **Pretreatment photographs** are taken (see Introduction and Foundation Concepts, Aesthetic Consultation section).
- **Avoidance of direct sun exposure** and daily use of a broad-spectrum **sunscreen** with SPF 30 prior to and throughout the course of treatment is advised.
- **Lightening background skin** may be considered dark Fitzpatrick skin types (IV–VI) to reduce risks of pigmentary changes such as PIH. Topical prescription skin-lightening products can be used such as hydroquinone cream 4–8% or over-the-counter cosmeceutical products containing kojic acid, arbutin, niacinamide, and azelaic acid (which are less effective) once or twice daily for 1 month prior to treatment.
- **Test spots** may be considered for patients with dark Fitzpatrick skin types (IV–VI) prior to the initial treatment. Test spot parameters are selected based on the patient's Fitzpatrick skin type and pigment characteristics following the manufacturer's guidelines for wavelength, spot size, fluence, and pulse width. Test spots are placed discretely near the intended treatment area (e.g., under the chin, behind or inferior to the ear) and pulses overlapped to simulate the technique used with treatment. Test spots are viewed 3–5 days after placement for evidence of erythema, blister, crust, or other adverse effect. Patients should be informed that lack of an adverse reaction with test spots does not ensure that a side effect or complication will not occur with a treatment.
- **Antiviral medication** may be given prophylactically for a history of herpes simplex or varicella zoster in or near the treatment area 2 days prior to the procedure and continued for 3 days postprocedure (e.g., valacyclovir/famciclovir 500 mg 1 tablet twice daily). Patients with a remote history of HSV infection have a lower risk of reactivation and an antiviral may instead be started on the day of treatment and continued for 5 days.
- **Hair in the treatment area** is shaved prior to treatment to reduce the risk of epidermal thermal injury.
- **Written pre-procedure instructions** are provided to patients (see Pigmented Lesion Before and After Instructions for Laser Treatments, Appendix 3b).

## Anesthesia

Anesthesia is not typically required for laser treatment of pigmented lesions. In addition, anesthesia can interfere with patient feedback, an important component for selecting appropriate treatment parameters. For patients with low pain thresholds, consider an oral analgesic such as tramadol (Ultram™) 50 mg 1–2 tablets 1 hour prior to procedure.

## Procedure for Laser Treatment of Pigmented Lesions

The following procedural recommendations for treatment of benign pigmented lesions, including the sections on selecting initial laser parameters for treatment, general treatment technique, desirable clinical endpoints, undesirable clinical endpoints, aftercare, treatment intervals, subsequent treatments, and common follow-ups are based on using an IPL device (Cynosure/Palomar Icon™ with the MaxG handpiece) that is indicated for Fitzpatrick skin types I–IV. Manufacturer guidelines for the specific device used should be followed at the time of treatment.

## Selecting Initial Laser Parameters for Treatment

Many clinical factors influence laser parameter selection for treatment including:

- **Fitzpatrick skin type.** Dark Fitzpatrick skin types (i.e., IV) have a greater risk of epidermal injury. Conservative parameters of long pulse widths and low fluences are used for treatments. Light skin types (I–III) can tolerate more aggressive parameters of short pulse widths and high fluences. For example, a patient with Fitzpatrick skin type IV with numerous lentigines may initially be treated using a pulse width of 30 ms and fluence of 26–28 J/cm$^2$. A patient with Fitzpatrick skin type II with many lentigines may initially be treated using a pulse width of 15 ms and fluence of 34–36 J/cm$^2$.
- **Pigmentation characteristics.** Treatment areas containing a lot of target (i.e., dark lentigines or a high density of lentigines) typically require conservative parameters of long pulse widths and low fluences. Treatment areas with less target (i.e., light-colored lentigines or sparse lentigines) usually require more aggressive parameters of high fluences and short pulse widths (Fig. 3). For example, an initial treatment for a patient with Fitzpatrick skin type II having numerous dark brown lentigines may use a pulse width of 20 ms and fluence of 30 J/cm$^2$. A patient having the same Fitzpatrick skin type with sparse light brown lentigines may use a pulse width of 15 ms and fluence of 34–36 J/cm$^2$.
- **Other chromophores in the treatment area.** When assessing the skin it is important to take all chromophores that are potentially targeted by the wavelength used

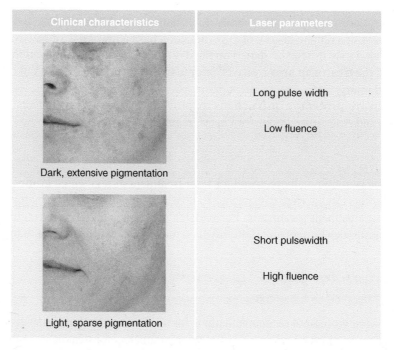

| Clinical characteristics | Laser parameters |
|---|---|
| Dark, extensive pigmentation | Long pulse width<br>Low fluence |
| Light, sparse pigmentation | Short pulsewidth<br>High fluence |

*FIGURE 3* ● Pigmented lesion characteristics and laser parameters. (Courtesy of R. Small, MD.)

into account. In addition to pigmented lesions, photodamaged skin often has red vascular lesions and may also have dark hair present.

- If **red vascular lesions** are present in the area being treated for pigment, more conservative parameters of long pulse widths and low fluences are used due to the greater amount of overall target in the skin. For example, if the treatment area has sparse, faintly pigmented lesions that overlie intense erythema, conservative laser parameters are used.
- If **dark hair** is present in the area being treated for pigment, it is advisable to use conservative parameters or avoid confluent IPL treatment by performing spot treatments to specific pigmented lesions only. For example, if the treatment area has sparse, faintly pigmented lentigines that overlie an area with dense dark hair such as a man's beard, the discrete lentigines can be spot treated using an opaque paper "mask" to cover skin surrounding the lentigines. In addition, hair is shaved prior to treatment to reduce excessive heating from singed hair on the skin surface. Treating over darkly colored hair may cause permanent hair reduction and patients need to be informed of this risk prior to treatment.

- **Size of treatment area.** Large flat areas such as the chest and extremities can be treated with fast repetition rates (e.g., 0.6 Hz), which shorten treatment times. Contoured areas such as the face usually require moderately slow rates (e.g., 0.4 Hz) to help ensure careful placement and complete contact between the skin and IPL tip.
- **Nonfacial areas.** Areas such as the extremities, neck and chest are treated using more conservative parameters than the face, due to slower healing times and greater risk of complications.

## General Treatment Technique

- IPL treatments on the face are performed outside of the orbit: above the supraorbital ridge (roughly where the eyebrows sit) and below the inferior orbital rim. Figure 14 in Introduction and Foundation Concepts shows the nontreatment areas of the face. Initially, it is advisable to avoid lips and as skill improves, providers may choose to treat lips for lesions such as lentigines.
- The face is typically broken down in to sections that are treated sequentially to help ensure complete coverage. Figure 14 in the Introduction and Foundation Concepts shows once possible sequence for IPL treatment of the full face, starting with section 1 and progressing to section 6.
- When preparing to pulse the laser, the IPL tip is placed firmly on the skin surrounded by a thin layer of gel. It remains in contact with the skin throughout the treatment.
- The IPL tip is held perpendicular to the skin and is moved toward the provider, which allows for good visualization of the handpiece tip on the skin (Fig. 16a, Introduction and Foundation Concepts).
- IPL pulses are placed adjacently with approximately 20% overlap of each pulse. Each section is covered confluently with pulses before moving onto the next section.
  **TIP: Areas requiring additional treatment, such as a lentigo that has not shown a desirable clinical endpoint, can be returned to and pulsed again after the full face is treated.**
  **TIP: The most sensitive areas are the upper lip (philtrum) and adjacent to the alar groove. When treating the upper lip, discomfort can be reduced by having the patient place their tongue over their teeth while keeping their lips closed.**

## Desirable Clinical Endpoints

When optimal parameters are used for treatment of pigmented lesions, one or more of the following clinical endpoints may be observed on the skin:

- **Darkening of the lesion and enhanced demarcation against** the background skin (Fig. 4b)
- **Perilesional erythema** (Fig. 4b)
- **Background erythema** (Figs. 4b and 5)
- **Gray or black discoloration of the lesion** may occur with aggressive treatment (Fig. 5)

    **Light Fitzpatrick skin types (I–III)** have clinical endpoints that are clearly visible and are seen immediately after or within a few minutes of pulsing the IPL. Lentigines and mottled pigmentation along with close-up views are shown in Figure 4 before (A) and immediately after (B) IPL treatment with clinical endpoints of lesion darkening and demarcation, perilesional erythema, and background erythema. Lesion blackening and intense erythema are indicators of an aggressive treatment (Fig. 5).

    **Dark skin types (IV)** are treated with conservative settings. Endpoints are subtle, typically consisting of slight lesion darkening and enhanced demarcation without erythema, and have a delayed appearance of 5–10 minutes after the IPL pulse.

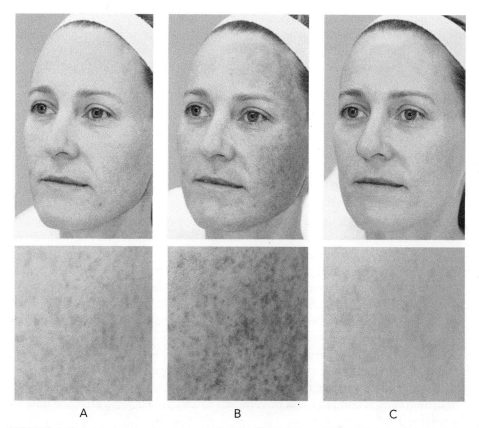

A                          B                          C

*FIGURE 4* ● Lentigines and mottled pigmentation before **(A)**, immediately after treatment showing clinical endpoints and close-up views of pigmented lesion darkening, border demarcation, and perilesional erythema **(B)**, and one month after treatment **(C)**, using intense pulsed light. (Courtesy of R. Small, MD.)

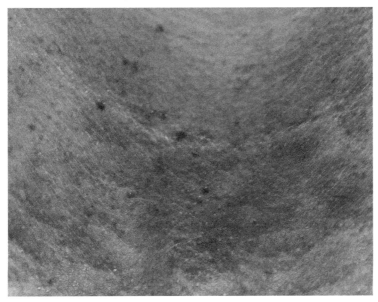

**FIGURE 5** ● Clinical endpoints of lesion blackening and background erythema immediately after treatment using intense pulsed light. (Courtesy of R. Small, MD.)

## Undesirable Clinical Endpoints

When overly aggressive laser parameters are used for treatment, one or more of the following undesirable clinical endpoints may be observed on the skin:

- **Severe whitening**
- **Blistering**

## Performing Laser Treatment for Pigmented Lesions

The following recommendations are guidelines for treatment of benign pigmented lesions associated with photoaging using an IPL device. These treatment steps are specific to the Cynosure/Palomar Icon™ system using the MaxG handpiece. Providers are advised to follow manufacturer guidelines specific to the device used at the time of treatment.

1. Inquire about sun exposure and sunscreen prior to treatment. If the patient is recently sun exposed or has tanned skin in the treatment area, it is advisable to wait 1 month before treating to reduce the risk of complications.
2. Remove jewelry that may reflect laser light.
3. Position the patient comfortably on the treatment table, prone or supine, to allow for exposure of the treatment area.
4. Shave the treatment area if dark hair is present.
5. Cleanse the skin with a nonalcohol wipe.
6. Tattoos and permanent makeup are covered (e.g., with wet gauze) and it is advisable to keep the laser tip approximately 1 inch away from the tattoo during treatment. **TIP: Full-thickness burns may result from treating over tattoos.**
7. Provide wavelength-specific protective eyewear to everyone in the treatment room. If working on the face provide the patient with extraocular lead goggles and have the patient remove contact lenses.
8. Always operate the laser in accordance with your clinic's laser safety policies and procedures and the manufacturer's guidelines.

9. The laser technician is comfortably positioned, usually seated, to allow for precise manipulation of the handpiece while depressing the foot pedal.

10. Select the pulse width and fluence based on the patient's Fitzpatrick skin type and pigmented lesion characteristics in the treatment area taking into account lesion darkness and density; and the presence of other targets in the treatment area such as vascularities and dark hair (see Selecting Initial Laser Parameters for Treatment section).

11. Select the repetition rate based on the size and contour of the treatment area (see Selecting Initial Laser Parameters for Treatment section).
    **TIP: Care must be taken to keep pulses adjacent when fast repetition rates are used to avoid skipping areas.**

12. Apply a thin layer of clear colorless gel to the skin.

13. Place the device treatment tip firmly on the skin, making certain that the handpiece is perpendicular to the skin surface and the entire tip is in contact with the skin.

14. Perform a single pulse at the lateral margin of the treatment (e.g., anterior to the ear) area and assess for patient tolerance and clinical endpoints (see above). In general, there should be subtle endpoints with initial treatments and pain should be less than or equal to 6 on a scale of 1–10. Allow a few minutes for endpoints to evolve for light skin types (I–III) and up to 10 minutes for darker skin types (IV). If no endpoints are observed, gradually increase the fluence in small increments as tolerated by the patient until desirable clinical endpoints are achieved.

15. Cover the entire treatment area confluently with IPL pulses, using approximately 20% overlap.

16. Continually assess laser–tissue interaction and clinical endpoints throughout the treatment and adjust settings accordingly.
    - If **undesirable endpoints** occur discontinue treatment in the area and cool the skin using wrapped ice packs for 15 minutes. Decrease fluence and/or increase pulse width to achieve desirable endpoints in the remaining treatment areas.

17. After the treatment area has been confluently covered with pulses, assess the pigmented lesions within the treated area for clinical endpoints.
    - If areas with **mottled pigmentation** do not have adequate endpoints, consider performing a second pass to the whole area with the same settings, or same pulse width and slightly lower fluence to enhance the clinical endpoints.
    - If discrete lesions such as **lentigines and ephelides** do not have adequate endpoints, spot treat the lesions and modify settings accordingly to achieve clinical endpoints. A lesion mask (Fig. 8, Chapter 3) may be used to specifically target the discrete lesions.

18. Ice packs wrapped in a towel may be applied immediately after treatment for 15 minutes and soothe the treatment area and reduce erythema and edema.

19. Hydrocortisone cream may be applied topically to erythematous areas: 1% for mild erythema and 2.5% for moderate erythema.

20. A broad-spectrum sunscreen (SPF 30 with zinc oxide or titanium dioxide) is applied to treatment areas that are sun exposed.

## Aftercare

- **Mild swelling and erythema** are expected and typically resolve within a few hours to a few days after treatment. Instruct patients to apply a wrapped ice pack 15 minutes every 1–2 hours and 1–2.5% hydrocortisone cream 2–3 times per day for a few days or until resolved. Patients are advised to contact their provider if erythema persists for more than 5 days as prolonged erythema may require evaluation to rule out complications (see Complications, section).

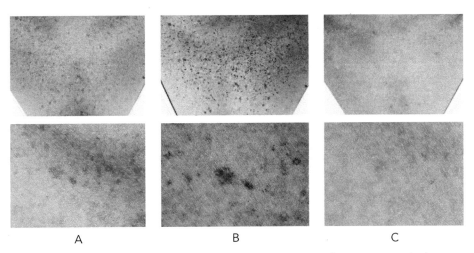

A                    B                    C

*FIGURE 6* ⬤ Chest lentigines and ephelides with close-up views before (**A**), one week after treatment showing pigmented lesion darkening due to microcrust formation (**B**), and two weeks after treatment (**C**), using intense pulsed light. (Courtesy of R. Small, MD.)

- **Mild sunburn-like sensation** in the treated area may also occur, and this typically resolves within a day and can be relieved with ice.
- **Pigmented lesion darkening** continues for 1–2 days after treatment and represents microcrust formation (Fig. 6b). The lesions demonstrate microscopic qualities of a crust; however, they are not palpable. Microcrusts flake off 1–2 weeks after treatment, exposing lightened or resolved lesions (Fig. 6c).
- **Postprocedure products** that are soothing and hydrating are used for 2 weeks post treatment including a broad-spectrum sunscreen of SPF 30 containing zinc oxide or titanium dioxide (see Introduction and Foundation Concepts, Postprocedure Skin Care Products for Laser Treatments section).
- **Direct sun exposure** is avoided for 4 weeks after treatment to minimize the risk of undesired pigmentary changes.
- **Written aftercare instructions** are provided to patients (see Pigmented Lesion Before and After Instructions for Laser Treatments, Appendix 3b).

## Common Follow-Ups

- **Pruritic, dry skin** is not uncommon in the 2 weeks following treatment. Use of a topical skin care regimen that provides hydration and does not have any active ingredients such as retinoids and hydroxy acids usually prevents itchiness and facilitates healing (see Introduction and Foundation Concepts, Postprocedure Skin Care Products section). Hydrocortisone 1–2.5% may be used daily or twice daily for pruritis as needed and an ointment-based product (e.g., Hydrabalm™ by SkinCeuticals) may be used instead of a cream moisturizer to provide additional hydration. Care should be taken to use occlusive products on the face for a limited time (less than 5 days) as these products can cause milia and acne.
- **Delayed exfoliation of microcrusts** with tiny specs of darkened pigmentation that persist for 3–4 weeks can occur, particularly with treatments on extremities. This can also occur in treatment areas where the skin is too dry. After 3 weeks patients may gently exfoliate the treated area to facilitate removal of microcrusts with either an over-the-counter microbead scrub (e.g., Micro-Exfoliating Scrub™ by SkinCeuticals) or a microdermabrasion treatment.

## Treatment Intervals

Treatment of benign epidermal pigmented lesions typically requires a series of 3–5 IPL procedures at monthly intervals for optimal results, depending on the severity of photodamage. Nonfacial areas are slower to exfoliate and heal and require longer intervals between treatments up to 8 weeks. One annual follow-up treatment is recommended for patients to maintain results.

## Subsequent Treatments

- **Lighter, sparse pigmented lesions** are observed over the course of a treatment series. Fluence is increased and pulse width decreased at subsequent visits in accordance with manufacturer's guidelines to appropriately match the pigmented lesion characteristics. It is recommended that only one parameter be changed to intensify treatments at any given visit. Typically, the fluence is increased initially for a few treatments (by 2-4 J/cm$^2$ each visit) and pulse width is decreased in later treatments.
- **Treat the entire area** at each visit.
- **Delay treatment** by 2 weeks if microcrusts are visible at the subsequent, and consider using microdermabrasion or an exfoliating scrub to speed lesion resolution.

## Results

Many factors influence treatment results of benign pigmented lesions, but in general, patients with light Fitzpatrick skin types that have dark epidermal pigmented lesions such as lentigines and ephelides have the most dramatic improvements with the fewest number of treatments. Faintly colored epidermal lesions and dermal lesions such as melasma, PIH, and Poikiloderma of Civatte tend to be more challenging.

- Figure 4 shows lentigines and mottled pigmentation on the face before (A), immediately after (B), and two months after (C), one treatment using an IPL (Icon™ with MaxG handpiece, Cynosure/Palomar).
- Figure 6 shows lentigines on the chest with close-up views before (A), one week after (B), and two weeks after (C), one treatment using an IPL. Note lentigines darkened and flaking one week after treatment (B) due to microcrust formation, and significant improvement in pigmentation at two weeks (C).
- Figure 7 shows lentigines and mottled pigmentation on the face before (A) and after (B) a series of five treatments using an IPL (StarLux™ with LuxG handpiece, Cynosure/Palomar).
- Figure 8 shows lentigines on the hand before (A) and after (B) a series treatments using an IPL (StarLux™ with LuxG handpiece, Cynosure/Palomar).
- Figure 9 shows lentigines on the arm before (A) and after (B) one treatment using an IPL (BBL™ with 515 nm filter, Sciton).
- Figure 10 shows lentigines and under-eye hyperpigmentation before (A) and after (B) two treatments using a QS 532 nm laser (RevLite™, Cynosure/ConBio).
- Figure 11 shows ephelides on the face before (A) and after (B) one treatment using a QS 532 nm laser (Laser Peel™, Medlite™ Cynosure/ConBio).
- Figure 12 shows ephelides on the face before (A) and after (B) one treatment using a fractional 1927 nm laser (Fraxel™, Solta).
- Figure 13 shows postinflammatory hyperpigmentation in a patient with Fitzpatrick VI skin type before (A) and after (B) a series of treatments using a QS 1064 nm laser (Medlite™, Cynosure/ConBio).
- Figure 14 shows melasma on the face before (A) and after (B) six treatments using a QS 1064 nm laser (RevLite™, Cynosure/ConBio).
- Figure 15 shows melasma on the face before (A) and after (B) four treatments using a fractional 1550 nm laser (Fraxel™, Solta).

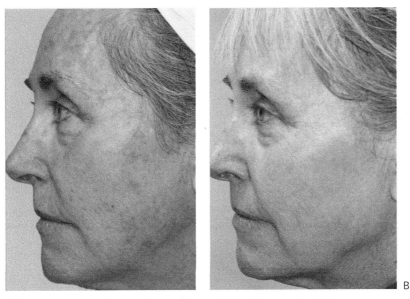

*FIGURE 7* ● Lentigines and mottled pigmentation before **(A)** and after **(B)** five treatments using intense pulsed light. (Courtesy of R. Small, MD.)

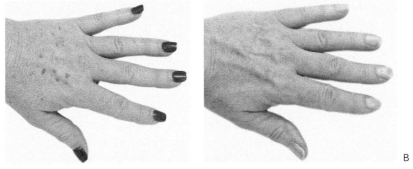

*FIGURE 8* ● Hand lentigines before **(A)** and after **(B)** a series of treatments using intense pulsed light. (Courtesy of R. Small, MD.)

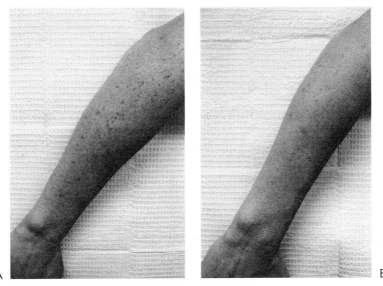

*FIGURE 9* ● Arm lentigines and mottled pigmentation before **(A)** and after **(B)** one treatment using intense pulsed light. (Courtesy of T. Mann, MD and Sciton.)

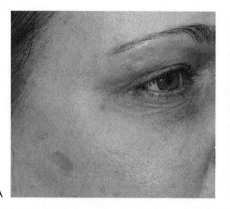
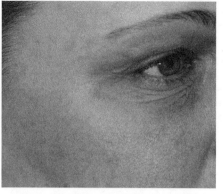

A                                                                                                                          B

*FIGURE 10* ● Lentigines and dark under eye "circles" before **(A)** and after **(B)** two treatments using a Q-switched 532 nm laser. (Courtesy of R. Small, MD.)

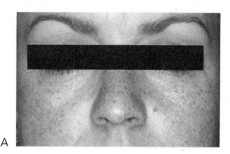
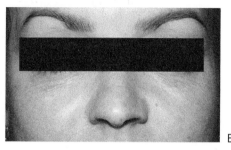

A                                                                                                                          B

*FIGURE 11* ● Ephilides before **(A)** and after **(B)** one treatment using a Q-switched 532 nm laser. (Courtesy of B. Saal, MD and Cynosure/ConBio.)

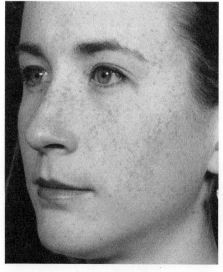
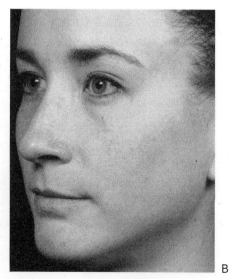

A                                                                                                                          B

*FIGURE 12* ● Ephilides before **(A)** and after **(B)** two treatments using a fractional 1927 nm laser. (Courtesy of Solta.)

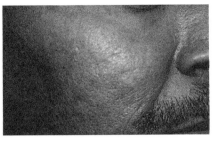
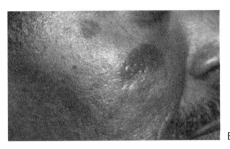

A B

FIGURE 13 ● Postinflammatory hyperpigmentation in a dark Fitzpatrick skin type patient before (A) and after (B) a series of treatments using a Q-switched 1064 nm laser. (Courtesy of J. Garden, MD and Cynosure/ConBio.)

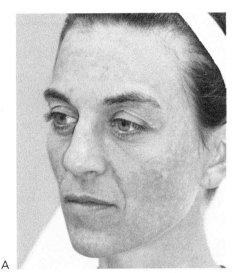
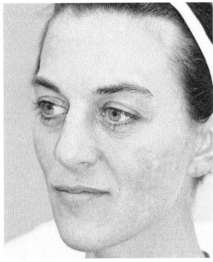

A B

FIGURE 14 ● Melasma before (A) and after (B) a series of treatments using a Q-switched 1064 nm laser. (Courtesy of R. Small, MD.)

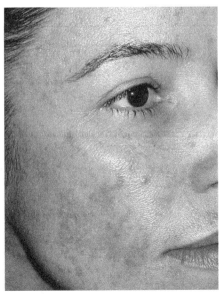
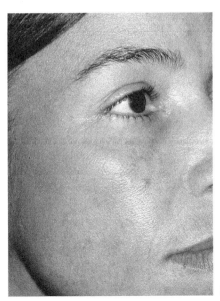

A B

FIGURE 15 ● Melasma before (A) and after (B) four treatments using a fractional 1550 nm laser. (Courtesy of H. Conn, MD and Solta.)

## Complications

- Pain
- Prolonged erythema
- Prolonged edema
- Urticaria
- Contact dermatitis
- Infection
- Milia
- Petechiae and purpura
- Visible skin patterns or striping
- Hyperpigmentation
- Hypopigmentation
- Burn
- Tattoo alteration
- Scarring
- Nonresponse, incomplete clearance, recurrence or worsening of unwanted pigmentation (e.g., worsening of melasma)
- Hair reduction in or adjacent to the treatment area
- Ocular injury

While serious complications are rare with laser treatment of benign pigmented lesions, knowledge of the potential complications and their management helps ensure the best possible outcomes. Complications associated with overtreatment such as burns, hyperpigmentation, and hypopigmentation occur most often with the use of aggressive treatment parameters: short wavelengths, short pulse widths, high fluences, and inadequate epidermal cooling. Patients with dark Fitzpatrick skin types (IV–VI) and those with light skin types (I-III) that have diffuse dyschromia such as actinic bronzing, tanned skin, and severely sun-damaged skin with extensive lentigines have the highest risk of these complications. The following discussion of complications focuses on those seen with nonablative lasers used for treatment of benign pigmented lesions; complications associated with ablative lasers are discussed in Chapter 6.

**Temporary erythema, edema, mild pruritis, and mild sunburn-like** discomfort after treatment are common, typically last for a few hours to several days, and are not considered complications.

**Pain** is usually only reported during treatment and is mild to moderate (less than 6 on a standard pain scale of 1–10) depending on the treatment area. Pain is more significant with fractional lasers, typically 5–6, and patients often require cooling with ice or a cool blower immediately after treatment for comfort. Complaint of pain several days postprocedure is uncommon and evaluation is advisable, particularly to assess for thermal injury due to overtreatment and infection.

**Prolonged erythema and edema** lasting up to 5 days can result from aggressive treatment of the cheeks, particularly with fractional lasers and pulsed dye lasers. Erythema and edema can be treated with application of wrapped ice packs applied for 15 minutes a few times per day, sleeping with the head elevated, an oral antihistamine such as cetirizine (Zyrtec®) 10 mg or diphenhydramine (Benadryl®) 12.5–25 mg daily, and a topical corticosteroid twice daily such as a low-potency steroid (e.g., hydrocortisone 2.5%) or a medium-potency steroid (e.g., triamcinolone acetonide 0.1%) depending on the severity. Prolonged erythema and edema lasting more than 5 days is not typical, and may be an indication of thermal injury due to overtreatment, contact dermatitis, or infection.

**Urticaria** in the treatment area may be seen immediately after treatment and is managed similarly (Fig. 14, Chapter 5). Once identified, patients who form hives in response to laser treatments may be pretreated with an antihistamine 1 hour prior to procedure to attenuate the histamine response.

**Contact dermatitis** is uncommon with nonablative lasers but is a consideration in patients who develop worsening erythema and pruritis after treatment. If contact dermatitis is suspected, postprocedure topical products are discontinued and a topical corticosteroid is used (per instructions for prolonged erythema and edema).

**Infections** after laser treatment of pigmented lesions are uncommon and require treatment specific to the pathogen. Reactivation of viral infections in the treatment area such as **herpes simplex** (and zoster) is one of the most common infectious complications, and pretreatment with an oral antiviral medication (e.g., valacyclovir/famciclovir 500 mg 1 tablet twice daily begun 2 days prior to the procedure and continued for 3 days postprocedure) in patients with a known history reduces this risk. **Bacterial infections** are rare (apart from acne), and if they occur usually result from streptococcus or staphylococcus. Figure 16 shows a bacterial infection in a shaved area on the leg 2 weeks after treatment with an IPL. Notice that microcrusts were removed in the shaved area. Treatment options include either topical antibiotics such as mupirocin (Bactroban®) or oral antibiotics such as doxycycline 100 mg twice daily for 1 week; local resistance patterns should be considered in

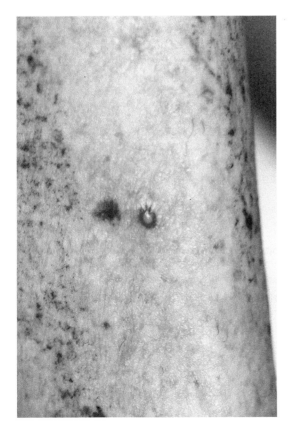

FIGURE 16 ● Bacterial infection on the leg in an area shaved two weeks after intense pulsed light treatment. (Courtesy of R. Small, MD.)

antibiotic selection. **Acne vulgaris** is relatively common after fractional laser treatments. It typically develops within the first few weeks and resolves spontaneously. If acne persists, an oral antibiotic such as doxycycline or minocycline (e.g., 100 mg 1 tab twice daily for 2 weeks) may be used.

**Milia** result from occlusion of sebaceous glands and most often occurs with fractional nonablative lasers. Ointments used to hydrate skin postprocedure can occlude sebaceous glands and contribute to milia formation. Milia do not usually resolve spontaneously and require lancing with a 20-gauge needle and extraction (i.e., gentle squeezing with cotton-tipped applicators) for removal.

**Petechiae and purpura** represent bleeding underneath the skin and usually appear a few minutes after treatment (Fig. 9, Chapter 3). Petechiae and purpura are common with QS lasers and short wavelength lasers (e.g., 532 nm), particularly when short pulse widths and high fluences are used. Petechiae typically take 3–5 days to resolve and purpura can take up to 2 weeks. Utilizing large spot sizes, low fluences, and skin compression if treating over erythema can reduce the incidence of purpura with lasers that are prone to purpura formation. Topical products such as arnica and vitamin K may be of limited use in treating purpura.

**Hyperpigmentation and hypopigmentation** are pigmentary complications resulting from alteration to background skin color. Patients with dark Fitzpatrick skin types (IV–VI) and light Skin types (I-III) with diffuse dyschromia such as severely photodamaged skin, actinic bronzing, and a recent tan have the highest risk of pigmentary complications. They occur most often with use of aggressive treatment parameters such as short wavelengths (e.g., 532 nm) and short pulse widths (e.g., QS lasers). Pigmentary changes can appear as discrete areas usually in the shape of the treatment tip, or as visible patterns and striping. **Patterns and striping** are common with IPL treatments, particularly in light Fitzpatrick skin types with diffuse dyschromia. These patterns can be the result of careful treatments with appropriate overlap of pulses, where the dark stripes represent the regions of overlap. In other cases, these patterns can result from removal of pigmentation in the shape of the treatment tip, where the darkened stripes represent untreated skin surrounding the footprint of the laser tip. Figure 17 shows a light Fitzpatrick skin type patient's chest with actinic bronzing before **(A)**, five days after treatment with hyperpigmentation and crusting in the shape of the IPL tip (B), and one month after one IPL treatment with resultant hypopigmented striping that represents lightened skin surrounded by untreated skin (C). Figure 18 shows stripes of hypopigmentation on the chest of a patient with a dark Fitzpatrick skin type resulting from treatment utilizing an IPL handpiece that was inappropriate for the patient's skin type.

**Hyperpigmentation** associated with laser treatments is primarily due to upregulation of melanin synthesis and deposition in the epidermis as a result of inflammation, referred to as **postinflammatory hyperpigmentation (PIH).** Prolonged erythema posttreatment combined with direct sun exposure is associated with PIH, particularly in dark skin types. Patients with undiagnosed **melasma** can also have worsened hyperpigmentation a few weeks after treatment, and this occurs most often in the setting of repetitive laser treatments at short intervals (e.g., 1-2 week intervals). Hyperpigmentation usually resolves spontaneously over several months, although in rare instances may be permanent. Sun protection including application of a broad-spectrum sunscreen with SPF 30 containing zinc oxide or titanium dioxide and sun avoidance are preventative measures for PIH. PIH can be treated using a topical lightening agent such as hydroquinone cream 4–8% twice daily in the PIH area, and superficial exfoliation procedures such as microdermabrasion and light chemical peels 1 month after treatment, and sun protection. Pretreatment of dark

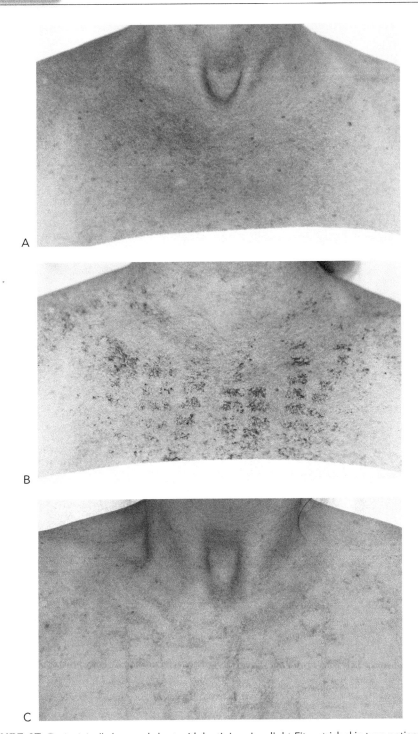

A

B

C

**FIGURE 17** ● Actinically bronzed chest with lentigines in a light Fitzpatrick skin type patient before **(A)**, five days after with crusting **(B)**, and one month after with striping **(C)**, one treatment using intense pulsed light. (Courtesy of R. Small, MD.)

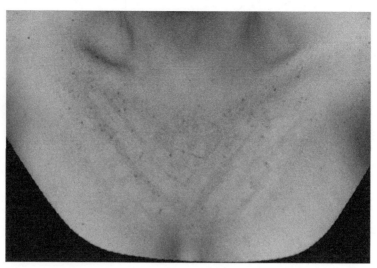

**FIGURE 18** ● Hypopigmented chest in a dark Fitzpatrick skin type patient three months after one treatment using intense pulsed light. (Courtesy of R. Small, MD.)

skin types with hydroquinone for 1 month may also aid in preventing hyperpigmentation. **Hypopigmentation** is a more significant complication that is usually temporary, but may be permanent. There are few treatment options for hypopigmentation, but it may repigment with exposure to ambient light sunlight, excimer laser (308 nm), and narrow band UVB treatment. Skin surrounding hypopigmented areas can be lightened with laser treatments in an attempt to blend the demarcation between background skin and hypopigmented areas.

**Burns** can result from aggressive treatment parameters, particularly with short wavelengths (e.g., 532 nm). Prompt application of a wrapped ice pack to areas suspected of overtreatment at the time of treatment that are intensely erythematous and painful may reduce the area of injury. Blisters and crusting are managed with application of an occlusive ointment such as Aquaphor™ or bacitracin, and covered with a gauze dressing and tape. Patients are monitored over the next few weeks for formation of bullae, intense prolonged erythema, induration, and scarring. **Tattoos and permanent makeup** have concentrated ink pigments and treatment over these can result in full-thickness skin burns.

**Scarring** is very rare but may occur with overly aggressive treatments, particularly in areas predisposed to scarring such as the sternum, or with treatments complicated by burns and infection. In addition, recent use of isotretinoin, previous radiation therapy in the treatment area, and a history of keloid formation are also risk factors for hypertrophic scarring. Persistent intense erythema can be an indicator of impending scar formation. Interventions for persistent intense erythema to reduce the risk of scarring and management of scarring are discussed in the Scarring section, Chapter 6.

**Nonresponse of pigmented lesions** can result from treatment parameters that are too conservative. Keratotic lesions such as seborrheic keratoses may lighten in color but do not flatten in response to nonablative lasers; they can be treated with resurfacing lasers and liquid nitrogen.

**Reduced hair** in or adjacent to the treatment area may occur. It is advisable to fully discuss this risk if hair is present, especially if treating over men's facial hair.

**Ocular injury** can be avoided by wearing appropriate laser-safe eyewear at all times during treatment, directing the laser tip away from the eye and treating outside of the eye orbit. Laser light on the retina can destroy retinal melanin, resulting in blindness.

## Special Populations and Additional Considerations

- **Pregnant and nursing.** Women who are pregnant or nursing typically do not undergo elective procedures such as lasers for treatment of red vascular lesions. One possible complication in nursing women is inhibition of lactation due to pain associated with a prolonged painful laser treatment.
- **Dark Fitzpatrick skin types.** Patients with dark skin types (IV–V) are treated using conservative settings with long pulse widths and low fluences. Treatment parameters are increased gradually to reduce the risk of complications. Patients may not experience the same degree of reduction in unwanted pigmentation that lighter Fitzpatrick skin types can achieve due to these restrictions.
- **Pediatric patients.** Pediatric patients are not generally candidates for cosmetic photorejuvenation treatments.
- **Nonfacial areas.** Nonfacial areas have fewer pilosebaceous units, which serve as sites of re-epithelialization that facilitate healing. These areas have delayed healing relative to the face, with a greater risk of overtreatment and scarring, and should be treated conservatively.
- **Melasma.** Results from laser treatments of melasma may be variable and in some cases, hyperpigmentation may be worsened, particularly with repetitive IPL treatments.

## Learning Techniques for Laser Treatment of Pigmented Lesions

Consider performing initial treatments in patients with light Fitzpatrick skin types (I-III) on the face using conservative parameters: high IPL cutoff filters (e.g., 560 nm), long pulse widths, and low fluences. Aiming for subtle clinical endpoints of pigmented lesion darkening with minimal perilesional erythema is advisable initially. As procedural skill is gained, modify settings to achieve standard clinical endpoints and consider advancing to treatment of nonfacial areas.

## Current Developments

**Fractional resurfacing** is one of the newest areas of laser medicine with many rejuvenation benefits including reduction of pigmentation. New applications for this technology, new wavelengths, and new device modifications are rapidly becoming available. Some of the latest techniques, for which there are limited clinical studies, involve combining fractional resurfacing with other laser technologies to achieve more comprehensive improvements for photoaged skin (see Introduction and Foundation Concepts, Combining Aesthetic Procedures section).

    **Over-the-counter fractional nonablative devices** are being developed with company claims of improving benign pigmented lesions in addition to treating other signs of photoaging such as wrinkles and skin texture. The ReAura (by Philips) is a nonablative fractional diode laser (1435 nm) that claims to improve photoaged skin. This laser penetrates 200 μm in depth, while in-office nonablative fractional lasers penetrate up to 1500 μm. Another home device offered in the United States for skin rejuvenation is

VISS (by Narian, Korea), an IPL 430–1200 nm with limited data available. Although modest improvements may be seen with home devices, their clinical effects are unlikely to be comparable to office-based technologies.

## Financial Considerations

Laser treatment of pigmented lesions is not reimbursable. The charges for treatment vary, and are largely determined by local prices. Individual treatment prices range from $350–$500 for a single treatment to a large area such as the face or chest, and $150–$250 for a small area such as the hands or neck. Several treatments are typically required to achieve maximal benefits and a series of 3 or 5 treatments may be offered to patients.

## Chapter 3

# Vascular Lesions

Rebecca Small, M.D.

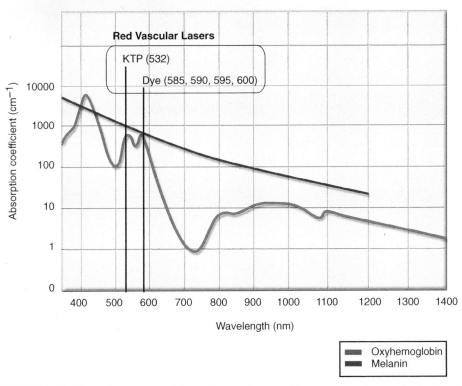

**FIGURE 1** ● Absorption spectra of tissue chromophores and lasers commonly used for treatment of red vascular lesions.

The most common vascular lesions associated with photoaging are telangiectasias, erythema, and cherry angiomas. In addition, certain skin conditions are also associated with or exacerbated by exposure to ultraviolet light such as poikiloderma of Civatte and rosacea. This chapter reviews laser* principles as they relate to treatment of red vascular lesions and conditions seen in photoaged skin and provides a step-by-step approach to treatment.

---

*Laser refers to both lasers and intense pulsed light devices, unless otherwise specified.

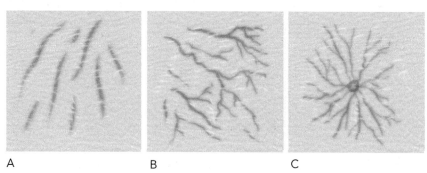

A                              B                              C

*FIGURE 2* ● Telangiectasias linear **(A)** and arborizing **(B)**, and spider angioma **(C)**.

## Anatomy

**Telangiectasias** are dilated vessels located in the superficial dermis, ranging in size from 0.1–1.0 mm, which usually appears in linear or arborizing configurations (Figs. 2A and 2B). Telangiectasias arising from dilated arterioles and venules have larger diameters, and those arising from capillaries may be discernible as fine lacy red vessels or **erythema.** **Rosacea** type I (erythematotelangiectatic rosacea) presents with telangiectasias and background erythema on the convexities of the face (i.e., cheeks, nose, chin, glabella) (Figs. 7 and 12) and symptoms of flushing. Rosacea type II (acne rosacea) has acne papules in addition to the lesions found in type I. Telangiectasias are also associated with long-term topical steroid use, radiation, medical conditions such as lupus erythematosus, hereditary hemorrhagic telangiectasia, and collagen vascular diseases including CREST syndrome (calcinosis, Raynaud syndrome, esophageal dysmotility, sclerodactyly, telangiectasia), and hyperestrogenic states such as pregnancy and liver failure.

    **Spider angiomas** have a central erythematous papule with radiating vessels (Fig. 2C). They can result from skin trauma, sun exposure, and hyperestrogenic states related to pregnancy and liver disease but are usually idiopathic.

    **Poikiloderma of Civatte** is a mottled discoloration of the skin consisting of erythema, telangiectasias (Fig. 3), and in some cases hyperpigmentation (Fig. 4), on

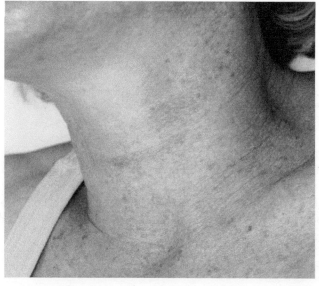

*FIGURE 3* ● Poikiloderma of Civatte with red coloration. (Courtesy of R. Small, MD.)

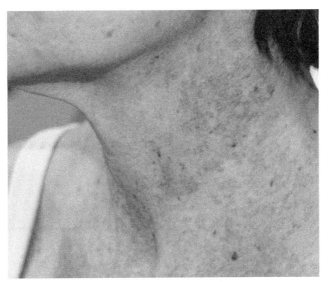

FIGURE 4  ● Poikiloderma of Civatte with red and brown coloration. (Courtesy of R. Small, MD.)

sun-exposed areas of the lateral neck, cheeks, and upper chest. Poikiloderma of Civatte is most common in women, and while chronic sun exposure is the chief etiologic factor, photosensitizing chemicals in perfumes and cosmetics may also be causative, as well as hormonal changes related to menopause.

**Cherry angiomas** are small, benign, erythematous dome-shaped papules (Fig. 14A), ranging in size from 0.5–3 mm, which result, from proliferation of capillaries in the superficial dermis. These lesions tend to appear after age 30 and may have a hereditary component.

## Laser Principles

Laser treatment of red vascular lesions is based on the principle of selective photothermolysis, the conversion of laser energy to heat, which selectively destroys vascular lesions. To achieve removal of vascular lesions, laser energy is applied to the skin and absorbed by **oxyhemoglobin,** the target chromophore found in red blood. Oxyhemoglobin strongly absorbs light between 400 and 600 nm, and has absorption peaks at 418, 542 and 577 nm (Fig. 4, Key References). Laser energy is converted to heat in red blood, causing vessel wall and perivascular damage, that results in vessel closure and reduced erythema. The surrounding skin minimally absorbs energy and remains unaffected.

## Laser Parameters for Treatment of Red Vascular Lesions

By adjusting laser parameters of wavelength, fluence, pulse width and spot size, maximal efficacy and safety can be achieved with laser treatments of red vascular lesions (also see Introduction and Foundation Concepts, Laser Parameters section).

- **Wavelength.** Wavelength is selected to target oxyhemoglobin. Lasers targeting oxyhemoglobin that are used to treat red vascular lesions are shown in Figure 1 and include **KTP (532 nm)** and **pulsed dye (585 nm, 590 nm, 595 nm, 600 nm). Intense pulsed light (IPL)** devices used for treatment of red vascular lesions emit

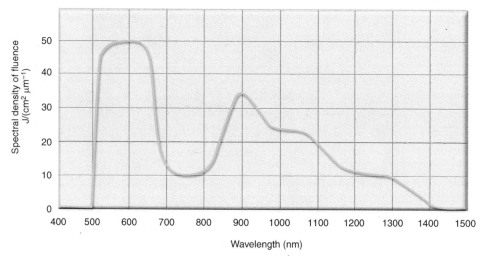

**FIGURE 5** ● Emission spectrum for an intense pulsed light handpiece used for treatment of red vascular lesions.

wavelengths that also target oxyhemoglobin. Figure 5 shows an emission spectrum from an IPL handpiece used for vascular lesions (MaxG, Palomar/Cynosure) with peaks at 500–670 nm and 870–1200 nm.

- **Fluence.** High fluences are used when less target chromophore is present either due to sparse blood vessels or faintly colored vessels. Lower fluences are used when more target chromophore is present either due to dense blood vessels or intensely colored vessels.
- **Pulse width.** Pulse width selection is based on vessel size and depth, and erythema intensity. Short pulse widths are used to treat small, superficial red vessels that are faintly colored. Longer pulse widths are used to treat large, deep vessels that are intensely colored. In addition, the deeper cutaneous penetration of long pulse widths makes them safer on the epidermis and preferable for treating darker Fitzpatrick skin types (IV–VI). Very short pulse widths can result in abrupt heat transfer that can ruptures vessels, causing petechiae and purpura.
- **Spot size.** Large spot sizes have deeper penetration of laser energy compared to small spot sizes. Large spot sizes are used to treat deeper vessels. Smaller spot sizes are used to treat small superficial red vessels.
- **Repetition rate.** Fast repetition rates allow for more rapid coverage of large treatment areas and can shorten treatment times. Slower repetition rates aid in precise placement of laser pulses and are useful for treatment of discrete lesions.
- **Pulse modes.** Some IPL devices have variable pulse modes. Multipulse modes with long delays between pulses (e.g., triple-pulsed mode) are typically used for treatment when more target chromophore is present. Multipulse modes with long delays are safer for the epidermis as they allow thermal energy to dissipate and are preferred in darker skin types. Single pulse mode is more aggressive and is used for treatment when less target chromophore is present and in lighter skin types.
- **Cooling.** Cooling protects the epidermis against thermal injury. Overcooling may blanch vessels decreasing the available target and reducing treatment efficacy.

Laser treatment parameters are often described as **aggressive or conservative.** Aggressive treatment parameters refer to the use of short wavelengths, short pulse widths, high fluences, and small spot sizes. Conservative treatment parameters refer to the use of long wavelengths, long pulse widths, low fluences, and large spot sizes (Fig. 3, Key References).

## Patient Selection

**Light Fitzpatrick skin types (I–III)** are the best candidates for treatment of red vascular lesions because these patients have a high contrast between background skin and target lesions. Red vascular lesions are less apparent in patients with **dark Fitzpatrick skin types (IV–VI)** and are a less common aesthetic complaint in this population. While dark Fitzpatrick skin type patients are candidates for vascular laser treatment, melanin in the background skin competes with chromophore in the target lesion and these patients have a greater risk of complications such as hyperpigmentation, hypopigmentation, and burns.

## Patient Expectations

Laser treatment of red vascular lesions may be performed on virtually any body region where red vascular lesions are present. The face, neck, and chest are the most commonly treated areas as they are chronically sun exposed. Noticeable results are evident with a single treatment in properly selected candidates, but a series of 3–5 laser treatments is usually necessary for optimal results. Rosacea patients should be counseled that, while erythema and telangiectasias will improve with treatments, laser is not a cure for rosacea and maintenance treatments are required to sustain results (see Treatment Intervals section).

Large red facial vessels demonstrate the most dramatic and rapid improvements with laser treatments. Small red vessels and diffuse erythema also respond to lasers, but usually require more treatments. Vessels on the ala of the nose can be resistant to laser treatments and may require more aggressive settings and repetitive visits for improvements. Discrete lesions such as cherry angiomas typically resolve without recurrence after 1 or 2 treatments.

## Indications

- Telangiectasias
- Erythema
- Cherry angiomas
- Spider angiomas
- Poikiloderma of Civatte
- Rosacea (Types I and II)

Vascular lasers are also used to treat other dermatologic conditions that have a vascular component such as erythematous acne scars, hypertrophic scars, and striae rubra (see Special Populations and Additional Considerations section). Congenital vascular anomalies such as infantile hemangiomas and port-wine stains (i.e., capillary vascular malformations) are advanced indications for treatment with vascular lasers and outside of the scope of this chapter.

## Alternative Therapies

**Electrosurgery** may be used for large telangiectasias and cherry angiomas but can result in hypopigmentation and scarring. **Photodynamic therapy (PDT)** utilizing topical photosensitizing medication activated by light (e.g., light-emitting diodes) has also been used for treatment of red vascular lesions (see Introduction and Foundation Concepts, Photodynamic Therapy section). Treatment cost is higher with PDT due to the medications used (e.g., levulinic acid), there is more downtime with intense erythema and crusting, and PDT requires strict avoidance of ambient sunlight posttreatment for 48 hours since it can lead to extended photosensitizer activation and associated complications.

## Devices Currently Available for Treatment of Red Vascular Lesions

| Laser | Wavelength (nm) |
|---|---|
| Potassium titanyl phosphate (KTP) laser | 532 |
| Pulsed dye lasers | 585, 590, 595, 600 |
| Intense pulsed light (IPL) | 500–1200 |

**KTP laser (532 nm)** is highly absorbed by oxyhemoglobin and is very effective for treating superficial small vessels, angiomas, and rosacea. The 532 nm is also highly absorbed by melanin, making it useful for treatment of superficial pigmented lesions. However, absorption by epidermal melanin limits 532 nm use to lighter skin types (I–III), and due to the short wavelength, 532 nm lasers can be associated with petechiae and purpura. Newer 532 nm devices with longer pulse widths (e.g., up to 100 ms) allow for slower vessel heating, making vessel rupture and purpura uncommon. Treatments are uncomfortable compared to other vascular lasers and can be associated with postprocedure pigmentary changes, and atrophic scarring particularly in the nasal area.

**Pulsed dye lasers (585 nm, 590 nm, 595 nm, 600 nm)** are also highly absorbed by oxyhemoglobin and are very effective for treatment of red vascular lesions found in photodamaged skin. They are the standard of care for treatment of congenital vascular lesions such as port-wine stains and infantile hemangiomas. Immediate posttreatment purpura is common with devices using small spot sizes, short pulse widths, and high fluences. Newer devices with longer pulse widths (e.g., 40 ms), larger spot sizes (12 mm), and contact skin cooling have reduced discomfort associated with treatment and less purpura than earlier devices. Like the KTP laser, these lasers are also associated with postprocedure pigmentary changes and are used primarily in lighter skin types (I–III).

**Intense pulsed light (IPL)** devices emit a spectrum of wavelengths and employ filters to refine the energy output, selecting for wavelengths that are absorbed by the target lesions. Figure 5 shows an IPL handpiece used to red vascular lesions that has emission peaks at 500–670 nm and at 870–1200 nm. Both melanin and oxyhemoglobin are targeted with these wavelengths. Lesions at different depths are also targeted where shorter wavelengths target more superficial lesions and the longer wavelengths target deeper lesions. In this way, a single IPL device can be used to treat both vascular and pigmented lesions at a variety of depths in the skin. IPLs can be used to treat large photodamaged areas confluently and many devices also have modified treatment tips that can be used to target discrete lesions. High quality devices use built in cooling for epidermal protection which provides some anesthesia as well. Due to large spot sizes, IPLs have relatively short treatment times but, IPL handpieces are bulkier and heavier than laser handpieces and precise placement on the skin can be more challenging.

Treatments with IPLs may cause pigmentary alterations such as patterning of the skin, or striping, which is usually temporary. Depending on the device, most IPLs can be used for Fitzpatrick skin types I-IV and some for skin types V.

**Argon (510 nm)** lasers were one of the first lasers used for treatment of vascular lesions. Due to their short wavelengths with strong melanin absorption, they have a high incidence of hypopigmentation and are not commonly used today for treatment of vascular lesions.

**Alexandrite (755 nm), diode (800–940 nm), and Nd:YAG (1064 nm) lasers** have some absorption by oxyhemoglobin and may be used for deep, large caliber red telangiectasias. However, they are primarily used for treatment of blue vascularities such as spider veins and reticular leg veins located in the deeper dermis. The longer wavelengths of these lasers allow for deeper penetration to reach these targets and they are well absorbed by deoxyhemoglobin and methemoglobin, the main chromophores in veins. In addition to deep penetration, the 1064 nm laser has low melanin absorption making it safe for use in the darkest Fitzpatrick skin types (V and VI).

See Supply Sources, Appendix 6 for laser manufacturers.

## Contraindications

### General Laser Contraindications

- Active infection in the treatment area (e.g., herpes simplex, pustular acne, cellulitis)
- Dermatoses in the treatment area (e.g., vitiligo, atopic dermatitis)
- Melanoma, or lesions suspected for melanoma in the treatment area
- Deep chemical peel, dermabrasion, or radiation therapy in the treatment area within the preceding 6 months
- Keloidal scarring[‡]
- Bleeding abnormality (e.g., thrombocytopenia, anticoagulant use)
- Impaired healing (e.g., immunosuppressive medications, poorly controlled diabetes mellitus)
- Peripheral vascular disease
- Seizure disorder
- Uncontrolled systemic condition
- Cardiac pacemaker
- Skin atrophy (e.g., chronic oral steroid use, genetic syndromes such as Ehlers–Danlos syndrome)
- Livedo reticularis, a vascular disease associated with mottled skin discoloration of the arms or legs exacerbated by heat exposure
- Erythema ab igne, a rare acquired reticular erythematous or pigmented rash exacerbated by heat exposure
- Direct sun exposure within the preceding 4 weeks resulting in reddened or tanned skin
- Self-tanning product within the preceding 4 weeks
- Topical prescription retinoid within the preceding week
- Isotretinoin (Accutane™) within the preceding 6 months
- Gold therapy (e.g., used for treatment of arthritis)
- Photosensitizing medications (e.g., tetracyclines, St. John's wort, thiazides)
- Photosensitive disorder (e.g., systemic lupus erythematosus)
- Pregnant or nursing

---

[‡]*Caution should be used in patients with hypertrophic scarring.*

- Unrealistic patient expectations
- Body dysmorphic disorder
- Treatment inside the eye orbit (i.e., without intraocular eye shields)

## Contraindications Specific to Laser Treatment for Red Vascular Lesions

- Skin type IV with some devices
- Skin type V with most devices
- Skin type VI with all devices except 1064 nm

## Advantages of Laser Treatment for Red Vascular Lesions

- Dramatic improvements in a relatively short amount of time
- Lower risks of scarring compared to electrocautery

## Disadvantages of Laser Treatment for Red Vascular Lesions

- Darker Fitzpatrick skin types (IV and above) have risks of hyperpigmentation, hypopigmentation, and scarring
- High equipment expense relative to nonlaser treatments

## Equipment

- Laser device appropriate for vascular lesion treatments
- Laser-safe eyewear for the patient and provider specific to the wavelength being used
- Nonalcohol facial wipes
- Clear colorless gel for treatment if indicated by the manufacturer
- Gauze $4 \times 4$ in
- Nonsterile gloves
- Ice packs
- Hydrocortisone cream 1% and 2.5%
- Sunscreen that is broad spectrum with SPF 30 containing zinc oxide or titanium dioxide
- Alcohol wipes for cleaning laser tip
- Germicidal disposable wipes for sanitizing the device

## Preprocedure Checklist

- **Aesthetic consultation** is performed to review the patient's medical history including photosensitive disorders such as lupus or abnormal scarring, medications that may worsen erythema such as topical steroids and niacin, contraindications to treatment, as well as previous methods for treating photodamaged skin and results. See also Introduction and Foundation Concepts, Aesthetic Consultation section.
- **Fitzpatrick skin type** is determined (Introduction and Foundation Concepts, Aesthetic Consultation section).
- **Examination of the treatment area** is performed. The presence of vascular lesions indicated for treatment is documented. Lesions suspicious for neoplasia are biopsied

or referred if indicated and negative biopsy results received before proceeding with laser treatments.

- **Informed consent** is obtained (see Introduction and Foundation Concepts, Aesthetic Consultation section). An example of a consent form is provided in Appendix 4c.
- **Pretreatment photographs** are taken (see Introduction and Foundation Concepts, Aesthetic Consultation section).
- **Avoidance of direct sun exposure** and daily use of a broad-spectrum **sunscreen** with SPF 30 prior to and throughout the course of treatment is advised.
- **Lightening background skin** may be considered in dark Fitzpatrick skin types (IV–VI) to reduce risks of pigmentary changes such as postinflammatory hyperpigmentation (PIH). Topical skin-lightening products may be used once or twice daily for 1 month prior to treatment such as prescription-strength hydroquinone cream 4–8% or over-the-counter cosmeceutical products containing kojic acid, arbutin, niacinamide, and azelaic acid (which are less effective).
- **Test spots** may be considered for patients with dark Fitzpatrick skin types (IV–VI) prior to the initial treatment. Test spot parameters are selected based on the patient's skin type and lesion characteristics following the manufacturer's guidelines for wavelength, spot size, fluence, and pulse width. Test spots are placed discretely near the intended treatment area (e.g., under the chin, behind or inferior to the ear) and pulses overlapped to simulate the technique used with treatment. Test spots are viewed 3–5 days after placement for evidence of erythema, blister, crust, or other adverse effect. Patients should be informed that lack of an adverse reaction with test spots does not ensure that a side effect or complication will not occur with a treatment.
- **Antiviral medication** may be given prophylactically for a history of herpes simplex or varicella zoster in or near the treatment area 2 days prior to the procedure and continued for 3 days postprocedure (e.g., valacyclovir 500 mg or acyclovir 400 mg 1 tablet twice daily). Patients with a remote history of HSV infection have a lower risk of reactivation and an antiviral may instead be started on the day of treatment and continued for 5 days.
- **Hair in the treatment area** is shaved prior to treatment to reduce the risk of epidermal thermal injury.
- **Written preprocedure instructions** are provided to patients (see Vascular Lesion Before and After Instructions for Laser Treatments, Appendix 3c).

## Anesthesia

Anesthesia is not typically required for laser treatment of red vascular lesions. Topical anesthetics in particular are discouraged, as they often contain vasoconstrictive agents that can reduce vascular targets and decrease treatment efficacy. Anesthesia can also interfere with patient feedback, an important component for selecting appropriate treatment parameters. For patients with low pain thresholds, consider an oral analgesic such as tramadol (Ultram™) 50 mg 1–2 tablets 1 hour prior to procedure (see Introduction and Foundation Concepts, Anesthesia section).

## Procedure for Laser Treatment of Red Vascular Lesions

The following procedural recommendations for treatment of red vascular lesions in photodamaged skin, including the sections on selecting initial laser parameters for treatment, general treatment technique, desirable clinical endpoints, undesirable clinical endpoints, aftercare, treatment intervals, subsequent treatments, and common follow-ups are based on using an IPL device (Cynosure/Palomar Icon™ with the MaxG handpiece) indicated for Fitzpatrick skin types I–IV. Manufacturer guidelines for the specific device used should be followed at the time of treatment.

## Selecting Initial Laser Parameters for Treatment

Many clinical factors influence laser parameter selection for the initial treatment including:

- **Fitzpatrick skin type.** Dark Fitzpatrick skin types (IV) have a greater risk of epidermal injury and conservative parameters of long pulse widths (e.g., 30 ms) and low fluences (e.g., 28–30 J/cm$^2$) are used for treatment. Lighter skin types (I–III) can tolerate more aggressive parameters of shorter pulse widths (e.g., 15 ms) and higher fluences (e.g., 36–38 J/cm$^2$).
- **Erythema characteristics.** Treatment areas containing a lot of target (i.e., intense erythema and dense vessels) typically require conservative parameters of long pulse widths and low fluences. Treatment areas with less target (i.e., faint erythema and sparse vessels) require more aggressive parameters of short pulse widths and high fluences (Fig. 6). For example, an initial treatment for a patient with Fitzpatrick skin type II having intense background erythema may use a pulse width of 20 ms and fluence of 32 J/cm$^2$. Treatment of a patient having the same Fitzpatrick skin type with faint background erythema may use a pulse width of 10 ms and fluence of 36 J/cm$^2$.
- **Discrete telangiectasias.** Discrete telangiectasias are commonly seen on the nasal ala and cheeks. Large telangiectasias are located deep in the dermis and are treated using long pulse widths and high fluences to enhance laser penetration and treatment efficacy. Small telangiectasias are usually located superficially in the dermis and are

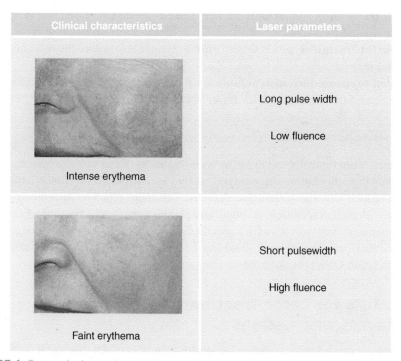

| Clinical characteristics | Laser parameters |
| --- | --- |
| Intense erythema | Long pulse width<br><br>Low fluence |
| Faint erythema | Short pulsewidth<br><br>High fluence |

*FIGURE 6* ● Vascular lesion characteristics and laser parameters. (Courtesy of R. Small, MD.)

treated with short pulse widths and usually also require high fluences. For example, treatment of a patient with Fitzpatrick skin type II with large, deep telangiectasias may use a pulse width of 100 ms and fluence of 50 J/cm$^2$. Treatment of a patient having the same Fitzpatrick skin type with small, superficial telangiectasias may use a pulse width of 15 ms and fluence of 40 J/cm$^2$.

- **Other chromophores in the treatment area.** When assessing the treatment area it is important to take all chromophores that are potentially targeted by the wavelength used into account. In addition to vascular lesions, photodamaged skin often has benign pigmented lesions and may also have dark hair present.
  - If **pigmented lesions** are present in the area being treated for red vascularities, more conservative parameters of long pulse widths and low fluences are used due to the greater amount of overall target in the skin. For example, if the treatment area has sparse, faint telangiectasias that overlie numerous dark lentigines, then conservative laser parameters are used.
  - If **dark hair** is present in the area being treated for red vascularities, it is advisable to use conservative parameters or avoid confluent IPL treatment by performing spot treatments to specific vessels only. For example, if the treatment area has faint, sparse telangiectasias that overlie an area with dense dark hair such as a man's beard, the discrete telangiectasias can be spot treated using an opaque paper "mask" to cover skin surrounding the vessels. In addition, hair is shaved prior to treatment to reduce excessive heating from singed hair on the skin surface. Treating over darkly colored hair may cause permanent hair reduction and patients need to be informed of this risk prior to treatment.
- **Size of treatment area.** Large flat areas such as the chest and extremities can be treated with fast repetition rates (e.g., 0.6 Hz), which shortens treatment times. Contoured areas such as the face usually require moderately slow rates (e.g., 0.4 Hz) to help ensure careful placement and complete contact between the skin and IPL tip.
- **Nonfacial areas.** Areas such as the neck and chest are treated using more conservative parameters than the face due to slower healing times and greater risk of complications.

## General Treatment Technique

- IPL treatments on the face are performed outside of the orbit; above the supraorbital ridge (roughly where the eyebrows sit) and below the inferior orbital rim. Figure 14 in Introduction and Foundation Concepts shows the nontreatment areas of the face.
- The face is typically broken down into sections that are treated sequentially to help ensure complete coverage. Figure 14 in the Introduction and Foundation Concepts shows one possible sequence for IPL treatment of the face, starting with section 1 and progressing to section 6.
- When preparing to pulse the laser, the IPL tip is placed firmly on the skin surrounded by a thin layer of gel. It remains in contact with the skin throughout the treatment.
- The IPL tip is held perpendicular to the skin and is moved toward the provider which allows for good visualization of the handpiece tip on the skin (Fig. 12A, Introduction and Foundation Concepts).
- IPL pulses are placed adjacently with approximately 20% overlap of each pulse. Each section is covered confluently with pulses before moving onto the next section.

TIP: Areas requiring additional treatment, such as telangiectasias that have not shown desirable clinical endpoints, can be returned to and pulsed again after the full face is treated using settings that are optimal for the telangiectasias.

TIP: The most sensitive areas are the upper lip philtrum and adjacent to the alar groove. When treating the upper lip, discomfort can be reduced by having the patient place their tongue over their teeth while keeping their lips closed.

## Desirable Clinical Endpoints

When optimal parameters are used for treatment of vascular lesions, one or more of the following clinical endpoints may be observed on the skin:

### Telangiectasias

- **Increased erythema** (Fig. 7B)
- **Vessel clearance** (referred to as blanching) (Fig. 8B)
- **Darkening with a grayish discoloration**
- **Purpura** (Fig. 9)

### Background Erythema

- **Increased erythema** (Fig. 7B)

### Spider and Cherry Angiomas

- **Darkening with a purplish discoloration**

**Light Fitzpatrick skin types (I–III)** have clinical endpoints that are clearly visible and are seen immediately after or within a few minutes of pulsing the IPL. Telangiectasias and erythema along with close-up views are shown in Figure 7 before (A) and

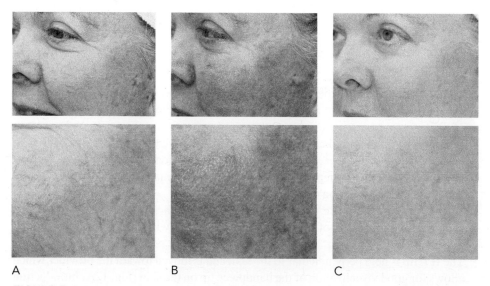

A                                      B                                      C

*FIGURE 7* ● Rosacea with erythema and telangiectasias before **(A)**, immediately after treatment showing clinical endpoints of increased erythema and vessel clearance **(B)**, and one month after treatment showing reduced erythema and vessel clearance **(C)**, using intense pulsed light. (Courtesy of R. Small, MD.)

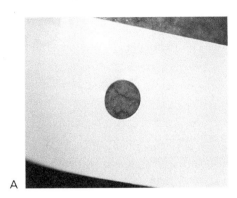 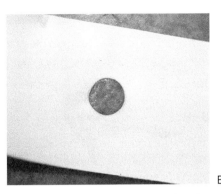

A                                                                                    B

FIGURE 8 ● Telangiectasia before (A) and immediately after (B) treatment showing clinical endpoint of vessel clearance using intense pulsed light with a lesion mask to cover the surrounding skin. (Courtesy of R. Small, MD.)

immediately after (B) IPL treatment with clinical endpoints of increased erythema and clearance of discrete vessels. Figure 8 shows a telangiectasia before (A) and immediately after (B) IPL treatment with clinical endpoints of vessel clearance. In rare instances, short pulse widths and high fluences may cause a vessel to rupture resulting in purpura (Fig. 9). Purpura is an aggressive endpoint with IPL. Patients must be reassured and informed that resolution can take up to 2 weeks. Angiomas may darken and change to a purplish color.

**Dark skin types (IV)** tend to be treated with conservative settings and have more subtle endpoints, typically consisting of minimal erythema and sluggish refill of telangiectasias. Increased erythema, if visible at all, is usually delayed and appears 5–10 minutes after the IPL pulse.

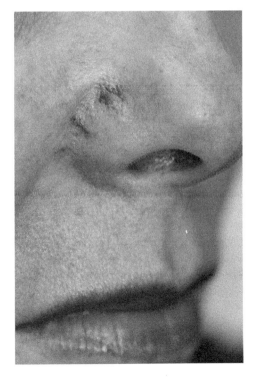

FIGURE 9 ● Purpura on the nasal ala immediately after a treatment of telangiectasias using intense pulsed light. (Courtesy of R. Small, MD.)

## Undesirable Clinical Endpoints

When overly aggressive laser parameters are used for treatment, the following undesirable clinical endpoint may be observed on the skin:

- **Blistering**

## Performing Laser Treatment for Red Vascular Lesions

The following recommendations are for treatment of red vascular lesions using an IPL device. These treatment steps are specific to the Cynosure/Palomar Icon™ system using the MaxG handpiece. Providers are advised to follow manufacturer guidelines for the specific device used at the time of treatment.

1. Inquire about sun exposure and sunscreen use at every visit. If the patient is recently sun exposed or has tanned skin in the treatment area, it is advisable to wait 1 month before treating to reduce the risk of complications.
2. Remove jewelry that may reflect laser light.
3. Position the patient supine on a flat procedure table. The physician is seated comfortably at the head of the patient.
4. Shave the treatment area if dark hair is present.
5. Cleanse the skin with a nonalcohol wipe.
6. Cover tattoos and permanent makeup (e.g., with wet gauze) and keep the laser tip approximately 1 inch away from the tattoo during treatment.
   **TIP: Full-thickness burns may result from treating over tattoos.**
7. Provide wavelength-specific protective eyewear to everyone in the treatment room. If working on the face provide the patient with extraocular lead goggles and have the patient remove contact lenses.
8. Always operate the laser in accordance with your office's laser safety policies and the manufacturer's guidelines.
9. Select the pulse width and fluence based on the patient's Fitzpatrick skin type and vascular lesion characteristics taking into account intensity, lesion density, and the presence of other targets in the treatment area such as pigmentation and dark hair (see Selecting Initial Laser Parameters for Treatment section).
10. Select the repetition rate based on the size and contour of the treatment area (see Selecting Initial Laser Parameters for Treatment section).
    **TIP: Care must be taken to keep pulses adjacent when fast repetition rates are used to avoid skipping areas.**
11. Apply a thin layer of clear colorless gel to the skin.
12. Place the laser tip firmly on the skin, making certain that the handpiece is perpendicular to the skin surface and the entire tip is in contact with the skin.
    **TIP: Avoid excessive downward pressure as this can cause vessels to blanch, diminishing target for the laser and reducing treatment efficacy.**
13. Perform a single pulse at the lateral margin of the treatment area (e.g., anterior to the ear) and assess for patient tolerance and clinical endpoints (see above). In general, there should be subtle endpoints with initial treatments and pain should be less than or equal to 6 on a scale of 1–10. Allow a few minutes for endpoints to evolve for light skin types (I–III) and up to 10 minutes for darker skin types (IV). If no endpoints are observed, gradually increase the fluence in small increments as tolerated by the patient until desirable clinical endpoints are achieved.

> **TIP: If there is no apparent change to a vessel, compress the vessel using a finger tip and observe for vessel blanching and refilling once pressure is removed. Adequately treated vessels will not blanch. Partially treated vessels will refill sluggishly.**

14. Cover the entire treatment area confluently with IPL pulses, using approximately 20% overlap.

15. Continually assess laser–tissue interaction and clinical endpoints throughout the treatment and adjust settings accordingly.
    - **If undesirable endpoints occur** discontinue treatment in the area and cool the skin using wrapped ice packs for 15 minutes. Decrease fluence and/or increase pulse width to achieve desirable endpoints in remaining treatment areas.

16. After the treatment area has been confluently covered with pulses, assess the vascular lesions within the treated area for clinical endpoints.
    - If areas with **rosacea** or **background erythema** do not have adequate endpoints, consider performing a second pass with the same settings, or use a shorter pulse width and slightly lower fluence, to enhance clinical endpoints in those areas.
    > **TIP: Areas receiving two passes, particularly the cheeks, often have more postprocedure edema.**
    - If discrete lesions such as **telangiectasias** or **angiomas** do not have adequate endpoints, modify settings accordingly and spot treat the lesions to achieve clinical endpoints. A lesion mask (Fig. 8) may be used to specifically target the discrete lesions.
    > **TIP: Telangiectasias on the ala can be resistant and often require repetitive pulsing with high settings.**

17. Ice packs wrapped in a towel may be applied immediately after treatment for 15 minutes to soothe the treatment area and reduce erythema and edema.

18. Hydrocortisone cream may be applied topically to erythematous areas: 1% for mild erythema and 2.5% for moderate erythema.

19. A broad-spectrum sunscreen (SPF 30 with zinc oxide or titanium dioxide) is applied to treatment areas that are sun exposed.

## Aftercare

- **Mild swelling and increased erythema** are expected and typically resolve within a few hours to a few days after treatment. Instruct patients to apply a wrapped ice pack 15 minutes every 1–2 hours and 1% hydrocortisone cream 2–3 times per day for a few days or until resolved. Patients are advised to contact their provider if erythema persists for more than 5 days as prolonged erythema may require evaluation to rule out complications (see Complications section).
- **Mild sunburn-like sensation** in the treated area may also occur which typically resolves within a day and can be relieved with ice.
- **Telangiectasias** that do not immediately resolve at the time of treatment tend to fade gradually during the week following treatment.
- **Cherry angiomas** gradually regress in size and fade over 1–2 weeks following treatment.
- **Purpura** can take up to 3 weeks to resolve.
- **Postprocedure products** that are soothing and hydrating are used for 2 weeks post-treatment including a broad-spectrum sunscreen of SPF 30 containing zinc oxide or

titanium dioxide (see Introduction and Foundation Concepts, Postprocedure Products section).

- **Direct sun exposure** is avoided for 4 weeks after treatment to help minimize the risk of undesired pigmentary changes.
- **Written aftercare instructions** are provided to patients (see Vascular Lesion Before and After Instructions for Laser Treatments, Appendix 3c).

## Common Follow-ups

- **Prolonged low-grade erythema and edema** are not uncommon, particularly in the cheek and infraocular areas following aggressive treatments, which can persist for 2 weeks following treatment. Prolonged erythema is undesirable, particularly in patients predisposed to hyperpigmentation such as those with darker skin types (IV–VI), as it can lead to postinflammatory hyperpigmentation. Erythema and edema can be treated with application of wrapped ice packs applied for 15 minutes a few times per day, sleeping with the head elevated, an oral antihistamine such as cetirizine (Zyrtec®) 10 mg or diphenhydramine (Benadryl®) 12.5–25 mg daily, and a topical corticosteroid twice daily such as a low potency steroid (e.g., hydrocortisone 2.5%) or a medium potency steroid (e.g., triamcinolone acetonide 0.1%) depending on the severity.
- **Recurrence of telangiectasias,** particularly on the ala is not uncommon. Settings are intensified at subsequent treatments to target vessels more aggressively.

## Treatment Intervals

Treatment of red vascular lesions and erythematous conditions usually requires 3–5 IPL procedures at bimonthly or monthly intervals for optimal results. Some vascular lesions, such as telangiectasias, can gradually recur over time, particularly in patients with rosacea, active lifestyles and frequent activities that cause flushing such as regular sauna and hot tub use. Biannual follow-up treatments are recommended to maintain results. Discrete lesions such as cherry angiomas typically resolve without recurrence after 1 or 2 treatments.

If pigmented lesions are present in the treatment area, subsequent treatments must be delayed until all darkened pigmentation has flaked off. Exfoliation of darkened pigment is usually complete by 4 weeks on the face and up to 8 weeks in nonfacial areas, and treatments can be resumed at that time.

## Subsequent Treatments

- **Less intense erythema and fewer vascular lesions** are observed over the course of a treatment series. Fluence is increased and pulse width decreased at subsequent visits to appropriately match the erythema and vascular lesion characteristics, in accordance with manufacturer's guidelines. It is recommended that only one parameter be changed to intensify treatments at any given visit. Typically, the fluence is increased initially for a few treatments (by 2–4 $J/cm^2$ each visit) and pulse width is decreased (by 5 ms each visit) in later treatments.
- If patients report **prolonged edema with prior treatments** lasting more than 5 days, consider increasing the fluence in small increments (e.g., 2 $J/cm^2$) and pretreating with an antihistamine such as cetirizine (Zyrtec) 10 mg or diphenhydramine (Benadryl) 12.5–25 mg 1 hour prior to treatment.

- **Treat the entire area** at each visit.
- If microcrusts are visible at the subsequent visit, delay treatment by 2 weeks.

## Results

Many factors influence treatment results of vascular lesions, but in general, large intensely erythematous vessels and angiomas in patients with light Fitzpatrick skin types are the easiest to treat while fine vessels and faintly colored erythema tend to be more challenging.

- Figure 7 shows rosacea and telangiectasias with close-up views before (A), immediately after (B), and one month after treatment (C), using an IPL (StarLux™ with LuxG handpiece, Cynosure/Palomar).
- Figure 10 shows telangiectasias on the nose before (A) and after (B) a series of treatments using an IPL (StarLux™ with LuxG handpiece, Cynosure/Palomar).
- Figure 11 shows telangiectasias on the chin before (A) and after (B) a series of treatments using an IPL (StarLux™ with LuxG handpiece, Cynosure/Palomar).
- Figure 12 shows rosacea on the face before (A) and after (B) five treatments using an IPL (ICON™ with MaxG handpiece, Cynosure/Palomar).

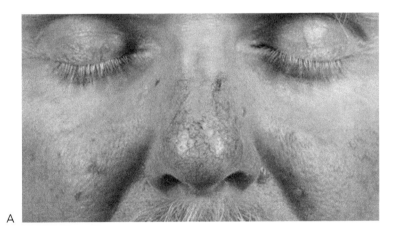

A

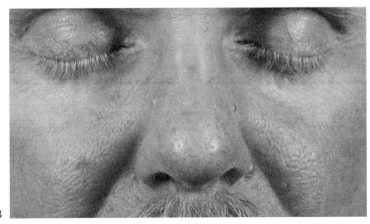

B

*FIGURE 10* ● Telangiectasias on the nose before **(A)** and after **(B)** a series of treatments using intense pulsed light. (Courtesy of M. Sinclair, MD.)

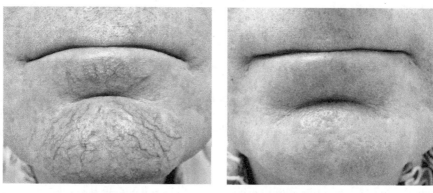

*FIGURE 11* ● Telangiectasias on the chin before **(A)** and after **(B)** a series of treatments using intense pulsed light. (Courtesy of M. Sinclair, MD.)

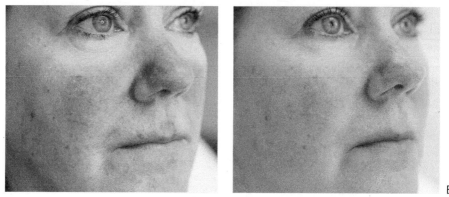

*FIGURE 12* ● Rosacea before **(A)** and after **(B)** five treatments using intense pulsed light. (Courtesy of R. Small, MD.)

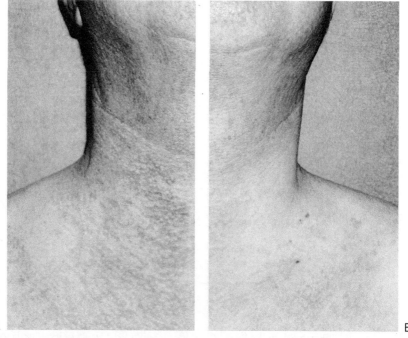

*FIGURE 13* ● Poikiloderma of Civatte on the neck before **(A)** and after **(B)** two treatments using intense pulsed light. (Courtesy of J. Wire, MD and Sciton.)

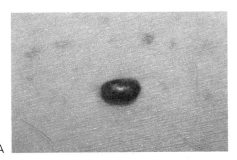 

A        B

*FIGURE 14* ● Cherry angioma before **(A)** and after **(B)** two treatments using intense pulsed light. (Courtesy of Cynosure/Palomar.)

- Figure 13 shows Poikiloderma of Civatte on the neck before (A) and after (B) two treatments using an IPL (BBL™ with 560 nm filter, Sciton).
- Figure 14 shows a cherry angioma before (A) and after (B) two treatments using an IPL (StarLux™ with LuxG handpiece, Cynosure/Palomar).

## Complications

- Pain
- Prolonged erythema
- Prolonged edema
- Contact dermatitis
- Infection
- Petechiae and purpura
- Visible skin patterns or striping
- Hyperpigmentation
- Hypopigmentation
- Burn
- Scarring
- Nonresponse, incomplete clearance, recurrence or worsening of erythematous skin conditions, and benign vascular lesions
- Tattoo alteration
- Urticaria
- Hair reduction in or adjacent to the treatment area
- Ocular injury

While serious complications are rare with laser treatment of vascular lesions, knowledge of the potential complications and their management is important to help ensure the best possible outcomes. Complications associated with overtreatment such as burns, hyperpigmentation, and hypopigmentation occur most often with the use of aggressive treatment parameters: short wavelengths, short pulse widths, high fluences and inadequate epidermal cooling. Patients with dark Fitzpatrick skin types (IV–VI) and those with light skin types (I-III) that have diffuse dyschromia such as actinic bronzing, tanned, and severely sun-damaged skin with extensive lentigines have the highest risk of these complications.

**Temporary erythema, edema, mild pruritus, and mild sunburn-like discomfort** after treatment are common, lasting a few hours to several days, and are not considered complications.

**Pain** is usually only reported during treatment and is mild to moderate (less than 6 on a standard pain scale of 1–10) depending on the treatment area. Treatments in the nasal and upper lip areas are usually more uncomfortable, typically 6–8. Complaint of pain several days postprocedure is uncommon and evaluation is advisable, particularly to assess for thermal injury due to overtreatment and infection.

**Prolonged erythema and edema** lasting 1–2 weeks is most often due to an aggressive treatment and may occur in patients with erythematous skin conditions such as rosacea, and patients prone to swelling. Aggressive treatment in the upper cheek at the level of the eyelids can produce edema in the periocular area and eyelids (see Common follow-ups section for management of erythema and edema). Rarely, prolonged erythema and edema may be indicators of thermal injury due to overtreatment, contact dermatitis, or infection.

**Contact dermatitis** is uncommon with nonablative laser treatments but is a consideration in patients who develop worsening erythema and pruritus after treatment. If contact dermatitis is suspected, postprocedure topical products are discontinued and a topical corticosteroid is used (per instructions for prolonged erythema and edema).

**Infections** postprocedure with laser treatment of red vascular lesions are rare, and require treatment specific to the pathogen. Reactivation of viral infections in the treatment area such as **herpes simplex** (and zoster) is one of the most common infectious complications, and pretreatment with an oral antiviral medication (e.g., valacyclovir/famciclovir 500 mg 1 tablet twice daily begun 2 days prior to the procedure and continued for 3 days postprocedure) in patients with a known history reduces this risk. Bacterial infections are rare but may occur any time the skin barrier is disrupted (see discussion of infections in Chapter 2, Complications Section).

**Petechiae and purpura** (Fig. 8) are due to rupture of superficial blood vessels and represent bleeding underneath the skin. They are usually seen a few minutes after treatment and most commonly occur with short wavelength lasers such as 532 nm, and use of aggressive treatment parameters such as short pulse widths, high fluences and small spot sizes. Petechiae typically take 3–5 days to resolve and purpura can take up to 2 weeks. Purpura can be distressing for patients and showing it to the patient and providing expectations for resolution are reassuring. Topical products such as arnica and vitamin K may be of limited use in treating purpura.

**Visible skin patterns or striping**, though rare, can be observed in severely erythematous skin. These patterns typically represent reduced vasculature in the shape of the treatment tip surrounded by untreated skin. Vascular skin patterns and striping typically occur after the initial treatment and resolve within a few days but may persist longer. They usually blend with subsequent treatments; however, there is a small risk that these patterns may be permanent.

**Hyperpigmentation and hypopigmentation** are pigmentary complications resulting from alteration to background skin color and are most commonly seen in patients with dark Fitzpatrick skin types (IV–VI), severely photodamaged skin, actinic bronzing, tanned skin, and with the use of aggressive laser parameters. They can appear as discrete areas usually in the shape of the treatment tip, or as visible patterns and striping. Prolonged erythema posttreatment combined with direct sun exposure is associated with PIH, particularly in dark skin types. **Hyperpigmentation** usually resolves spontaneously over several months, although in rare instances may be permanent. Sun protection including the application of a broad-spectrum sunscreen with SPF 30 containing zinc oxide or titanium dioxide and sun avoidance are preventative measures for PIH. PIH can be treated using a topical lightening agent such as hydroquinone cream 4–8% twice daily in the PIH area, superficial exfoliation procedures such as microdermabrasion and light chemical peels 1 month after treatment, and sun protection. Pretreatment of dark skin types with hydroquinone for 1 month may also aid in preventing hyperpigmentation. **Hypopigmentation** is a more significant complication that is usually temporary but may be permanent. There are few treatment options for hypopigmentation, but it may repigment with exposure to ambient light sunlight, excimer laser (308 nm), and narrow band UVB treatment. Alternatively, skin surrounding hypopigmented areas can be lightened to blend skin color and reduce the demarcation between background skin and hypopigmented areas.

**Burns** can result from aggressive treatment parameters, particularly with lasers that utilize short wavelengths (e.g., 532 nm). Prompt application of a wrapped ice pack to areas suspected of overtreatment at the time of treatment that are intensely erythematous and painful may reduce the area of injury. Blisters and crusting are managed with application of an occlusive ointment such as Aquaphor™ or bacitracin, and covered with a gauze dressing and tape. Patients are monitored over the next few weeks for formation of bullae, intense prolonged erythema, induration, and scarring. **Tattoos and permanent makeup** have concentrated ink pigments and treatment over these can result in full-thickness skin burns.

**Scarring** is rare. It is associated with aggressive treatment parameters including pulse stacking (where the laser is repeatedly pulsed over a lesion while keeping the treatment tip on the skin), and is most often seen with treatments complicated by burns and infection. Certain locations such as the anterior neck and sternum are more susceptible to scarring. The 532 nm laser is associated with atrophic scarring adjacent to the nasal ala, as the vessels here often require aggressive treatment parameters. In addition, recent use of isotretinoin, previous radiation therapy in the treatment area, and a history of keloid formation are also risk factors for hypertrophic scarring. Persistent intense erythema can be an indicator of impending scar formation. Interventions for persistent intense erythema to reduce the risk of scarring and management of scarring are discussed in Chapter 6, Scarring section.

**Urticaria** in the treatment area may be seen immediately after treatment (Fig. 14, Chapter 5). Urticaria can be managed with ice, oral antihistamines, and topical corticosteroids (see Common Follow-ups section). Once identified, patients who form urticaria in response to laser treatments may be pretreated with an antihistamine 1 hour prior to procedure to attenuate the histamine response.

**Reduced hair** in or adjacent to the treatment area may occur. This risk should be discussed if hair is present, especially if treating over men's facial hair.

**Ocular injury** can be avoided by wearing appropriate laser-safe eyewear at all times during treatment, directing the laser tip away from the eye and treating outside the eye orbit. Laser light on the retina can destroy retinal melanin, resulting in blindness.

## Special Populations and Additional Considerations

- **Pregnant and nursing.** Women who are pregnant or nursing typically do not undergo elective procedures such as lasers for treatment of red vascular lesions. One of the complications in nursing women is possible inhibition of lactation due to pain associated with a prolonged treatment.
- **Dark Fitzpatrick skin types.** Patients with dark skin types (IV) are treated using conservative settings with long pulse widths and low fluences. Treatment parameters are increased gradually to reduce the risk of complications. Patients may not experience the same degree of reduction in vascular lesions that lighter Fitzpatrick skin types can achieve due to these restrictions.

- **Pediatric patients.** Pediatric patients can present with congenital vascular anomalies such as port-wine stains and hemangiomas, which are indicated for treatment with vascular lasers but are outside the scope of this book.
- **Nonfacial areas.** Nonfacial areas such as the neck and chest are commonly treated for red vascular lesions. These areas have delayed healing relative to the face due to fewer pilosebaceous units, which serve as sites of reepithelialization that facilitate healing. Nonfacial areas have a greater risk of overtreatment and scarring, and it is advisable to treat conservatively compared to the face.
- **Erythematous scars.** Hypertrophic scars, acne scars, and striae rubra can all exhibit erythema and sometimes telangiectasias. Conservative settings with long wavelengths, low fluences, and long pulse widths are used for treatment as fibrotic and atrophic tissue is more prone to blistering and further scar formation.

## Learning Techniques for Laser Treatment of Red Vascular Lesions

It is advisable to perform treatments initially in patients with light Fitzpatrick skin types (I–III) on the face using conservative laser parameters such as high IPL cutoff filters (e.g., 560 nm), long pulse widths, and low fluences. Conservative clinical endpoints with sluggish vessel refill after compression are desirable when getting started with treatment of vascular lesions.

## Current Developments

**Nonablative fractional lasers** such as 1550 nm have been shown to reduce erythema and hyperpigmentation associated with poikiloderma of Civatte, and while more commonly used for reduction of wrinkles, acne scars and pigmented lesions, their use for treatment of erythematous lesions is being explored.

**Multimodality devices** such as IPL combined with radiofrequency are being used to simultaneoulsy target pigmentation, vascularities, and skin texture.

**Long wavelength lasers**, such as 940 and 980 nm diode lasers, are being used to target red facial vessels. In addition, a new 1064 nm Nd:YAG laser utilizing microsecond pulse widths (0.65 ms) has recently been shown to safely and effectively treat telangiectasias.

## Financial Considerations

Laser treatment of red vascular lesions associated with photoaging is usually not reimbursable; however, some insurance companies may cover treatment of rosacea. Charges for treatment vary, and are largely determined by local prices. Individual treatment prices range from $350–$550 for a single treatment to a large area such as the face or chest, and $150–$300 for a small area such as the hands or neck. Several treatments are typically required to achieve maximal benefits and a series of 3 or 5 treatments may be offered to patients.

## Chapter 4

# Tattoo Removal

Rebecca Small, M.D.

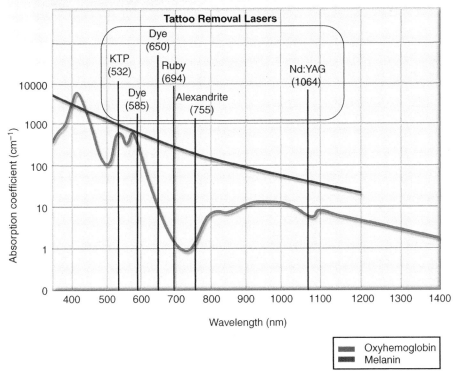

**FIGURE 1** ● Absorption spectra of tissue chromophores and tattoo removal lasers.

The prevalence of tattoos has steadily increased, and consequently, demand for tattoo removal has also grown. Reasons cited for tattoo removal vary; many patients report career changes, stigmatization, or feelings of embarrassment and low self-esteem. Early tattoo removal methods relied on nonspecific mechanical or chemical destruction such as dermabrasion and chemical peels, often with unsatisfactory results and complications of scarring and inadequate ink removal that left "tattoo ghosts" seen as a permanent haze of ink (Fig. 2). Q-switched lasers, which are the current standard of practice, target tattoo ink, and offer a safer, more effective means for removing tattoos. This chapter reviews the physiology of tattoo placement, laser principles as

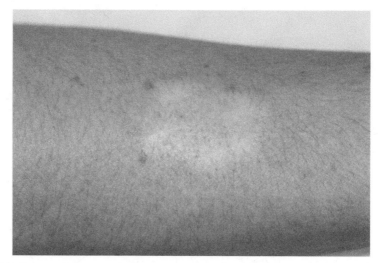

FIGURE 2 ● Dermabrasion results for tattoo removal showing scarring, hypopigmentation, and residual ink. (Courtesy of R. Small, MD.)

they relate to tattoo removal, and provides a step-by-step approach for tattoo removal using Q-switched lasers.

## Tattoos

Tattoos are placed by injecting ink particles (ranging in size from 20–400 nm) into the dermis. During the tattooing process, the epidermis and upper papillary dermis are homogenized, and ink particles are distributed extracellularly and intracellularly. After 2–3 months, the skin layers reestablish and the ink remains concentrated within fibroblasts beneath a layer of scar tissue in the dermis (Fig. 3). Tattoo inks are not regulated by the Food and Drug Administration (FDA), and most patients do not know the constituents of their tattoos.

There are many different types of tattoos. Decorative tattoos are the most common and are the focus of this book. They are categorized as either amateur or professional, based on their method of placement.

- **Amateur decorative** tattoos are typically tapped by hand into the skin using a wire or needle resulting in a low density of ink particles that are located superficially in the skin. These are usually black in color and composed of carbon-based inks such as pen ink or burnt wood.
- **Professional decorative** tattoos are placed with a "tattoo gun." These devices have a single needle or group of needles that rapidly oscillate in and out of the skin. Professional tattoos usually contain organic dyes mixed with heavy metals to give vibrant colors. For example, red is often made from mercury, yellow from cadmium, green from chromium, and blue from cobalt.
- **Cosmetic** tattoos are commonly referred to as "permanent makeup." They are typically applied to eyelash margins, eyebrows, and lips to simulate makeup, and are usually combinations of colors containing pink and flesh tone inks that may be mixed with white. Flesh tones often contain iron oxide, and white commonly contains titanium dioxide or zinc oxide. When pulsed with a tattoo laser, these inks can turn black or brown becoming darker and more noticeable after the initial treatment.

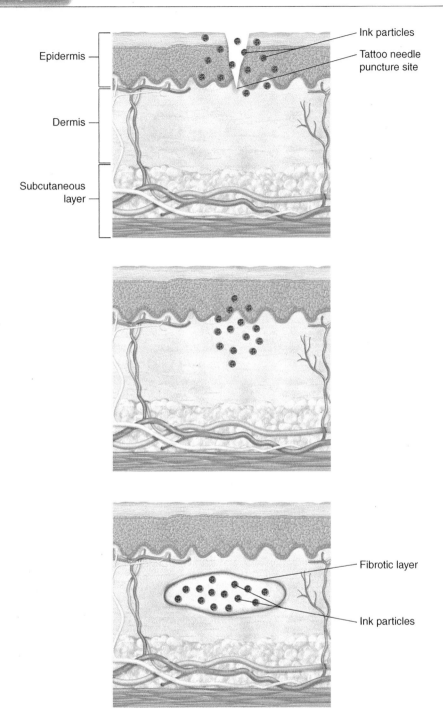

*FIGURE 3* ● Tattoo ink placement.

- **Traumatic** tattoos result from deposition of pigment in the skin by abrasion. Common causes include trauma from gravel referred to as "road rash," pencil graphite, or by explosive forces as with shrapnel and fireworks. These materials become lodged in the dermis after reepithelialization of the wound and result in blue/black tattoos.
- **Medical** tattoos are placed as markers for radiation therapy. These are usually black, carbon-based inks.

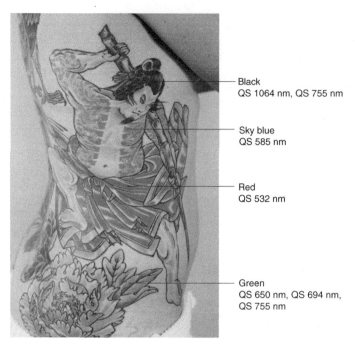

Black
QS 1064 nm, QS 755 nm

Sky blue
QS 585 nm

Red
QS 532 nm

Green
QS 650 nm, QS 694 nm,
QS 755 nm

*FIGURE 4* ● Laser wavelengths used for different tattoo colors. (Courtesy of R. Small, MD.)

## Laser Principles

Laser tattoo removal is based on the principle of selective photothermolysis, the conversion of laser energy to heat, which selectively destroys tattoo ink. **Tattoo ink** is the target chromophore in tattoos. Different ink colors are preferentially absorbed by specific wavelengths of light as shown in Figure 4. When laser energy is applied to skin it is converted to heat within ink particles, causing fragmentation of large particles and rupture of fibrous capsules surrounding the ink. Smaller ink particles are then eliminated through epidermal extrusion, lymphatic drainage, and macrophage phagocytosis (Fig. 5). The surrounding skin minimally absorbs energy and remains unaffected. Laser-treated ink particles also have altered optical properties rendering ink that remains in the skin less visible to the eye.

**Q-switched** lasers that generate high-power pulses with very short widths in the nanosecond range (and more recently mode-locking lasers that generate picosecond pulse widths) are used for tattoo removal. In addition to selective photothermolysis, these lasers operate under the principle of photoacoustic vibration where oscillation of ink particles facilitates fragmentation and removal (see also Introduction and Foundation Concepts, Very Short Pulse Lasers section).

## Laser Parameters for Tattoo Removal Treatments

Laser parameters (also referred to as settings) such as wavelength, pulse width, spot size, and fluence can be modified at the time of treatment to maximize tattoo ink removal and minimize thermal damage to surrounding tissue (also see Introduction and Foundation Concepts, Laser Parameters section).

- **Wavelength.** Wavelength is selected to target the appropriately colored ink. Lasers used for tattoo removal are shown in Figure 1 and include **QS 1064, QS 755, QS**

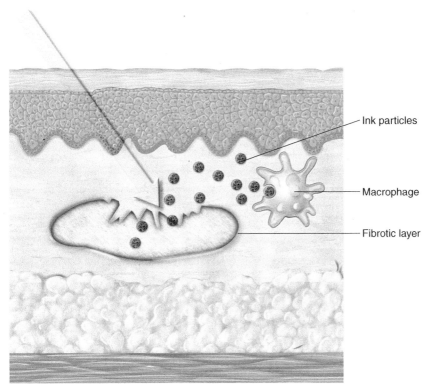

Ink particles

Macrophage

Fibrotic layer

*FIGURE 5* ● Laser tattoo removal.

**694, QS 650, QS 585, and QS 532 nm**. The 1064 nm wavelength penetrates deeply, is less absorbed by epidermal melanin than other wavelengths and is, therefore, the safest tattoo removal wavelength that causes the least epidermal injury.

- **Fluence.** Fluence settings should be sufficient to produce immediate whitening during treatment without bleeding or blistering. High fluences are used when less target chromophore is present with faintly colored amateur tattoos. Lower fluences are used when more target chromophore is present with intensely colored professional tattoos and 'cover-up' tattoos.
- **Pulse width.** Q-switched lasers have fixed nanosecond (one billionth of a second, $10^{-9}$ second) pulse widths that cannot be adjusted. A mode-locking tattoo removal laser with a picosecond (one trillionth of a second, $10^{-12}$ second) pulse width has recently become available.
- **Spot size.** Large spot sizes have less photon scatter of the laser beam resulting in deeper penetration. Deeper penetration maximizes delivery of laser energy to the dermal ink and reduces epidermal injury. Larger spot sizes (e.g., 4–8 mm) are preferable for tattoo treatment as long as sufficient fluence can be obtained to achieve desired clinical endpoints. Smaller spot sizes (e.g., 2–3 mm) have greater scattering of photons, deliver energy less efficiently, and have greater risk of epidermal injury.
- **Repetition rate.** Slower repetition rates (e.g., 2–5 Hz) allow for more control of the laser handpiece and are helpful with very small tattoos that require precision pulsing. Faster repetition rates (e.g., 10 Hz) allow for rapid treatment of medium and large tattoos ($\geq 10$ in$^2$).

Laser treatment parameters are often described as aggressive or conservative. **Aggressive** treatment parameters refer to the use of short wavelengths (e.g., 532 nm), high fluences (e.g., $\geq 8$ J/cm$^2$ with 1064 nm), and small spot sizes (e.g., 2–3 mm). Aggressive parameters are often necessary to target lighter ink as laser treatments progress over time, and they can be associated with a greater risk of epidermal injury. **Conservative** laser parameters refer to the use of long wavelengths, low fluences, and large spot sizes.

## Patient Selection

Patients of **all Fitzpatrick skin types (I–VI)** are candidates for laser tattoo removal. However, patients with darker skin types (IV–VI) are at greater risk for side effects, including hypopigmentation and hyperpigmentation. Additionally, patients of Asian and African decent may have a greater predisposition to hypertrophic and keloidal scarring. Fitzpatrick skin type VI patients have the greatest risk of complications with any aesthetic procedure and treatment of this skin type is an advanced laser application, outside the scope of this book.

## Patient Expectations

Multiple laser tattoo removal treatments are needed to achieve satisfactory results. Due to variation in tattoo ink depth, density, composition, and techniques used for placement, estimating the number of treatments needed for removal can be challenging. However, some generalizations about the number of treatments can be made based on patient and tattoo characteristics (Table 1). Professionally placed tattoos have greater ink density and typically require 12–16 and sometimes up to 20 treatments; whereas amateur tattoos typically require 4–8 treatments. Faded, older tattoos on paler skin types in proximal locations tend to be removed with fewer treatments than intense, multicolored tattoos on darker skin types in distal locations. A "cover-up" is a tattoo that has one tattoo placed on top of another, rendering a very high density of ink in the skin and requires more treatments for removal. Prior tattoo removal methods that create scar tissue, such as abrasion and caustic chemical agents, can make laser tattoo removal less successful.

Q-switched lasers only treat ink and are not intended to improve the texture of the skin. If a tattoo is palpable prior to laser treatment, it will usually be palpable when the treatment series is completed.

## TABLE 1

**Factors Affecting the Number of Treatments Needed for Tattoo Removal**

| Characteristics | Fewer Number of Treatments | Greater Number of Treatments |
| --- | --- | --- |
| Tattoo type | Amateur, traumatic | Professional, cosmetic |
| Color | Black | Multicolored |
| Ink intensity | Faded | Dark |
| Cover-up | No | Yes |
| Age of tattoo | Old | New |
| Prior removal method | No | Yes |
| Location | Proximal[a] | Distal |
| Scarring | No | Yes |
| Fitzpatrick skin type | I–III | IV–VI |

[a]Proximal (or axial) location refers to being near the center of the body.

Laser tattoo removal is painful. However, treatment of smaller tattoos (e.g., $\leq 9$ in$^2$) is fast, in the order of 5 minutes, and due to the rapidity of treatment can usually be performed without anesthesia. Treatment of larger tattoos such as confluent arm tattoos, referred to as a "sleeve," can take 20–30 minutes and may require anesthesia.

Results from laser tattoo removal treatments are cumulative. Ink intensity gradually fades over the month following treatment. Fading from some treatments is more noticeable than others, and it is helpful to inform patients of this so they are not concerned with this variability. In addition, tattoos can change color as treatments progress due to removal of constituent inks.

Patients often ask what the end result will look like after completion of laser tattoo removal treatments. While there is no standardized definition for tattoo removal, when viewed from 3–4 ft away, it is unlikely that onlookers will be able to detect the presence of a prior tattoo. When scrutinized up-close, patients may be able to discern where the tattoo was due to variations in skin pigmentation and in some cases, textural changes.

## Indications

- Amateur tattoos
- Professional tattoos
- Cosmetic tattoos
- Traumatic tattoos
- Medical tattoos

## Alternative Therapies

Alternative treatment options for tattoo removal include, continuous-wave lasers (e.g., CO2, argon), dermabrasion (a surgical procedure, different from microdermabrasion), salabrasion (scrubbing with salt), chemical peels (e.g., trichloroacetic acid), cryotherapy (liquid nitrogen) and electrocautery. These alternative therapies are not generally recommended as they usually have unsatisfactory results with incomplete resolution of ink. In addition, they have increased risks of adverse outcomes such as scarring, hypopigmentation, hyperpigmentation, pain, prolonged healing time, infection, textural changes and, unpredictable outcomes. Surgical excision may be recommended as a last resort in certain situations if Q-switched laser tattoo removal has failed and patients are adamant about removal.

## Devices Currently Available for Tattoo Removal

| Tattoo Ink Color | Laser Wavelength for Removal (nm) |
| --- | --- |
| Black | QS 1064, QS 755 |
| Red, orange, yellow | QS 532 |
| Green | QS 650 , QS 694 , QS 755 |
| Sky blue | QS 585 |

QS, Q-switched.

Q-switched lasers are widely regarded as the gold standard for laser tattoo removal. Devices differ in their wavelengths, spot sizes, and peak powers. In general, devices adequate for tattoo removal have a range of spot sizes that includes both small (e.g., 2–3 mm) and large (e.g., 4–8 mm) sizes, and can achieve adequate power with the large spot sizes (e.g., a 1064 nm Q-switched laser with a 4-mm spot size should have fluence settings greater than 3 J/cm$^2$).

**Q-switched Nd:YAG lasers (QS 1064 nm, QS 532 nm, QS 585 nm, QS 650 nm).** Nd:YAG lasers primarily produce a **1064 nm** wavelength that is ideal for treating black and dark-colored inks and is preferable for treating darker-skinned patients. A primary disadvantage of 1064 nm is its limited efficacy in removing yellow and green inks. However, many Nd:YAG devices can also produce a **532 nm** wavelength, which treats red, orange, and yellow inks. This process of converting 1064 nm to 532 nm is called harmonic doubling, and involves passing the 1064 nm wavelength through a potassium titanyl phosphate (KTP) crystal that doubles the frequency and halves the wavelength. Some devices can also generate **585 nm**, which is used for treatment of sky blue ink, and **650 nm** used for treatment of green ink, by passing 532 nm through additional handpieces containing dye-impregnated polymers.

**Q-switched alexandrite laser (QS 755 nm).** This wavelength has good absorption by black, green, and dark blue, but poor absorption by red ink. A **picosecond alexandrite laser** that is not Q-switched has recently become available and is discussed in the Current Developments section at the end of this chapter.

**Q-switched ruby laser (QS 694 nm).** This wavelength works well for darker colors (black, blue black, green) but poorly on yellow and red ink. Although more effective for green ink than the Nd:YAG, higher rates of hypopigmentation and hyperpigmentation are reported.

See Supply Sources, Appendix 6 for laser manufacturers.

# Contraindications

## General Laser Contraindications

- Active infection in the treatment area (e.g., herpes simplex, pustular acne, cellulitis)
- Dermatoses in the treatment area (e.g., vitiligo, psoriasis, atopic dermatitis)
- Melanoma, or lesions suspected for melanoma in the treatment area
- Deep chemical peel, dermabrasion or radiation therapy in the treatment area within the preceding 6 months
- Keloidal scarring[‡]
- Bleeding abnormality (e.g., thrombocytopenia, anticoagulant use)
- Impaired healing (e.g., immunosuppressive medications and poorly controlled diabetes mellitus)
- Peripheral vascular disease
- Seizure disorder
- Uncontrolled systemic condition
- Cardiac pacemaker
- Skin atrophy (e.g., chronic oral steroid use, genetic syndromes such as Ehlers–Danlos syndrome)
- Livedo reticularis, a rare autoimmune vascular disease associated with mottled skin discoloration of the arms or legs exacerbated by heat exposure with laser treatments
- Erythema ab igne, a rare acquired reticular erythematous rash exacerbated by heat exposure with lasers
- Direct sun exposure within the preceding 2 weeks resulting in reddened or tanned skin

[‡]Caution should be used in patients with hypertrophic scarring.

- Self-tanning product within the preceding 2 weeks
- Topical prescription retinoid within the preceding week
- Isotretinoin (Accutane™) within the preceding 6 months
- Gold therapy (e.g., used for treatment of arthritis)
- Photosensitizing medications (e.g., tetracyclines, St. John's wort, thiazides)
- Photosensitive disorder (e.g., systemic lupus erythematosus)
- Pregnant or nursing
- Unrealistic patient expectations
- Body dysmorphic disorder
- Treatment inside the eye orbit (i.e., without intraocular eye shields)

Certain dermatoses such as vitiligo, psoriasis and atopic dermatitis can erupt at sites of trauma (referred to as koebnerization), and an active dermatosis in the treatment area is a contraindication. Patients with a history of koebnerizing dermatoses in nontreatment areas should be treated with caution as these conditions may develop at laser treatment sites.

## Contraindications Specific to Tattoo Removal

- Tattoo ink allergy

An allergic reaction to tattoo ink at the time of placement is a contraindication to laser tattoo removal. After laser tattoo treatment, ink is disseminated systemically through the lymphatic system and patients with a prior reaction may be at risk for allergic reactions at the time of removal. Ink allergy presents with signs of an allergic dermatitis (erythema, edema, pruritus, and induration), and rarely inflammatory nodules and granulomas. Allergic reactions are most commonly seen with bright-colored inks such as red (Fig. 20) and less commonly with yellow, green, and blue inks.

## Advantages of Laser Tattoo Removal

- Considered the "gold standard" for tattoo removal
- Individual treatments are relatively quick
- Provides the best cosmetic result when compared to other forms of tattoo removal

## Disadvantages of Laser Tattoo Removal

- Expensive
- Uncomfortable
- Multiple treatments required
- Risk of hyperpigmentation, hypopigmentation, textural changes, and scarring

## Equipment

- Q-switched laser device
- Topical anesthetic
- Gauze $4 \times 4$ in
- Nonalcohol wipe to cleanse skin
- Protective eyewear for patient and laser operator that is specific to the wavelength used
- Ice packs

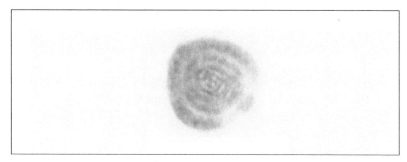

*FIGURE 6* ● Concentric rings seen with pulsing a Q-switched 1064 nm tattoo removal laser on white paper representing good internal mirror alignment. (Courtesy of R. Small, MD)

- Nonsterile gloves
- Sunscreen that is broad spectrum with SPF 30 containing zinc oxide or titanium dioxide
- Alcohol wipes to clean the laser tip
- Germicidal disposable wipes for sanitizing the device
- Face shield for laser operator (optional)
- Masks for laser operator (optional)

Q-switched lasers, like any laser device, have fragile components. They usually have long articulated arms with multiple internal mirrors that can become misaligned when bumped or during transportation. If there is a concern that the mirrors have become misaligned, perform a test pulse on a moist wooden tongue depressor or thick white paper using manufacturer-recommended settings to observe for concentric circles (Fig. 6). If this pattern is not evident, the equipment requires servicing by the manufacturer.

Q-switched lasers can aerosolize tissue and rarely, rupture blood vessels. The laser operator may wear a plastic face shield and/or mask, and use a cone-shaped distance guide on the laser tip for protection against tissue and blood contact (Fig. 7).

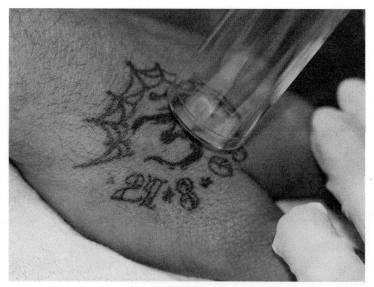

*FIGURE 7* ● Cone distance guide on the laser tip reduces exposure to tissue debris. (Courtesy of R. Small, MD.)

# Preprocedure Checklist

- **Aesthetic consultation** is performed to review the patient's medical history including contraindications to treatment (particularly active dermatoses such as psoriasis and vitiligo), history of postinflammatory hyperpigmentation, and abnormal scarring. See also Introduction and Foundation Concepts, Aesthetic Consultation section.
- **Tattoo history** is reviewed including:
  - Tattoo type: amateur, professional, cosmetic, traumatic
  - Colors at the time of placement, including the presence of flesh tone and white inks
  - Number of years present
  - Whether it is a cover-up
  - Use of prior methods for tattoo removal and which methods
  - Allergic reaction at the time of placement
- **Tattoos are examined** for:
  - Colors, including the presence of flesh tone and white inks
  - Intensity of ink color
  - Body location
  - Presence of raised scarring or textural change. Some patients present with tattoos that are slightly raised, which is considered a textural change. Document the presence of textural changes and scarring prior to treatment and inform the patient that these will not improve and may worsen with treatment.
- **Fitzpatrick skin type** is determined (Introduction and Foundation Concepts, Aesthetic Consultation section).
- **Informed consent** is obtained (see Introduction and Foundation Concepts, Aesthetic Consultation section). Lesions suspicious for neoplasia are biopsied or referred if indicated, and negative biopsy results received before proceeding with laser treatments. An example of a consent form is provided in Appendix 4d.
- **Pretreatment photographs** are taken (see Introduction and Foundation Concepts, Aesthetic Consultation section).
- **Avoidance of direct sun exposure** and daily use of a broad-spectrum sunscreen with SPF 30 prior to and throughout the course of treatment is advised.
- **Lightening background skin** may be considered dark Fitzpatrick skin types (IV–VI) to reduce risks of pigmentary changes such as PIH. Topical skin-lightening products may be used once or twice daily for 1 month prior to treatment such as prescription-strength hydroquinone cream 4–8% or over-the-counter cosmeceutical products containing kojic acid, arbutin, niacinamide, and azelaic acid (which are less effective).
- **Test spots** are rarely performed prior to the initial treatment but may be considered for patients with dark Fitzpatrick skin types (IV–VI). Test spot parameters are selected based on the patient's skin type and tattoo characteristics following the manufacturer's guidelines for wavelength, spot size, and fluence. Test spots may be placed on part of the tattoo. Test spots are viewed 3–5 days after placement for evidence of erythema, blister, crust, or other adverse effect. Patients should be informed that lack of an adverse reaction with test spots does not ensure that a side effect or complication will not occur with a treatment.
- **Antiviral medication** may be given prophylactically for a history of herpes simplex or zoster in or near the treatment area 2 days prior to the procedure and continued for 3 days postprocedure (e.g., valacyclovir 500 mg or acyclovir 400 mg 1 tablet twice daily). Patients with a remote history, of HSV infection have a lower risk of

reactivation, and an antiviral may instead be started on the day of treatment and continued for 5 days.

- **Hair in the treatment area** is shaved prior to treatment to reduce the risk of epidermal thermal injury.
- **Snacks** such as granola bars or juice can be offered on the day of treatment to help raise blood sugar and avert hypoglycemia if patients have not eaten for a prolonged period and have a relatively large tattoo.
- **Written preprocedure instructions** are provided to patients (see Tattoo Removal Before and After Instructions for Laser Treatments, Appendix 3d).

## Anesthesia

Tattoo treatments are painful but can be performed relatively quickly. The use of anesthesia depends on the patient's pain threshold as well as the size and location of the tattoo. Smaller tattoos (e.g., $\leq 9$ in$^2$) and those on fleshier areas rarely require anesthesia and patients can typically manage pain by squeezing a stress ball and breathing slowly during the procedure as treatment times are very fast, in the order of a few minutes. Larger tattoos (e.g., covering an arm) and those in sensitive areas such as boney prominences like the sacrum or wrist may require anesthesia. In addition, treatments performed on the face often require anesthesia due to sensitivity and the need for absolute immobility.

A topical anesthetic cream such as benzocaine:lidocaine:tetracaine (BLT), lidocaine (L-M-X™), or lidocaine/prilocaine (EMLA™) may be applied to the tattoo and occluded with plastic wrap to enhance penetration for 30–45 minutes prior to the laser treatment (Appendix 6). If patients are intolerant of treatment, complete anesthesia may be obtained by using small volumes of 1% lidocaine with epinephrine injected subdermally. However, most tattoos are too large for injectable lidocaine to be considered practical or safe (see Introduction and Foundation Concepts, Anesthesia for Laser Procedures section).

Oral analgesics such as tramadol (Ultram™) 50 mg 1–2 tablets taken 1 hour prior to procedure or stronger opioids such as hydrocodone/acetaminophen (Vicodin™) and oxycodone/acetaminophen (Percocet™) are other options. Patients using stronger opioids may require assistance with getting home postprocedure.

## Laser Tattoo Removal Procedure

The following procedural recommendations for tattoo removal including the sections on selecting initial laser parameters for treatment, general treatment technique, desirable clinical endpoints, undesirable clinical endpoints, aftercare, treatment intervals, subsequent treatments, and common follow-ups are based on using a Q-switched laser (RevLite™, Cynosure/ConBio) that is indicated for all Fitzpatrick skin types (I–VI). As mentioned in the Patient Selection section above, treatment of Fitzpatrick skin type VI is an advanced laser application and is not within the scope of this book. Manufacturer guidelines specific to the device used should be followed at the time of treatment.

### Selecting Initial Laser Parameters for Treatment

Many clinical factors influence laser parameter selection for the initial treatment including the following:

- **Fitzpatrick skin type.** Dark Fitzpatrick skin types (IV and V) are treated with large spot sizes (e.g., 6–8 mm) and low fluences for initial treatments. Light skin types

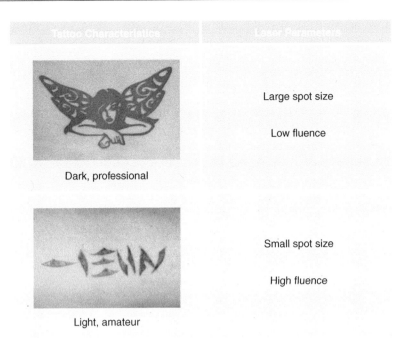

Tattoo Characteristics          Laser Parameters

Dark, professional

Large spot size

Low fluence

Light, amateur

Small spot size

High fluence

FIGURE 8 ● Tattoo characteristics and laser parameters. (Courtesy of R. Small, MD.)

(I–III) are treated with smaller spot sizes (e.g., 4–6 mm) and higher fluences. For example, a black tattoo on a patient with Fitzpatrick skin type V may initially be treated with an 8-mm spot size and fluence of 1.5 J/cm$^2$; whereas the same tattoo on a patient with Fitzpatrick skin type II may initially be treated with a 6-mm spot size and 2.5 J/cm$^2$.

- **Ink color.** Initial laser tattoo removal treatments are typically performed with QS 1064 nm regardless of the color, and as treatments progress wavelengths specific to the presenting ink color are used. Tattoo artists often combine several colors to create unique shades, and these constituent colors may not be discernible when looking at the tattoo. A dark green tattoo for example, may contain black ink as well as green. It is safest to use QS 1064 nm for the initial treatments to remove the darkest ink and assess the tattoo's response to treatment.
- **Ink intensity.** Tattoos with a high concentration of ink such as dark, professional tattoos, require a large spot size and low fluence to achieve desirable clinical endpoints than tattoos with less ink such as light, amateur tattoos (Fig. 8). Tattoos with a low concentration of ink such as light, amateur tattoos, require more aggressive parameters with smaller spot sizes and higher fluences. For example, a patient with Fitzpatrick skin type III with a dark black tattoo may require a 6-mm spot size and 1.5 J/cm$^2$, whereas a faded black tattoo on the same patient may require a 4-mm spot size and 3.5 J/cm$^2$ to achieve desirable clinical endpoints.
- **"Cover-up" tattoos.** Cover-ups have a high density of ink and are initially treated with a large spot size and very low fluence to reduce the risk of overtreatment.
- **Tattoo size and location.** Medium to large tattoos can be treated with fast repetition rates (e.g., 10 Hz) to shorten treatment times. Small tattoos, particularly on facial areas, are treated with slower repetition rates (e.g., 2–5 Hz) for greater precision.

- **Nonfacial areas.** Areas with thin skin such as the neck, breast, inner arm and inner thighs are treated with conservative settings using large spot sizes and low fluences to decrease the risk of complications.

## General Treatment Technique

- Laser treatments on the face are performed outside of the orbit, the area above the supraorbital ridge (roughly where the eyebrows sit) and below the inferior orbital rim.
- Hold the laser tip perpendicular to the skin at all times
  **TIP: In the periocular area, angle the laser tip away from the eyes to reduce the risk of ocular injury and laser reflection off the patient's lead goggles.**
- The laser tip distance guide is in contact with the skin when pulsing the laser to maintain a uniform distance from the skin.
  **TIP: Holding the laser too far or too near to the skin can affect the focal length for some lasers (e.g., QS 585 and QS 650 nm dye handpieces), which can vary the spot size and fluence delivered to the skin. In other words, holding the laser too far from the skin with these dye handpieces can reduce the spot size resulting in overtreatment of the epidermis.**
- Move the laser tip smoothly over the tattoo in a painting motion, tracing the ink pattern in the skin.
- Cover the tattoo confluently by placing tattoo pulses adjacent to one another with minimal overlap (approximately ≤10%).
  **TIP: If areas are skipped, fill them in by pulsing the laser over any untreated areas.**
- For circumferential tattoos covering extremities, consider performing treatment to either the dorsal (outer) side or the volar (inner) side of the extremity at one visit and the opposite side at a subsequent visit to help avoid possible tourniqueting effect from circumferential limb edema.
- Universal precautions are used during and after the treatment due to possible tissue splatter and bleeding.

## Desirable Clinical Endpoints

When optimal parameters are used for laser tattoo removal treatments, one or more of the following desirable clinical endpoints may be observed:

- **Whitening** of tattoo ink. Immediately after Q-switched laser treatment, the tattoo has a white discoloration. This white color change represents formation of steam in the tissues in response to rapid heating and fades over 15–30 minutes after treatment. Patients may perceive this as reduction in ink and need to be informed that it is only temporary. Figure 9 shows a black tattoo with immediate whitening during treatment with a 1064 nm Q-switched laser.
- **Snapping,** both audible and palpable, is observed during laser pulses due to photoacoustic vibration.
- **Erythema** of the background skin and extension approximately 1 in around the tattoo occurs shortly after treatment.
- **Edema (swelling)** of the tattoo is seen immediately with treatment.
- **Petechiae and purpura** (Fig. 10) represent bleeding underneath the skin and usually appear a few minutes after treatment. They are defined based on size where petechiae are pinpoint dots less than 3 mm, purpura is 3–10 mm (and ecchymoses are greater than 10 mm). These findings are desirable endpoints and indicate that aggressive settings are being used.

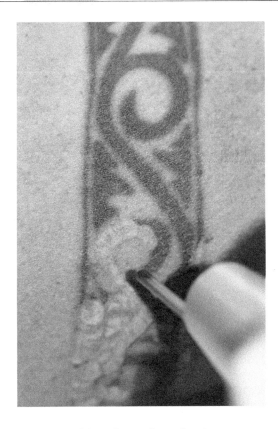

*FIGURE 9* ● Clinical endpoint of ink whitening immediately after Q-switched laser pulses. (Courtesy of R. Small, MD.)

## Undesirable Clinical Endpoints

When overly aggressive laser parameters are used for treatment, one or more of the following undesirable clinical endpoints may be observed on the skin:

• **Immediate blistering**
• **Frank bleeding**

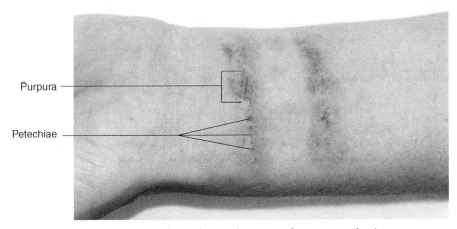

Purpura

Petechiae

*FIGURE 10* ● Clinical endpoint of petechiae and purpura a few minutes after laser tattoo removal treatment. (Courtest of R. Small, MD.)

## Performing Laser Tattoo Removal

The following recommendations are for tattoo removal treatments using a Q-switched laser. These treatment steps are specific to the Cynosure/ConBio RevLite™ system. Providers are advised to follow manufacturer guidelines for the specific device used at the time of treatment.

1. Inquire about sun exposure and sunscreen use. If the patient is recently sun exposed or has tanned skin in the treatment area, consider waiting 1 month before treating to reduce the risk of pigmentary complications.
2. Remove any jewelry that may reflect laser light.
3. Apply topical anesthetic (e.g., BLT) if necessary and remove after 30–45 minutes.
4. Position the patient comfortably on the treatment table, prone or supine to allow for exposure of the tattoo.
5. Shave the treatment area if dark hair is present.
6. Cleanse the treatment area with a wipe and allow to dry.
7. Provide wavelength-specific protective eyewear to everyone in the treatment room. If working on the face, provide the patient with extraocular lead goggles and have the patient remove contact lenses.
8. Always operate the device in accordance with your clinic's safety policies and procedures and the manufacturer's guidelines and recommended settings.
9. The laser technician is comfortably positioned, usually seated, to allow for precise manipulation of the handpiece while depressing the foot pedal.
10. Select the appropriate wavelength for the tattoo color. For the initial treatment Q-switched 1064 nm is selected. Different wavelengths will be selected for multicolored tattoos at subsequent treatments (see Subsequent Treatments for Multicolored tattoos section).
11. Select the appropriate spot size and fluence based on the patient's Fitzpatrick skin type, ink intensity and whether it is a cover-up (see Selecting Initial Laser Parameters for Treatment section).
12. Select the repetition rate based on the size and location of the tattoo (see Selecting Initial Laser Parameters for Treatment section).
13. Confirm again that everyone in the room is wearing appropriate eyewear and all doors are closed.
14. Instruct the patient not to move if they experience discomfort and to say "break" or "stop" if they need a short rest during the procedure.
    **TIP: Patients will experience discomfort even if topical anesthetic was used. Reminding patients to breathe and squeeze a stress ball during treatment will assist with pain management. Watch for vasovagal signs of lightheadedness, perspiration, and fatigue and discontinue treatment if these occur.**
15. Hold the handpiece at a 90-degree angle with the distance guide lightly touching the skin.
16. Perform a single pulse on the darkest area of the tattoo to achieve subtle endpoints.
    - **Subtle clinical endpoints for light Fitzpatrick skin types (I–III)** in the initial treatment are yellowing (as opposed to whitening), audible and palpable snapping, erythema, and edema without petechiae.
    - **Subtle clinical endpoints for dark Fitzpatrick skin types (IV and V)** in the initial treatment are erythema, edema, and palpable snapping.
17. Cover the entire tattoo confluently with the Q-switched 1064 nm laser using the same spot size and fluence that were used for test pulses.

18. Continually assess laser–tissue interaction and clinical endpoints throughout the treatment and adjust settings accordingly.
    - If undesirable clinical endpoints occur discontinue treatment in the area. **Blistered areas** are cooled using a wrapped ice pack applied for 15 minutes. **Bleeding** is managed with pressure and gauze until hemostatic. Decrease fluence and/or increase spot size before proceeding with treatment of other areas.
19. After treating the entire tattoo, assess the skin to determine if it is intact or not intact (i.e., has blisters or bleeding).
    - **If the skin is fully intact,** and in an area that will not be abraded, apply a broad-spectrum sunscreen containing zinc oxide or titanium dioxide with an SPF of 30 without a dressing.
    - **If the skin is not intact,** apply an occlusive ointment like Aquaphor™ or bacitracin, and loosely cover with a gauze dressing and tape.
20. Apply a wrapped ice pack to the skin for 15 minutes.

## Aftercare

- **Swelling, redness, and tenderness** at the site are expected after laser tattoo treatment and typically resolve within a few hours to a few days. Instruct patients to apply a wrapped ice pack for 15 minutes every 1–2 hours on the day of treatment to manage these symptoms and reduce the risk of blistering.
- **Tattoo darkening followed by crust formation** is commonly seen a few days after treatment. Crusts appear as thin darkened flakes of skin.
- **If the skin is intact** (i.e., does not have blisters or crusts) and is in an area that will not be abraded, a broad-spectrum sunscreen containing zinc oxide or titanium dioxide with an SPF of 30 or greater is applied daily without a dressing.
- **If the skin is not intact** (i.e., has bled, develops blisters or crusts) an occlusive ointment like Aquaphor or bacitracin is applied to the tattoo and loosely covered with a gauze and tape dressing that is changed daily to facilitate moist wound healing. Care should be taken not to macerate the treated area with excessive occlusion. Blisters will spontaneously rupture and form crusts that slough off over 1–2 weeks. Blisters and crusts should not be removed and patients cautioned against picking, as this increases the risk of scarring. Skin can be cleansed with a gentle, nonfragranced cleanser (e.g., Cetaphil™). Once the skin is intact, a daily broad-spectrum sunscreen is applied for the duration of the tattoo removal treatments and cleansed with mild soap and water.
- **Shiny skin** is a normal part of the healing process and can be seen up to 3 weeks, or longer, following treatment. Skin that is fully healed will appear dull like the surrounding untreated epidermis.
- **Pruritus** is also part of the healing process and is common during the first few weeks following treatment.
- **Topical silicone** can be used to facilitate healing and shorten recovery times. Silicone is available as gel sheets (e.g., ScarAway® and Mepitel®) or self-drying gel (e.g., bioCorneum®). The gel sheets cut to the size of the tattoo, or the self-drying gel, are applied daily for 12–24 hours once the skin is intact, usually 2 weeks after the laser treatment.
- **Strenuous exercise and exposure to water** are avoided until the skin is intact.
- **Written aftercare instructions** are provided to patients (see Tattoo Removal Before and After Instructions for Laser Treatments, Appendix 3d).

## Common Follow-Ups

- **Prolonged healing** of the tattoo with shiny skin persisting for 8 weeks or more can occur, particularly with tattoos on distal extremities and with aggressive laser parameters that result in crusts or blisters. Topical silicone (see Aftercare section) can be used to facilitate healing and shorten recovery times.
- **Postinflammatory hyperpigmentation** is common with laser tattoo removal treatments, particularly in patients with darker Fitzpatrick skin types (IV and V). PIH is usually apparent as an indistinct brown haze around the tattoo (Fig. 16). If PIH occurs, temporarily suspend laser treatments. Apply hydroquinone cream (4–8%) twice daily along with a broad-spectrum sunscreen daily once skin is intact, and consider covering the tattoo if the area is directly exposed to sun on a regular basis. With these measures, hyperpigmentation usually resolves within a few months, although resolution can be prolonged in some patients. Performing laser tattoo removal treatments on a tattoo that has PIH can result in hypopigmentation as the patient's native melanin is targeted and removed.
- **Small blisters** (Fig. 17) **and crusting** commonly occur, particularly toward the end of a treatment series when more aggressive parameters are used. Management of small blisters and crusts is discussed in the Aftercare section above. Intervals between treatments are lengthened to allow additional time for healing.

## Treatment Intervals

Laser tattoo removal treatments are 4–8 weeks apart to allow the skin to fully heal. Tattoos in proximal locations tend to heal faster than those located distally, and in areas that are abraded (such as wrists and hips). Treatment intervals may be extended without any reduction in efficacy, and in fact, treated tattoo ink may continue to fade slightly after 6 weeks. The tattoo is appropriate for retreatment once the skin is fully intact, without a shiny appearance or skin flaking. Patients commonly request shorter treatment intervals as they are usually highly motivated to remove their tattoos. However, treating too frequently may increase the risk of textural changes, scarring, and hypopigmentation.

   **Note:** If the laser has been recalibrated or serviced between treatments, perform test spots at the subsequent treatment with low fluences to avoid unintentional overtreatment in case the laser output is increased relative to its precalibration status.

## Subsequent Treatments for Black Tattoos

- **Ensure skin is healed.** Once the treated skin has returned to its baseline dull appearance the tattoo may undergo laser tattoo removal treatment again. If the skin is shiny or flaking additional time is needed for healing and treatment is delayed, usually by 2 weeks.
- **Intensify laser treatment parameters.** At subsequent visits tattoo ink will be lighter and the laser fluence will need to be increased and spot size reduced to achieve desired clinical endpoints. Typically, only one parameter is intensified in a given visit. The fluence is increased first, in small increments from 0.2–0.5 J/cm$^2$; usually no more than 1.5 J/cm$^2$ higher than the prior treatment, while keeping the spot size constant. After maximizing the fluence over several visits, the spot size is then decreased with an associated reduction in fluence.
   **TIP: A test spot is performed at each visit prior to initiating treatment to determine the appropriate settings.**

- **Example for laser parameter progression over a treatment series.** When treating a black tattoo on a patient with Fitzpatrick skin type II, treatments may be intensified and desirable clinical endpoints achieved with the following parameters over a treatment series:
  - Treatment 1 use 1064 nm Q-switched laser with 6-mm spot size and 2.5 J/cm$^2$.
  - Treatments 2–5: use 1064 nm Q-switched laser with 6-mm spot size and fluences of 3.0 J/cm$^2$ (Treatment 2), 3.5 J/cm$^2$ (Treatment 3) and so on up to 4.5 J/cm$^2$, which is the maximal fluence for 6 mm.
  - Treatment 6 use 1064 nm Q-switched laser and decrease the spot size to 4 mm in order to intensify the treatment. Perform test spots starting with slightly lowered fluences of 4.0 J/cm$^2$ and increase until endpoints are seen, which may be 5 J/cm$^2$ for example.
  - Treatments 7 and above, continue to increase fluence and decrease spot size as described above.
  - Once the ink color is lightened, and if there is minimal to no change with the Q-switched 1064 nm wavelength, shorter wavelengths such as QS 532 nm can be used instead of the QS 1064 nm to intensify treatments. Start with the largest spot size and lowest fluence to achieve a desirable clinical endpoint and progress as described above.
  TIP: **QS 532 nm pulses tend to make crisp white spots. Application of ice as part of aftercare on the day of treatment is particularly important with this short wavelength to reduce the risk of blistering.**

## Subsequent Treatments for Multicolored Tattoos

- **Ensure skin is healed.** Once the treated skin has returned to its baseline dull appearance and is no longer shiny, the tattoo may undergo laser tattoo removal treatment again.
- **Intensify laser treatment parameters.** Follow recommendations above for black tattoos.
  TIP: **A test spot is performed at each visit prior to initiating treatment to determine the appropriate settings.**
- **Example for laser parameter progression over a treatment series.** When treating a multicolored tattoo on a patient with Fitzpatrick skin type II, treatments may be intensified and desirable clinical endpoints achieved with the following parameters over a treatment series:
  - Treatment 1 use 1064 nm Q-switched laser regardless of the color of the tattoo. Use conservative settings with a large spot size such as 6 mm and low fluence such as 1.5–2.0 J/cm$^2$.
  - Treatment 2 and subsequent treatments: use 1064 nm Q-switched laser to treat the whole tattoo with largest spot size and lowest fluence to achieve desirable clinical endpoints. Over the treatment series, intensify settings by increasing the fluence and decreasing the spot size as described in Subsequent Treatments for Black Tattoos above.
  - Once there is minimal to no change in a particular color after treatment with the Q-switched 1064 nm, discontinue use of 1064 nm and select the wavelength specific to the tattoo ink color being targeted (Table 1 and Fig. 4). For example, a tattoo with black, green, red, and sky blue ink may have no change in the red and sky blue ink after the 4th treatment. Parameters for the 5th treatment might be as follows:

QS 1064 nm to the dark ink areas (black and green), QS 532 nm to the red areas, and QS 585 nm to the sky blue areas. If the green ink showed no reduction with that treatment, then the 6th treatment might be: QS 1064 nm to the black areas, QS 650 nm to the green areas, QS 532 nm to the red areas, and QS 585 nm to the sky blue areas. At the subsequent treatment, the fluence would continue to be increased and spot size decreased to intensify treatments as described above.

**TIP: Avoid treating one tattoo color with multiple wavelengths in the same visit as this excessive energy can cause epidermal injury. The patient in Figure 17 developed small blisters after treatment with Q-switched 1064 and 650 nm lasers that were pulsed over each other in the same areas; prolonged icing on unprotected skin then resulted in bullae formation.**

**TIP: Spot size varies with distance from the skin for QS 585 and QS 650 nm dye handpieces. The tendency is to pull the laser tip away from the skin and this decreases the spot size and thereby intensifies the treatment. It is important to keep the distance guide in contact with the skin surface to avoid epidermal injury.**

- Toward the end of a treatment series, multicolored tattoos often look "muddy" with indistinct colors. Shorter wavelengths such as Q-switched 532 nm can be used for the final stages of removal.

## Results

Many factors influence laser tattoo removal results, but in general, amateur black tattoos are the easiest to remove and professional multicolored tattoos tend to be more challenging.

- Figure 11 shows a black rose tattoo before (A) and after (B) six treatments with a Q-switched laser using the 1064 nm wavelength (Medlite™, Cynosure/ConBio).

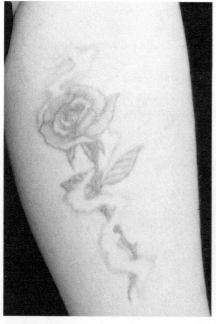 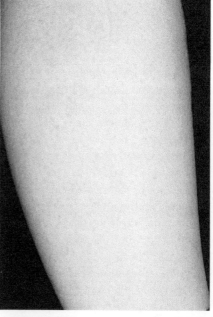

A                                                                                            B

*FIGURE 11* ● Black rose tattoo before **(A)** and after **(B)** six treatments with a Q-switched 1064 nm laser. (Courtesy of L. Chavez, MD and Cynosure/ConBio.)

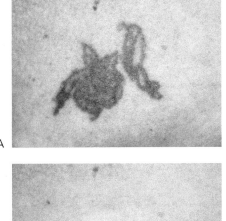

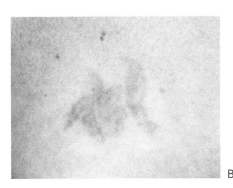

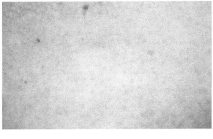

FIGURE 12 ● Black and green flower tattoo before (A), after four treatments (B), and after 14 treatments (C), with Q-switched 1064 nm and 650 nm lasers. (Courtesy of R. Small, MD.)

- Figure 12 shows a multicolored black and green flower tattoo before (A), after four treatments showing residual green ink (B), and after 14 treatments (C) with a Q-switched laser using 1064- and 650 nm wavelengths (RevLite™, Cynosure/ConBio).
- Figure 13 shows a black facial tattoo before (A) and after (B) ten treatments with a Q-switched 1064 nm laser (Spectra™, Lutronic).
- Figure 14 shows a black cross tattoo before (A) and after (B) four treatments with a picosecond laser using the 755 nm wavelength (PicoSure™, Cynosure/ConBio).
- Figure 15 shows cosmetic eyebrow tattoo before (A) and after (B) twelve treatments with a Q-switched laser using the 1064 nm wavelength (RevLite™, Cynosure/ConBio). Figure 15B also shows hair reduction as Q-switched 1064 nm lasers can remove fine dark hair. This eyebrow tattoo was lightened in order to replace it with differently shaped eyebrow tattoo.

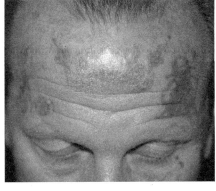

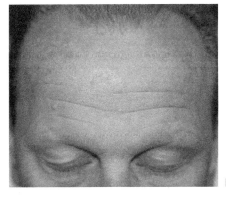

FIGURE 13 ● Black facial tattoo before (A) after (B) ten treatments with a Q-switched 1064 nm laser. (Courtesy of M. Werner, MD and Lutronic.)

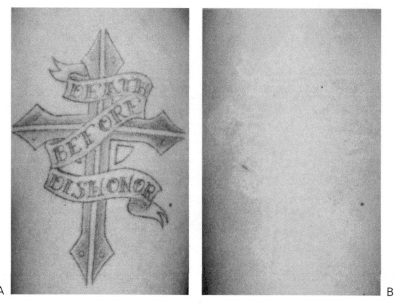

**FIGURE 14** ● Black cross tattoo before **(A)** after **(B)** four treatments with a picosecond 755 nm laser. (Courtesy of Cynosure.)

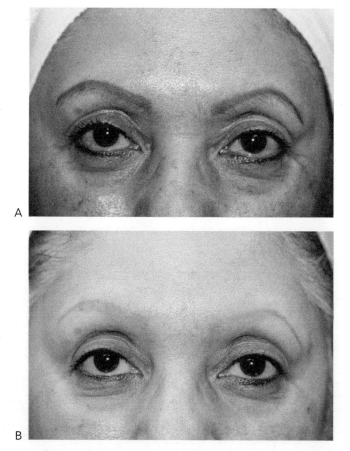

**FIGURE 15** ● Cosmetic eye brow tattoo before **(A)** and after **(B)** twelve treatments with a Q-switched 1064 nm laser. (Courtesy of R. Small, MD.)

# Complications

- Pain
- Hyperpigmentation
- Hypopigmentation
- Blisters and bullae
- Bleeding
- Prolonged healing
- Textural change
- Scarring
- Incomplete ink removal
- Infection
- Dermatosis exacerbation (e.g., psoriasis, atopic dermatitis)
- Allergic reactions
- Paradoxical tattoo darkening (common with cosmetic tattoos)
- Ignition of flammable debris (possible with traumatic tattoos)
- Vasovagal episode/syncope or hypoglycemia
- Compartment syndrome

There is a fine line between anticipated side effects (some of which are discussed in Common Follow-ups) and true complications from laser tattoo removal treatments. For example, discomfort, edema, crusts, itching, small blisters, and PIH are commonly associated with the laser tattoo treatments, but extreme pain, limb edema, bullae, intractable pruritus, and scarring are uncommon and are true complications from treatment. Complications associated with overtreatment such as burns and pigmentary changes (hyperpigmentation and hypopigmentation) are more likely to occur with aggressive laser parameters: short wavelengths, short pulse widths, high fluences in patients with dark Fitzpatrick skin types (IV–VI), or dyschromia such as actinic bronzing, recently tanned skin, and severely sun-damaged skin with extensive lentigines.

**Pain** is intense with tattoo removal treatments and the greatest discomfort is experienced while the laser is pulsing. Pain management is a more significant consideration with larger tattoos and therapeutic options such as topical anesthetics and oral pain medications are discussed in the Anesthesia section above. Pain, stress, and anxiety can precipitate a **vasovagal episode.** Vasovagal signs and symptoms include lightheadedness, fatigue, waning alertness, nausea, perspiration, tinnitus, and can progress to **syncope.** If symptoms are noted, discontinue the procedure and follow appropriate protocols for vasovagal emergencies. This may include laying the patient flat, elevating their legs, and rehydrating with water or juice. Administering 2–4 oral glucose tablets (approximately equivalent to 15 gm of glucose) can also be helpful as **hypoglycemia** can present similarly. Complaint of pain several days postprocedure is uncommon and evaluation is advisable, particularly to assess for thermal injury due to overtreatment and infection.

**Hyperpigmentation** (Fig. 16) **and hypopigmentation** (Fig. 14B) result from alteration to background skin color and are seen in nearly half the patients treated with Q-switched lasers for tattoo removal. These pigmentary changes usually resolve in 6–12 months but in some cases are permanent. The risk of hyperpigmentation and hypopigmentation is greatest with dark Fitzpatrick skin types (IV–VI), tanned skin, actinic bronzing, severely photodamaged skin, and with aggressive laser parameters. Unprotected direct sun expo-

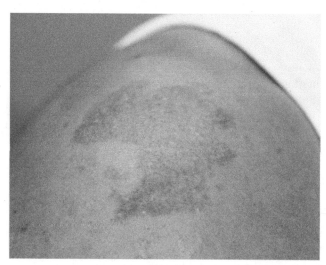

**FIGURE 16** ● Postinflammatory hyperpigmentation seen as a haze of brown around green tattoo ink one month after treatment with a Q-switched 1064 nm laser in a patient with dark Fitzpatrick skin type. (Courtesy of R. Small, MD.)

sure after treatment is associated with hyperpigmentation, particularly in dark skin types. **Hyperpigmentation** usually resolves spontaneously over several months, although in rare instances may be permanent. Sun protection including the application of a broad-spectrum sunscreen with SPF 30 containing zinc oxide or titanium dioxide and sun avoidance are preventative measures for PIH. PIH can be treated using a topical lightening agent such as hydroquinone cream 4–8% twice daily in the PIH area, superficial exfoliation procedures such as microdermabrasion and light chemical peels 1 month after treatment, and sun protection. **Hypopigmentation** is more common with short wavelengths (e.g., 532 nm) than longer wavelengths (e.g., 1064 nm). Hypopigmentation is usually temporary and may resolve spontaneously with exposure to ambient light sunlight, but in some cases it is permanent. There are few specific treatment options for hypopigmentation but it may respond to the excimer (308 nm) laser or narrow band UVB treatment. Alternatively, skin surrounding hypopigmented areas can be lightened to reduce the demarcation between background skin and hypopigmented areas.

**Small blisters** (Fig. 17) can occur within a few days of treatment, particularly with use of short wavelength such as 532 nm, and management is discussed above in the Aftercare section. **Bullae** (Fig. 18) are not an anticipated outcome. While they will rupture spontaneously, patients may prefer to have them lanced. Using clean technique, bullae can be lanced and incised with an 18-gauge needle, the serous fluid gently expressed, dressed with an occlusive ointment like Aquaphor™ or bacitracin, gauze, bandage, and taped firmly to minimize reaccumulation of fluid. Dressings are changed daily until the crust is gone revealing intact skin.

**Pinpoint bleeding,** while not a desired endpoint with laser tattoo removal treatment, is occasionally observed with the use of small spot sizes (e.g., 2 mm) and high fluences. **Frank bleeding** with gauze saturation is a complication. Management of nonintact skin is described in the Aftercare section above. Areas, which blister and bleed, usually have prolonged healing of 8 weeks or more. **Prolonged healing** can also be seen in treatment areas that are chronically abraded (e.g., hips and wearing jeans, wrists and

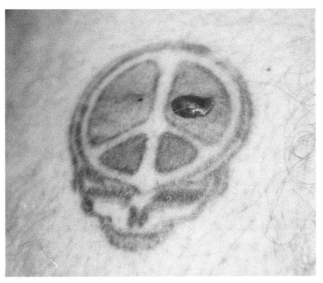

**FIGURE 17** ● Blister in the yellow portion of a multicolored tattoo after laser tattoo treatment with Q-switched 532 nm in the red/yellow and Q-switched 1064 nm in the green and black areas. (Courtesy of R. Small, MD.)

wearing bracelets) and in distal locations (e.g., ankles, fingers). Patients with bleeding, blistering, and prolonged healing are monitored for induration and scarring.

**Scarring**, including atrophic and hypertrophc scars (Fig. 19), and subtle textural changes can occur, particularly at sites treated aggressively that have blistered or bled. Patients prone to textural changes and scarring with trauma have an increased risk of scarring with laser tattoo removal. In addition, certain areas are more prone to

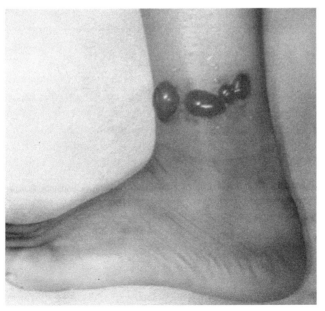

**FIGURE 18** ● Bullae in a green tattoo after treatment with Q-switched 1064 nm and 650 nm lasers sequentially pulsed in the same areas. (Courtest of R. Small, MD.)

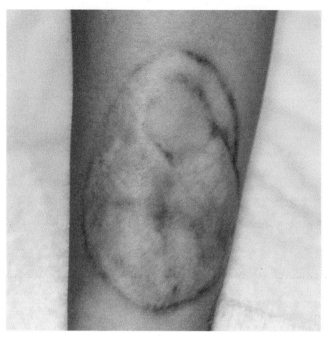

*FIGURE 19* ● Scarring after tattoo treatment using a Q-switched 1064 nm laser and 2-mm spot size with report of frank bleeding during treatment. (Courtesy of R. Small, MD.)

scarring such as the sternum. Textural changes are often transient and typically resolve spontaneously within a few months, however; textural changes and scarring may be permanent. Persistent intense erythema and induration can be an indicator of impending scar formation and early intervention may help avoid permanent scarring. If **impending scar formation** is suspected, a very high-potency topical corticosteroid ointment may be applied (e.g., clobetasol 0.05% or betamethasone dipropionate 0.05% twice daily), topical silicone (described in the Common Follow-ups section), and pulsed dye lasers (QS 585 and QS 595 nm) may be used to reduce scar formation. The appearance of **hypertrophic scars** may also be improved with the above therapies as well as injections of low-dose triamcinolone acetonide (Kenalog®-10, 10 mg/mL, using 1–2 mg). Injections may be repeated monthly, taking care not to overtreat, which can result in depressed atrophic scar formation. If hypertrophic scarring occurs, ink is not usually visible in the scarred area and additional tattoo laser treatments are rarely required. If atrophic scarring or textural changes occur, visible ink may persist; removal of the remaining ink is more challenging, and patients have an increased risk for further scarring. If, after being advised of the risks, patients elect to proceed with additional tattoo treatments, they will require more treatments and more time for tattoo removal than initially estimated as conservative treatment parameters must be used moving forward along with longer treatment intervals of 8 weeks or more for maximal healing time between treatments.

**Incomplete ink removal** is a disappointing complication. This is more common in tattoos that are scarred, either as a result of the tattooing process, as a result of nonlaser tattoo removal methods, or by laser tattoo removal treatments. Surgical excision is an option if the final result is unacceptable and patients are willing to tolerate a surgical scar.

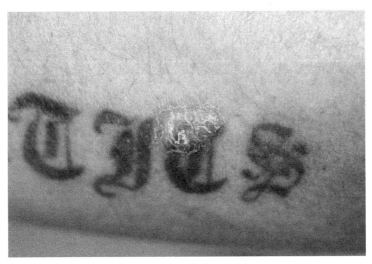

FIGURE 20 ● Psoriasis flare at the site of laser tattoo removal treatment. (Courtesy of R. Small, MD.)

**Infections** postprocedure with tattoo laser treatment are rare and require treatment specific to the pathogen. Reactivation of viral infections in the treatment area such as **herpes simplex** (and varicella zoster) is one of the most common infectious complications, and pretreatment with an oral antiviral medication (e.g., valacyclovir/famciclovir 500 mg 1 tablet twice daily begun 2 days prior to the procedure and continued for 3 days postprocedure) in patients with a known history reduces this risk.

**Dermatosis exacerbation** can occur at sites of trauma. For example, **atopic dermatitis** or **psoriasis** (Fig. 20) can be triggered by tattoo removal treatments.

**Allergic reactions** to tattoo ink have been reported at the time of tattoo placement and after Q-switched laser treatments. Reactions usually consist of local erythema, pruritus, and edema, and less commonly inflamed nodules and granulomas. Allergic reactions are most common with red tattoos (that may contain mercury sulfide) and have also been reported with yellow (cadmium sulfide), green (chromium), and blue (cobalt) inks. Figure 21 shows a red ink allergy 3 weeks after treatment with a Q-switched 532 nm laser. Treatment of mild reactions consists of topical medium-potency steroids (e.g., triamcinolone acetonide cream 0.1%), sunlight avoidance, and sunscreen use. In patients with more severe reactions, oral antihistamines or oral corticosteroids may also be used. Granulomas can be managed with intralesional steroid injections, or in some cases, surgical removal. **Systemic allergic reactions,** while extremely rare, can occur. Patients with allergic responses to ink at the time of tattoo placement may be at higher risk for allergic reactions with laser tattoo removal. Follow appropriate protocols for systemic allergic reactions, which may include medications such as epinephrine, diphenhydramine (Benadryl®), and methylprednisolone (Solu-Medrol®) when indicated.

**Paradoxical darkening** is darkening of tattoo ink after treatment with a laser for tattoo removal (Fig. 22). This routinely occurs with cosmetic tattoos. They usually contain white ink composed of zinc oxide or titanium dioxide pigments or flesh tone colors containing iron oxides, which can turn brown or black by Q-switched lasers. This darkened ink responds well to and is lightened with subsequent tattoo laser treatments, but the initial darkening can be disconcerting to patients as the tattoo looks more obvious

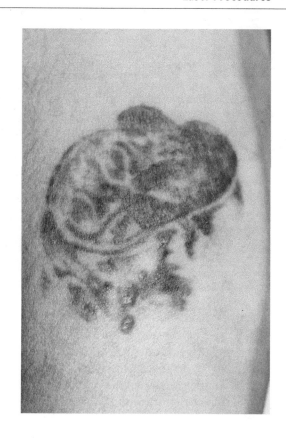

*FIGURE 21* ● Red ink allergy after
Q-switched 532 nm laser tattoo removal
treatment. (Courtesy of R. Small, MD.)

than it did prior to treatment. If paradoxical darkening occurs, the tattoo can be treated as if it were black ink using a Q-switched 1064 nm wavelength at the subsequent visits.

**Ignition of flammable debris** has been reported with treatment of a traumatic tattoo resulting from firework debris in the skin. This underscores the importance of obtaining a thorough history when treating traumatic tattoos. Most traumatic tattoos result from asphalt trapped in the skin after abrasion, referred to as "road rash," and can be effectively and safely treated with laser tattoo removal.

**Compartment syndrome** is a rare but serious complication, that can occur with circumferential treatment of an extremity. This requires evaluation and management in an urgent care setting with surgical consultation.

## Special Populations and Additional Considerations

- **Pregnant and nursing.** Women that are pregnant or nursing do not typically undergo elective procedures such as laser tattoo removal. One of the potential complications from pain during a tattoo treatment might be inhibition of lactation in women who are nursing.
- **Dark Fitzpatrick skin types.** Patients with dark skin types (IV and V) are treated using conservative settings with large spot sizes and low fluencies. Treatment parameters are increased slowly over the treatment series to reduce the risk of complications. Observe for PIH and hypopigmentation.
- **Pediatric patients.** Tattoos may be treated with patient and parental consent. Pain management is important with this population and age-appropriate analgesics and dosing is necessary.

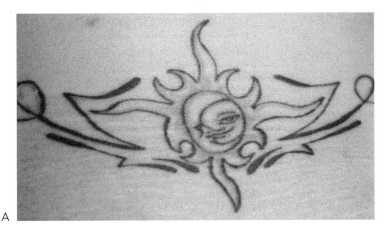

A

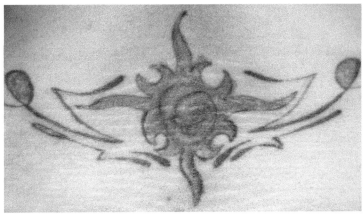

B

*FIGURE 22*  ⊕  Paradoxical darkening of yellow and pink inks shown before (A) and after (B) Q-switched 1064 nm laser tattoo removal treatment. (Courtesy of R. Small, MD.)

- **Nonfacial areas.** Nonfacial areas such as distal extremities have delayed healing relative to the face due to fewer pilosebaceous units, which serve as sites of reepithelialization and facilitate healing. Nonfacial areas have a greater risk of overtreatment and scarring, and it is advisable to treat conservatively compared to the face.
- **Cosmetic and traumatic tattoos** are most often treated with Q-switched 1064 nm. While initial treatment may be associated with paradoxical darkening, subsequent treatment with tattoo lasers are more predictable and consistent with decorative tattoo ink response to lasers. Cosmetic tattoos can be more challenging to remove than decorative tattoos, and providers may want to wait to perform these treatments until they are confident in their skill with decorative tattoo removal.

## Learning Techniques for Laser Tattoo Removal

Providers getting started can practice eye–hand coordination with the laser by drawing an image with a black marker on a large grapefruit or orange and treating with the laser using a low fluence. Treating patients with black tattoos and light Fitzpatrick skin types is advisable initially as complications are less common in this population and treatment parameters are more straightforward. Consider using low repetition rates (e.g., 2 or 5 Hz) initially for easier control of the laser handpiece. As skill level progresses providers can advance to treating multicolor tattoos and darker Fitzpatrick skin types.

## Current Developments

**Picosecond** alexandrite (755 nm) and most recently picosecond 532 nm lasers (e.g., PicoSure™ by Cynosure) are being used for tattoo removal with promising results. Early studies with this shorter pulse width have shown effective and rapid treatment of black, blue, and green tattoos with similar safety profiles compared to Q-switched lasers and potentially fewer treatments.

**Iridescent ink** is a newer form of tattoo ink that is only observable under a black light. Patients refer to these tattoos as "glow-in-the-dark." These tattoos should not be treated as their ink contains no chromophore for selective absorption by tattoo removal lasers.

**Infinitink™**, which is marketed as a tattoo ink that is easily removable, is used by a small number of tattoo artists. This ink is a bioresorbable dye encapsulated in polymethylmethacrylate transparent capsules that, according to the manufacturer (Freedom 2™), require fewer treatments with Q-switched lasers for removal.

## Financial Considerations

Tattoo removal is considered a cosmetic treatment and is not reimbursed by insurance companies. Fees can vary widely and are dependent on geographical regions. Most providers base their fee for tattoo removal on the size of the tattoo and presence or absence of multiple colors. For example, the fee for a single tattoo removal treatment of a black tattoo less than or equal to 9 in$^2$ may be \$200; 10–25 in$^2$ may be \$350; 26–49 in$^2$ may be \$500 and an additional \$100 may be added for treatment of tattoos containing challenging colors such as sky blue or green. Laser tattoo removal treatments are painful and can require 12–16 visits, or more in some cases. Some patients may become discouraged over time by the number of treatments necessary and the costs they incur. To help ensure that patients complete their treatment series and achieve satisfactory results, some providers may reduce the cost of treatments as the series progresses.

## Chapter 5

# Wrinkles—Nonablative Resurfacing

Rebecca Small, M.D.

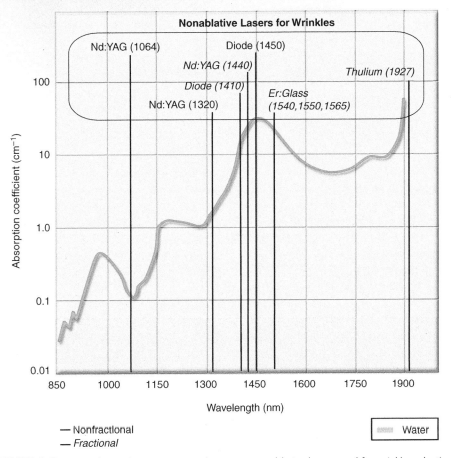

**FIGURE 1** ● Water absorption spectrum and common nonablative lasers used for wrinkle reduction.

Nonablative skin resurfacing lasers[*] offer a gentle means of improving skin texture and wrinkles with minimal downtime. They are versatile and can be combined with other lasers for treatment of pigmentation and vascularities, as well as other minimally invasive

---

*Laser refers to both lasers and intense pulsed light devices, unless otherwise specified.

procedures such as botulinum toxin and dermal fillers. Devices used for nonablative resurfacing are a heterogeneous group of technologies, but are all similar in that they induce dermal collagen remodeling with collagen synthesis while keeping the epidermis intact. Wrinkle reduction results are modest compared to ablative lasers; however, nonablative lasers are a good option for patients seeking gradual cosmetic improvements who want minimal or no disruption to daily activities. Common terms used for wrinkle reduction with nonablative lasers include: nonablative resurfacing, nonablative laser resurfacing, skin toning, and noninvasive laser rejuvenation. With recent advances in fractional devices that deliver higher energies and have deeper cutaneous penetration, nonablative lasers have become one of the primary modalities used for rejuvenation of photodamaged skin.

## Anatomy

**Wrinkles** are one of the most prominent characteristics of photoaged skin. Histologically, wrinkled skin is atrophied with a thinned cellular epidermis and has reduced structural proteins in the dermal extracellular matrix (ECM) such as collagen and elastin that give skin its firmness and elastic recoil. Synthesis of ECM components slows naturally with age, and ultraviolet (UV) light stimulates degradative enzymes that also breakdown and weaken these proteins. There is also diminished functioning of the sweat and oil glands, and fewer ECM glycosaminoglycans, which reduces skin hydration and suppleness. In certain cases of advanced photoaging, skin can have solar elastosis changes with tangled masses of damaged elastin protein in the dermis.

**Nonablative lasers used for skin resurfacing maintain an intact stratum corneum** while causing mild thermal injury to the dermis. A wound healing response ensues after treatment resulting in collagen shrinkage and fibroblast activation with synthesis of new collagen and other ECM components, referred to as dermal collagen remodeling. Expanding the ECM thickens the dermis and smoothes the skin, resulting in clinical reduction of wrinkles. In addition to wrinkle reduction, collagen remodeling effects with nonablative lasers also include improvement in atrophic scars, hypertrophic scars, pore size, striae, and rough skin texture.

Nonablative lasers used for skin resurfacing employ either a nonfractional or fractional method of delivering laser energy to the skin. **Nonfractional lasers** gently heat the dermis in bulk (Fig. 2A), evoking a mild collagen remodeling response. They typically penetrate to the papillary dermis, approximately 100–300 μm. **Fractional lasers** heat a portion of the skin creating microscopic columns of epidermal and dermal tissue damage (Fig. 2B). These columns are referred to as microthermal treatment zones (MTZs) and penetrate deeply to the reticular dermis, approximately 1500 μm. Tissue in the MTZs is coagulated while the stratum corneum is left intact. Untreated tissue between the MTZs serves as a reservoir for regenerative cells that migrate into the treated areas and facilitate rapid wound healing with neocollagenesis and collagen remodeling leading to wrinkle reduction. Fractional lasers also treat pigmented lesions such as solar lentigines, ephelides, other dyschromic conditions such as melasma and poikiloderma of Civatte, as well as actinic keratoses. Pigment removal with fractional lasers is nonspecific and results from extrusion of microscopic epidermal and dermal necrotic debris as part of the healing process. Fractional nonablative lasers induce a more profound wound healing response relative to other nonablative lasers and are associated with greater dermal collagen remodeling effects and more significant reduction of wrinkles, atrophic scars, hypertrophic scars, striae, and skin laxity.

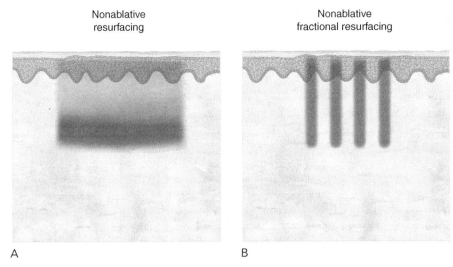

Nonablative
resurfacing

Nonablative
fractional resurfacing

A                                    B

*FIGURE 2* ● Nonablative laser patterns of cutaneous injury: nonfractional **(A)** and fractional **(B)**.

## Laser Principles

Most nonablative lasers used for skin resurfacing heat the dermis by targeting the **water chromophore,** and some work by targeting **melanin and oxyhemoglobin chromophores.** Water absorbs light between 950 and 11000 nm (Fig. 6, Key References). When skin is irradiated with a laser targeting water, the dermis is either gently warmed (with nonfractional lasers) or more aggressively heated and coagulated (with fractional lasers) depending on the method of laser energy delivery. Lasers that target melanin and oxyhemoglobin chromophores, while primarily used for treatment of pigmented lesions or vascular lesions according to their chromophore specificity, can also be used for skin resurfacing. These pigmented chromophores absorb light from 400–1200 nm (Fig. 4, Key References). Heating the dermis by absorbing laser energy with water, melanin, or oxyhemoglobin chromophores activates fibroblasts and stimulates a collagen remodeling response, which increase dermal thickness and reduce wrinkles.

### Laser Parameters for Nonablative Resurfacing Treatments

Nonablative laser devices are a diverse group of technologies and parameters vary widely based on the device used. Wrinkle reduction is primarily in response to dermal injury and some generalizations can be made about parameters that help achieve deep penetration to the dermis using these devices.

- **Wavelength.** Most lasers used for skin resurfacing target the **water chromophore,** which absorbs laser energy from approximately 950–11000 nm (Fig. 6, Key References). Lasers targeting water that are used for nonablative resurfacing are shown in Figure 1 and include **fractional (1410 nm, 1440 nm, 1540 nm, 1550 nm, 1565 nm, 1927 nm) and nonfractional (1064 nm, 1320 nm, 1450 nm).** The depth of penetration of these lasers (when using a similar method of delivery and other parameters being equal) is determined by their affinity for water, where short wavelengths have lower water absorption and deeper cutaneous penetration; longer wavelengths have higher water absorption and more superficial penetration. **Lasers that target melanin and oxyhemoglobin** are also used for skin resurfacing treatments and absorb light from 400–1000 nm and these devices include **532 nm, 585 nm, 595 nm, 755 nm, 1064 nm, and intense pulsed light** (Fig. 5, Key References). The depth of penetration of these lasers is determined by beam scatter and melanin and oxyhemoglobin absorption, where short wavelengths penetrate superficially and long wavelengths penetrate deeply.

- **Fluence.** Laser fluence is a major determinant of the depth of penetration, where higher fluences penetrate deeper in the skin.
- **Pulse width.** Longer pulse widths penetrate deeper in the skin and are safer for dark skin types.
- **Spot size.** Large spot sizes have greater absorption and deeper cutaneous penetration compared to small spot sizes. Larger spot sizes also cover more body area per pulse, which translates to shorter treatment times.
- **Repetition rate.** Fast repetition rates allow for more rapid coverage of large treatment areas and can shorten treatment times.
- **Scanners.** Some devices utilize scanners and computer software to "randomly" deliver pulses within a set pattern so that the pulses are not adjacent to one another. Delivering the pulses in this way allows for high energies to be used during treatment and reduces the risk of epidermal thermal injury.
- **Cooling.** Adequate cooling is required to protect the epidermis, while overcooling can reduce clinical effects. Excessive cooling can induce epidermal cold injury, particularly in darker Fitzpatrick skin types, resulting in postinflammatory hyperpigmentation (PIH).
- **Fractional lasers.**
  - **Spot size.** Spot sizes used with fractional devices are very small, ranging from 100–900 µm, and are not adjustable. These tiny spot sizes can penetrate very deeply (to 1.5 mm) and increasing penetration depth with increasing spot size does not hold true when considering the tiny spot sizes used with fractional lasers.
  - **Spot density.** Fractional devices also have a density setting which determines the percentage of skin that is treated with a pulse (that range from 5–50%). High-density settings are associated with more aggressive treatments, have longer healing times and greater improvements.
  - **Fluence.** High fluences are associated with deep penetration and large MTZs (i.e., skin treatment areas). High fluences are also associated with longer healing times.

Laser treatment parameters are often described as **aggressive or conservative.** Aggressive treatment parameters refer to the use of short wavelengths, short pulse widths, high fluences, and small spot sizes. Conservative laser parameters refer to the use of long wavelengths, long pulse widths, low fluences, and large spot sizes (Fig. 3, Key References).

## Patient Selection

Patient selection for skin resurfacing treatments with nonablative lasers is based on the severity of wrinkling, patient expectations for improvement, and tolerance for recovery time (Table 1). Patients seeking dramatic results from only 1 treatment are not ideal candidates for nonablative resurfacing treatments and may be better served by ablative skin resurfacing as they typically require fewer treatments for reduction of wrinkles (see Wrinkles—Ablative Resurfacing, Chapter 6).

## TABLE 1

### Patient Selection and Results with Nonablative Lasers for Skin Resurfacing

| Device (Chromophore) | Wrinkle Severity | Results | Discomfort | Downtime |
|---|---|---|---|---|
| Nonfractional (melanin and oxyhemoglobin) | + | + | + | + |
| Nonfractional (water) | + | + | + | + |
| Fractional (water) | ++ | ++ | ++ | ++ |

Nonfractional (melanin and oxyhemoglobin) = 532 nm, 585 nm, 595 nm, 755 nm, 1064 nm, IPL (500–1200 nm).
Nonfractional (water) = 1064 nm, 1320 nm, 1450 nm.
Fractional (water) = 1410 nm, 1440 nm, 1540 nm, 1550 nm, 1565 nm, 1927 nm.
+ mild; ++ moderate.

**Patients with mild to moderate wrinkles** such as Glogau types I–III (see Introduction and Foundation Concepts, Glogau Classification of Photoaging section) are appropriate candidates for all nonablative lasers. Patients who are willing to accept modest improvements and desire short visits with little to no downtime postprocedure are best suited to treatment with nonfractional lasers (Table 1). Patients with mild to moderate wrinkles seeking more dramatic reduction of wrinkles, who are willing to accept some procedural discomfort and postprocedure downtime, are good candidates for fractional lasers. Patients with severe wrinkling are better candidates for ablative lasers or surgery, especially if skin laxity is significant.

**Light Fitzpatrick skin types (I–III)** may be treated with all nonablative laser technologies including those with shorter wavelengths (e.g., 532 nm and pulsed dye lasers) as these patients have relatively lower risks of complications such as hyperpigmentation. **Dark Fitzpatrick skin types (IV–VI)** can be safely treated with nonfractional lasers that target water. While, fractional lasers that target water are also indicated for darker skin types, these technologies have greater risks of pigmentary alterations and may necessitate more conservative settings which can attenuate results.

## Patient Expectations

Skin resurfacing with nonablative lasers requires a series of treatments performed at monthly intervals to demonstrate visible results: 4–6 for fractional lasers and 6–8 for nonfractional lasers. Results with nonablative resurfacing treatments (even with a series) are slow and subtle compared to ablative lasers (see Chapter 6). Assessment of patients' expectations at the time of consultation and commitment to a series of treatments is essential to ensure success with these treatments.

**Nonfractional lasers that target water or melanin and oxyhemoglobin** result in mild wrinkle reduction. Results are typically seen 2–3 months after the initial laser treatment, and improvements may continue up to 6 months posttreatment. Relative to fractional nonablative lasers, skin resurfacing effects are less dramatic. However, these treatments have the advantage of requiring little to no recovery time, lower risks of complications, and are easily incorporated into patients' daily lives.

**Fractional lasers that target water** have faster results and more significant improvements than nonfractional lasers. Results are usually seen by 1 month posttreatment and, like nonfractional lasers, improvements may continue up to 6 months posttreatment. These laser treatments are more uncomfortable than other nonablative lasers and typically require topical anesthetic preprocedure and forced-air cooling during the procedure for treatment to be tolerable. Some patients require oral analgesics and anxiolytics. Postprocedure erythema and edema typically last for 3–4 days, and procedures can be associated with complications such as pigmentary alteration, acne exacerbations, and milia formation.

## Indications

- Mild static rhytids
- Rough skin texture
- Enlarged pores
- Superficial acne scars

### Additional Indications for Nonablative Fractional Lasers

- Moderate static rhytids
- Benign pigmented lesions (e.g., lentigines, ephelides)
- Melasma
- Scarring (atrophic and hypertrophic)
- Striae
- Actinic keratoses
- Hypopigmentation
- Poikiloderma of Civatte
- Telangiectasias and erythema

## Alternative Therapies

**Ablative lasers** (e.g., carbon dioxide and erbium lasers) are the gold standard for skin resurfacing. These more aggressive, deeper skin resurfacing procedures offer greater potential for static wrinkle reduction, but require longer recovery times and have greater risks of complications. Although fractional lasers have reduced recovery time and risk of complications, ablative laser treatments, whether fractional or nonfractional, create an open wound and have risks of scarring and infection.

**Nonlaser treatment options** for wrinkle reduction include superficial skin resurfacing with light **chemical peels** or **microdermabrasion,** and **topical skin care products** such as retinoids and exfoliants (e.g., hydroxy acids). More aggressive skin resurfacing has historically been performed with deeper chemical peels (e.g., phenol) and **dermabrasion,** which utilizes a motorized rotating wire bristle brush to abrade the skin, but these higher-risk procedures are uncommon today. Other available treatments for facial lines and wrinkles include **botulinum toxin** for dynamic wrinkles and **dermal fillers** for static lines, and these treatments are often performed in conjunction with laser procedures. For severe wrinkling with saggy lax skin, **surgery** is an option.

**Light-emitting diodes (LEDs)** emit a narrow range, or band, of low-intensity wavelengths without inducing epidermal or dermal damage. While these light-based devices have similarities to lasers and other light-based technologies, their results are extremely modest and are briefly discussed here. Red light LED devices (570–670 nm) have been used for mild wrinkle reduction and blue light LED devices (400–500 nm) for acne. They do not operate based on the theory of selective photothermolysis, but rather are based on the principle of photomodulation, where cellular activity is modulated through illumination by particular wavelengths of light. The main advantage of LEDs is their ease of use.

**Radiofrequency** technologies are used to reduce skin laxity and skin folds and to treat wrinkles. Reduction of skin laxity and folds to improve skin contour is commonly known as "skin tightening"; however, the term used by the U.S. Food and Drug Administration (FDA) is soft tissue coagulation. Radiofrequency devices (such as Thermage®, Solta) employ rapidly alternating current that creates heat when applied to the skin due to the skin's resistance to current flow. Tissue heating with radiofrequency devices is controlled by several factors, including the type of electrodes used (e.g., monopolar or bipolar), fluence, and cooling times. These technologies have been shown to improve laxity in areas such as the periocular region, nasolabial folds, jowls, neck, and abdomen. Newer radiofrequency devices are being used for fractional resurfacing (e.g., Matrix RF™, Syneron and Infini™, Lutronic). Fractional RF devices concentrate heat in the mid to deep dermis with limited epidermal disruption and these devices are therefore, referred to as subablative. Enhanced results have been seen for facial wrinkles and laxity. These devices also show promise for treatment of darker skin types due to the limited epidermal involvement, and may have lower risks of scarring. Some devices combine IPL with bipolar radiofrequency (e.g., Elos™, Syneron). Bipolar radiofrequency preferentially targets warmer tissue. This combination technology uses this property by utilizing the IPL to heat target colored chromophores and then the radiofrequency targets the heated tissue to stimulate collagen remodeling and reduce wrinkles. In addition to treatment of wrinkles and skin laxity, radiofrequency devices are also used for cellulite reduction.

**Broadband infrared devices** (e.g., Titan™, Cutera) emit wavelengths ranging from 1100–1800 nm with long pulse widths (of several seconds) and are also used for skin tightening and wrinkles.

**Photodynamic therapy (PDT)** has been used for skin rejuvenation to improve wrinkles, dyschromia, and vascular ectasias as well as actinic keratoses. PDT requires application of a photosensitive medication such as aminolevulinic acid (Levulan®). The medication is concentrated in particular tissues, such as sebaceous glands and actinically damaged cells and is activated by a light source (e.g., LED or IPL). Once activated, a cytotoxic reaction occurs targeting and destroying the areas with the highest medication concentration. PDT is currently approved by the FDA for treatment of nonhyperkeratotic actinic keratoses, and is used off label to enhance the results with nonablative lasers for photorejuvenation and wrinkle reduction.

## Devices Currently Available for Nonablative Resurfacing

| Target Chromophore | Laser |
|---|---|
| Water | Nonfractional: 1064 nm, 1320 nm, 1450 nm |
| | Fractional: 1410 nm, 1440 nm, 1540 nm, 1550 nm, 1565 nm, 1927 nm |
| Oxyhemoglobin or melanin | Nonfractional: 532 nm, 585 nm, 595 nm, 755 nm, 1064 nm, intense pulsed light (500–1200 nm) |

Nonablative resurfacing lasers can be broadly classified into two categories based on their target chromophore: (1) lasers targeting the water chromophore and (2) lasers targeting melanin and oxyhemoglobin chromophores.

## Lasers Targeting Water

- **Nonfractional** lasers that target water (1064 nm, 1320 nm, 1450 nm) were the first generation of nonablative lasers to be used for skin resurfacing and are still in common use today. The depth of penetration of these lasers is based on their affinity for water where shorter wavelengths such as 1320 nm have lower water absorption and deeper cutaneous penetration, while longer wavelengths such as 1450 nm have higher water absorption and more superficial penetration. These lasers can be used in all skin types.
- **Fractional** lasers that target water (1410 nm, 1440 nm, 1540 nm, 1550 nm, 1565 nm, 1927 nm) are the most recent addition to the class of nonablative lasers used for skin resurfacing and 1550 nm was the first fractional nonablative wavelength used for treatment of photoaged skin(see Introduction and Foundation Concepts, Fractional Lasers section). The depth of penetration of these lasers is also based on their affinity for water where shorter wavelengths such as 1550 nm have lower water absorption and deeper cutaneous penetration, which is associated with more significant dermal effects such as collagen remodeling and reduction of dermal dyschromia such as melasma. Longer wavelengths such as 1927 nm have higher water absorption with more superficial penetration and are used for treatment of epidermal pigmented lesions such as lentigines and ephelides. These lasers can be used in all skin types but caution is advised with darker skin types due to the risk of PIH. Fractional nonablative lasers are also used to treat dyschromia (see Chapter 2).

   Fractional lasers vary in how the fractionated beam is applied to the skin. One of the most commonly used types of fractional lasers uses a disposable roller on the tip that is continuously moved across the skin during treatment (e.g., Fraxel Re:Store™, Solta). Other devices utilize a stamping technique, where a lens inside the handpiece fractionates the beam each time the laser pulses and all pixels are created at once (e.g., Icon Max1540™, Cynosure/Palomar). Some devices utilize scanners to fractionate the beam where pixels are sequential, either in a fixed pattern or randomly distributed on skin that is treated during the pulse.

## Lasers Targeting Melanin and Oxyhemoglobin

- **Lasers that target melanin and oxyhemoglobin** (532 nm, 585 nm, 595 nm, 755 nm, 1064 nm, intense pulsed light) are all nonfractional. They are primarily used for treatment of vascular ectasias and/or pigmented lesions as they are highly absorbed by colored tissue chromophores. The 532 nm and pulsed dye 585 nm and 595 nm lasers have traditionally been used for treatment of vascular lesions. Recent technologic advancements in these devices (i.e., larger spot sizes and longer pulse widths) have enhanced cutaneous penetration and improved their safety profiles, expanding their application to include wrinkle reduction while reducing the risk of purpura. The 1064 nm (Nd:YAG) laser is the one of the most commonly used nonfractional lasers for skin resurfacing. While it targets multiple chromophores (water, melanin, and oxyhemoglobin), the long wavelength allows for deep penetration to the dermis, and it essentially bypasses epidermal melanin making it safe for all skin types. It is used in a long-pulsed mode (e.g., Laser Genesis™, Cutera) and very short-pulsed modes as Q-switched lasers (e.g., RevLite®, Cynosure/ConBio). Studies of 1064 nm lasers with both modes demonstrate histologic and clinical reduction of wrinkles, as well as other collagen remodeling effects, such as reduction of pore size, rough skin texture, and superficial acne scarring. In addition to dermal remodeling, Q-switched 1064 nm lasers are also commonly used for tattoo removal, reduction of dermal pigmentation such as melasma, and reduction of fine dark hair, due to melanin chromophore specificity. The diverse applications of 1064 nm and other colored chromophore–dependent lasers offer a means to address many aspects of photoaging simultaneously.

**Epidermal Cooling** is used with most nonfractional lasers to protect the epidermis from thermal injury. Some devices utilize cryogen spray coolants (e.g., 1320 nm) or contact cooling through the tip of the device (e.g., intense pulse light). Due to minimal epidermal energy absorption by 1064 nm and the relatively low fluences used for skin resurfacing (compared to leg veins for example), these devices do not typically utilize cooling for nonablative resurfacing treatments.

# Contraindications

## General Laser Contraindications

- Active infection in the treatment area (e.g., herpes simplex, pustular acne, cellulitis)
- Dermatoses in the treatment area (e.g., vitiligo, psoriasis, atopic dermatitis)
- Melanoma, or lesions suspected for melanoma in the treatment area
- Deep chemical peel, dermabrasion or radiation therapy in the treatment area within the preceding 6 months
- Keloidal scarring[‡]
- Bleeding abnormality (e.g., thrombocytopenia, anticoagulant use)
- Impaired healing (e.g., immunosuppressive medications, poorly controlled diabetes mellitus)
- Peripheral vascular disease
- Seizure disorder
- Uncontrolled systemic condition
- Cardiac pacemaker
- Skin atrophy (e.g., chronic oral steroid use, genetic syndromes such as Ehlers–Danlos syndrome)
- Livedo reticularis, a vascular disease associated with mottled skin discoloration of the arms or legs exacerbated by heat exposure
- Erythema ab igne, a rare acquired reticular erythematous and pigmented rash exacerbated by heat exposure
- Direct sun exposure within the preceding 2 weeks resulting in reddened or tanned skin
- Self-tanning product within the preceding 2 weeks
- Topical prescription retinoid within the preceding week
- Isotretinoin (Accutane™) within the preceding 6 months
- Gold therapy (e.g., used for treatment of arthritis)
- Photosensitizing medications (e.g., tetracyclines, St. John's wort, thiazides)
- Photosensitive disorder (e.g., systemic lupus erythematosus and polymorphous light eruption)
- Pregnant or nursing
- Unrealistic patient expectations
- Body dysmorphic disorder
- Treatment inside the eye orbit (i.e., without intraocular eye shields)

---

[‡]*Caution should be used in patients with hypertrophic scarring*

## Advantages of Nonablative Lasers for Wrinkles

- Minimal recovery time and minimal risk of complications relative to more aggressive resurfacing procedures, such as ablative carbon dioxide and erbium lasers.
- Treatments are readily incorporated into patients' daily lives and easily combined with other minimally invasive aesthetic procedures.
- Many technologies used for nonablative resurfacing are appropriate for darker skin types (IV and V) and some are even safe with skin type VI. More aggressive resurfacing procedures (e.g., ablative laser skin resurfacing and medium-depth chemical peels) are typically restricted to Fitzpatrick skin types I–III.

## Disadvantages of Nonablative Lasers for Skin Resurfacing

- Wrinkle reduction is slow and may require months before becoming clinically evident
- Results are subtle and can be challenging to demonstrate photographically
- Clinical results vary and some patients may not show demonstrable improvements

## Equipment

- Laser device appropriate for skin resurfacing treatments
- Eyewear for the patient and provider specific to the device being used
- Nonalcohol cleansing facial wipes
- Clear colorless gel for treatments if necessary per the manufacturer
- Nonsterile gloves
- Gauze $4 \times 4$ in
- Ice packs (or cool air blower device)
- Soothing nonocclusive topical product (e.g., Epidermal Repair™ by SkinCeuticals)
- Topical anesthetic such as EMLA or benzocaine:lidocaine:tetracaine (BLT) for fractional nonablative treatments
- Broad-spectrum sunscreen of SPF 30 containing zinc oxide or titanium dioxide
- Hydrocortisone cream 1% and 2.5%
- Alcohol wipes for cleaning laser tip
- Germicidal disposable wipes for sanitizing the laser

## Preprocedure Checklist

- **Aesthetic consultation** is performed to review the patient's medical history including contraindications to treatment, history of PIH, abnormal scarring, and photosensitizing medications (see Introduction and Foundation Concepts, Aesthetic Consultation section).
- **Fitzpatrick skin type** is determined (see Introduction and Foundation Concepts, Aesthetic Consultation section).
- **Examination of the treatment area** is performed. Wrinkle severity (see Introduction and Foundation Concepts, Glogau Classification of Photoaging section) and other indications for treatment are documented. Lesions suspicious for neoplasia are biopsied or referred if indicated and negative biopsy results received before proceeding with laser treatments.
- **Informed consent** is obtained (see Introduction and Foundation Concepts, Aesthetic Consultation section). An example of a consent form is provided in Appendix 4e.
- **Pretreatment photographs** are taken (see Introduction and Foundation Concepts, Aesthetic Consultation section).

- **Avoidance of direct sun exposure** and daily use of a broad-spectrum sunscreen with SPF 30 containing zinc oxide or titanium dioxide prior to and throughout the course of treatment is advised.
- **Lightening background skin** may be considered in dark Fitzpatrick skin types (IV–VI) to reduce risks of pigmentary changes such as PIH. Topical skin-lightening products may be used once or twice daily for 1 month prior to treatment such as prescription-strength hydroquinone cream 4–8% or over-the-counter cosmeceutical products containing kojic acid, arbutin, niacinamide, and azelaic acid (which are less effective).
- **Test spots** may be considered for patients with dark Fitzpatrick skin types (IV–VI) prior to the initial treatment, particularly with fractional treatments. Test spot parameters are selected based on the patient's skin type and lesion characteristics following the manufacturer's guidelines for wavelength, spot size, fluence, and pulse width. Test spots are placed discretely near the intended treatment area (e.g., under the chin, behind or inferior to the ear) and pulses overlapped to simulate the technique used with treatment. Test spots are viewed 3–5 days after placement for evidence of erythema, blister, crust, or other adverse effect. Patients should be informed that lack of an adverse reaction with test spots does not ensure that a side effect or complication will not occur with a treatment.
- **Antiviral medication** may be given prophylactically for a history of herpes simplex or zoster in or near the treatment area 2 days prior to the procedure and continued for 3 days postprocedure (e.g., valacyclovir 500 mg or acyclovir 400 mg 1 tablet twice daily). Patients with a remote history of HSV infection have lower risk of reactivation and an antiviral may instead be started on the day of treatment and continued for 5 days.
- **Dark hair in the treatment area** may be reduced with the 1064 nm laser. This is an advantage for women with fine dark facial hair. However, facial hair reduction may not be desirable in men and this possibility should be discussed prior to treatment.

See Before and After Instructions for Laser Treatment, Appendix 3e.

## Anesthesia

Anesthesia requirements vary according to the specific device being used and patients' pain tolerance.

**Nonfractional** laser treatments do not typically require anesthesia. Most nonfractional lasers have built-in cooling mechanisms, such as a cooled sapphire tip or a cryogen spray that maintain a constant epidermal temperature throughout treatment. This increases safety and provides some anesthesia.

**Fractional** lasers are more uncomfortable and patients typically require topical anesthetic pretreatment such as EMLA (prilocaine 2.5%:lidocaine 2.5%), ELA-Max (lidocaine 4%) or BLT (benzocaine 20%.lidocaine 6%:tetracaine 4%) and a cool air blower during treatment to improve treatment tolerability (see Supply Sources, Appendix 6). In some cases oral analgesics and anxiolytics may also be required (see Introduction and Foundation Concepts, Anesthesia for Laser Procedures section).

## Nonablative Laser Resurfacing Procedure for Wrinkle Reduction

The following procedural recommendations including selecting initial laser parameters for treatment, general treatment technique, desirable clinical endpoints, undesirable clinical endpoints, aftercare, treatment intervals, subsequent treatments, and common follow-ups are based on treatment of mild to moderate facial wrinkles using a Q-switched 1064 nm laser (RevLite®, Cynosure/ConBio) that is indicated for all Fitzpatrick skin types (I–VI). Manufacturer guidelines for the specific device used should be followed at the time of treatment.

## Selecting Initial Laser Parameters for Treatment

- **Fitzpatrick skin type.** Darker skin types (V and VI) are treated more conservatively with larger spot sizes (e.g., 8 mm) and lower fluencies (e.g., 1.5–2.0 $J/cm^2$) than lighter skin types which can initially be treated with smaller spot sizes (e.g., 6 mm) and higher fluencies (e.g., 2.0–3.0 $J/cm^2$).
- **Chromophores in the treatment area.** The treatment area is assessed for the presence of all chromophores that are targets for the wavelength being used. The 1064 nm wavelength is absorbed by water, melanin, and hemoglobin (e.g., in blue vessels). In addition to collagen remodeling effects such as reduction of wrinkles, acne scars, rough texture, and coarse pores, it is also used for dermal hyperpigmentation (such as melasma) and reduction of fine dark hair. If these pigmented targets are present in the area being treated for wrinkle reduction, more conservative settings with larger spot sizes and lower fluences are used due to the greater amount of target in the skin.
- **Size of treatment area.** Large areas such as the face are treated with fast repetition rates, which shorten treatment times.
- **Nonfacial areas.** Areas such as the neck and chest are treated using more conservative parameters than the face due to slower healing times and greater risk of complications in nonfacial areas.

## General Treatment Technique

- Laser treatments on the face are performed outside of the orbit, the area above the supraorbital ridge (roughly where the eyebrows sit) and below the inferior orbital rim. Figure 14 in Introduction and Foundation Concepts shows the nontreatment areas of the face.
- The face is typically broken down into sections to help ensure complete coverage of the entire face. One possible sequence for treating the face starting with section 1 and progressing to section 6 is shown in Figure 14, Introduction and Foundation Concepts.
- The handpiece for Q-switched 1064 nm lasers is held perpendicular to the skin, approximately 1 in above the skin, which is determined by the handpiece depth guide (Fig. 3). There is approximately 20% overlap of each pulse.
- It is advisable to start at the periphery of the face and progress medially, as the central face is more sensitive. The handpiece is moved in a painting motion across the face using long switch-back strokes (Fig. 12B, Introduction and Foundation Concepts). **TIP: The most sensitive facial area is the central upper lip (philtrum)**

## Desirable Clinical Endpoints

When optimal parameters are used for nonablative resurfacing treatments, one or more of the following clinical endpoints may be observed:

- **Mild to moderate erythema** (Fig. 4)
- **Pigmented lesion darkening** (especially dermal lesions, such as melasma) with enhanced demarcation against the background skin (Fig. 5)
- **Papular acne lesion erythema**

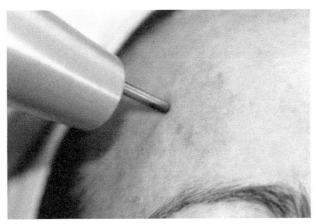

**FIGURE 3** ● Technique for nonablative skin resurfacing treatments using a Q-switched 1064 nm laser. (Courtesy of R. Small, MD.)

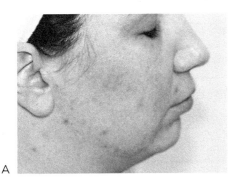
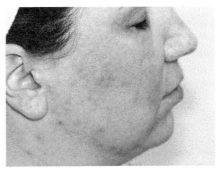

A
B

**FIGURE 4** ● Clinical endpoint of mild erythema before **(A)** and immediately after **(B)** nonablative skin resurfacing treatment using a Q-switched 1064 nm laser. (Courtesy of R. Small, MD.)

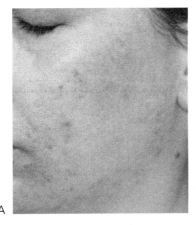
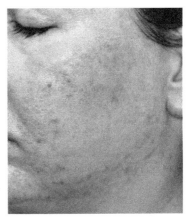

A
B

**FIGURE 5** ● Clinical endpoint of hyperpigmentation darkening before **(A)** and immediately after **(B)** nonablative wrinkle reduction treatment using a Q-switched 1064 nm laser. (Courtesy of R. Small, MD.)

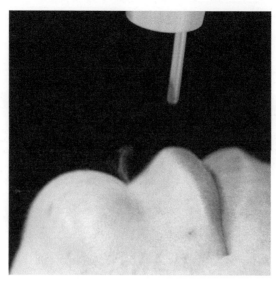

*FIGURE 6* ● Clinical endpoint of sebum vaporization on the chin during nonablative skin resurfacing treatment using a Q-switched 1064 nm laser. (Courtesy of R. Small, MD.)

- **Vaporization of sebum** in sebaceous facial areas such as the nose and chin, and areas with coarse pores and comedonal acne (Fig. 6)
- **Audible snapping** sound with laser pulses, loudest over sebaceous areas
- **Petechiae** (Fig. 13) may be seen with aggressive treatment parameters

## Undesirable Clinical Endpoints

When overly aggressive laser parameters are used for treatment, one or more of the following undesirable clinical endpoints may be observed on the skin:

- **Graying**
- **Severe whitening**
- **Blistering**

## Performing Nonablative Laser Skin Resurfacing Procedure for Wrinkle Reduction

The following guidelines are for nonablative skin resurfacing on the full face to treat mild/moderate facial wrinkles using a Q-switched 1064 nm laser. These treatment steps are specific to Cynosure/ConBio RevLite® system. Providers are advised to follow manufacturer guidelines for the specific device used at the time of treatment.

1. Inquire about sun exposure and sunscreen use. If the patient is recently sun exposed or has tanned skin, it is advisable to wait 1 month before treating to reduce the risk of pigmentary complications.
2. Remove jewelry that may reflect laser light.
3. Have the patient remove contact lenses.
4. Position the patient supine with the treatment table flat. The physician is seated comfortably at the head of the patient.
5. Cleanse the skin with a nonalcohol wipe.

6. Cover tattoos and permanent makeup (e.g., with wet gauze) and keep the laser tip approximately 1 inch away from the tattoo during treatment.
   **TIP: Treating over tattoos and permanent make-up can permanently alter their color.**

7. Provide the patient with extraocular lead goggles and provide wavelength-specific protective eyewear to everyone in the treatment room.

8. Always operate the laser in accordance with your office's laser safety policies and the manufacturer's guidelines.

9. Select the fluence and spot size based on the patient's Fitzpatrick skin type (see Selecting Initial Laser Parameters for Treatment section).

10. Hold the handpiece at a 90-degree angle to the skin surface with the distance guide lightly touching the skin.

11. Select the repetition rate based on the size (see Selecting Initial Laser Parameters for Treatment section).

12. Perform a few pulses at the lateral margin of the treatment area (e.g., anterior to the ear) and assess for patient tolerance and clinical endpoints which will be subtle or not visible. Pain should be less than or equal to 4 on a scale of 1–10.

13. Perform one "pass" to the entire face, by covering the entire treatment area confluently with pulses, using approximately 20–50% overlap.

14. Continually assess laser–tissue interaction and clinical endpoints throughout the treatment and adjust settings accordingly.
    - **Petechiae are indicative of aggressive parameters.** If petechiae occur during treatment, the fluence should be reduced or the spot size increased to reduce treatment intensity. The treatment may be continued but the petechial area should not receive additional passes.
    - **If undesirable endpoints occur** discontinue treatment in the area and cool the skin using wrapped ice packs for 15 minutes. Decrease fluence and/or increase spot size to achieve desirable endpoints in the remaining treatment areas.

15. After the treatment area has been confluently covered with pulses, assess the treated area for clinical endpoints. If there is mild to no erythema, perform a second pass to the treatment area. In areas with wrinkles, hyperpigmentation, papular acne or coarse pores, perform up to three to four additional passes, or until the desired endpoints are reached.

16. Immediately after treatment, ice packs wrapped in a towel may be applied for 15 minutes to soothe the treatment area and reduce erythema and edema. If no discomfort is reported it is advisable to avoid the use of ice as the desired thermal reaction in the skin continues for a short while after treatment and it is terminated upon application of ice.

17. Hydrocortisone cream may be applied topically to erythematous areas: 1% for mild erythema or 2.5% for moderate erythema.

18. A broad-spectrum sunscreen SPF 30 containing zinc oxide or titanium dioxide is applied to treatment areas that are sun exposed.

## Aftercare

- **Mild swelling and mild erythema** are expected and usually resolve within 15 minutes to 1 hour after treatment. If patients report areas that feel hot, or have more significant erythema, instruct patients to apply a wrapped ice pack for 15 minutes every 1–2 hours and hydrocortisone cream 1% two times per day for 3–4 days or until erythema resolves. Patients are advised to contact their provider if erythema persists for more than 5 days as PIH can occur with prolonged erythema.

- **Postprocedure products** that are soothing and hydrating are used for 2 weeks post procedure including a broad-spectrum sunscreen of SPF 30 containing zinc oxide or titanium dioxide (see Introduction and Foundation Concepts, Postprocedure Skin Care for Laser Treatments section).
- **Direct sun exposure** is avoided for 4 weeks after treatment to help minimize the risk of undesired pigmentary changes.
- **Written aftercare instructions** are provided to patients (see Before and After Instructions for Laser Treatments, Appendix 3e).

## Common Follow-Ups

In general, skin recovers rapidly and follow-up issues are rare with nonablative skin resurfacing treatments.

## Treatment Intervals

Nonablative laser treatments for skin resurfacing typically require a series of 6–8 treatments at monthly intervals for demonstrable improvements. Patients may consider repeating a treatment series every 2 years to maintain results. Alternatively, as these treatments are well tolerated and results are cumulative, patients may choose to incorporate nonfractional laser treatments as part of regular skin maintenance and undergo treatments at monthly or quarterly intervals.

## Subsequent Treatments

- **The intensity of treatments** may be increased at subsequent visits, by increasing fluence, decreasing spot size, and increasing the number of passes. In general, only one parameter is changed to intensify treatments in any given visit. Typically, the fluence or number of passes is increased initially for a few treatments to achieve desired clinical endpoints, and spot size is decreased in later treatments.
- Treat the **entire area** at each visit.

## Results

Reduction of mild to moderate wrinkles with nonablative lasers is subtle, and results vary based on the technology used and with individual patients. Treatments are performed in a series and results are usually evident 2–3 months after the initial treatment with nonfractional lasers, and 1 month after treatment with fractional lasers; improvements can continue to be seen with both procedures up to 6 months after the final treatment. Studies of nonablative lasers consistently show histologic improvements with increased numbers of fibroblasts and collagen deposition. However, clinical improvements are less predictable and do not always correlate with histologic changes. Fractional devices show more reliable and more significant clinical changes than nonfractional nonablative lasers. Below are before and after photos using some of the nonablative resurfacing technologies discussed in the chapter.

- Figure 7 shows facial rhytids before (A) and after (B) a series of six nonablative skin resurfacing treatments using a long pulse 1064 nm Nd:YAG laser (Laser Genesis™, Cutera).
- Figure 8 shows infraocular rhytids before (A) and after (B) a series of nonablative skin resurfacing treatments using a Q-switched 1064 nm Nd:YAG laser (RevLite®, Cynosure/ ConBio).
- Figure 9 shows cheek rhytids before (A) and after (B) two nonablative skin resurfacing treatments using a 1565 nm laser (ResurFX™, Lumenis).

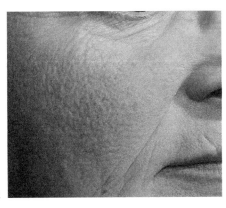
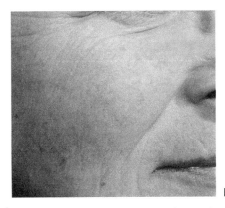

A

B

**FIGURE 7** ● Facial wrinkles before **(A)** and after **(B)** a series of six treatments using a long pulse 1064 nm laser. (Courtesy of K. Smith, MD and Cutera.)

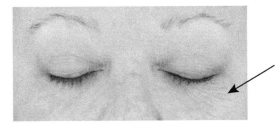

A

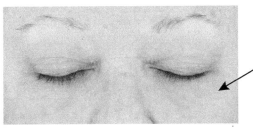

B

**FIGURE 8** ● Infraocular wrinkles before **(A)** and after **(B)** a series of treatments using a Q-switched 1064 nmYAG laser. (Courtesy of D. Goldberg, MD and Cynosure/ConBio.)

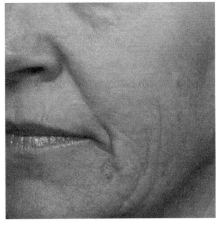
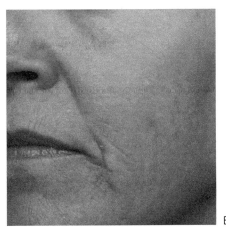

A

B

**FIGURE 9** ● Cheek wrinkles before **(A)** and after **(B)** nonablative fractional skin resurfacing treatments using a 1565 nm laser. (Courtesy of M. Palm, MD and Lumenis.)

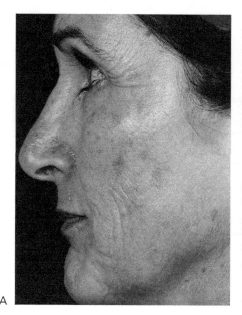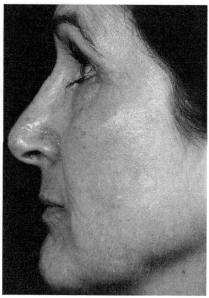

A                                                                                 B

*FIGURE 10* ● Cheek wrinkles, crow's feet, and hyperpigmentation before **(A)** and after **(B)** nonablative fractional skin resurfacing treatments using a 1550 nm laser. (Courtesy of Z. Rahman, MD and Solta.)

- Figure 10 shows cheek rhytids, crow's feet, and mottled pigmentation before (A) and after (B) a series of nonablative skin resurfacing treatments using a 1550 nm laser (Fraxel Re:store™, Solta).
- Figure 11 shows acne scars before (A) and after (B) a series of nonablative skin resurfacing treatments using a 1550 nm laser (Fraxel Re:store™, Solta).

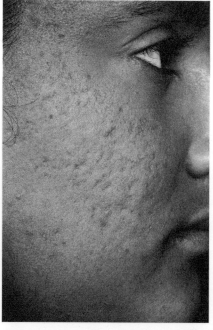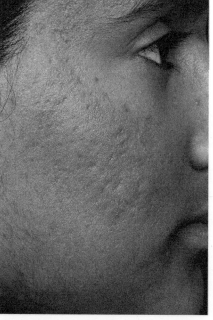

A                                                                                 B

*FIGURE 11* ● Acne scars before **(A)** and after **(B)** nonablative fractional skin resurfacing treatments using a 1550 nm laser. (Courtesy of Z. Rahman, MD and Solta.)

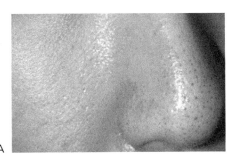 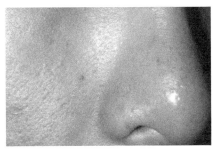

A                                                                                          B

**FIGURE 12** ● Enlarged pores before **(A)** and after **(B)** three treatments using a Q-switched
1064 nm laser. (Courtesy of G.S. Lee, MD and Lutronic.)

- Figure 12 shows enlarged pores before (A) and after (B) three nonablative skin resurfacing treatments using a Q-switched 1064 nm Nd:YAG laser (Spectra™, Lutronic).

## Complications

- Pain
- Prolonged erythema
- Prolonged edema
- Petechiae and purpura
- Urticaria
- Contact dermatitis
- Infection
- Milia
- Hyperpigmentation
- Hypopigmentation
- Burn
- Scarring
- Tattoo alteration
- Inadequate collagen remodeling effects including lack of reduction of wrinkles, folds, scars, or recurrence after completion of treatments
- Deeper than intended resurfacing
- Hair reduction in or adjacent to the treatment area
- Toxicity from topical anesthetic
- Dermal filler alteration
- Ocular injury

Nonablative laser treatments for skin resurfacing have minimal risks of side effects and complications. Though infrequent, complications occur more often with fractional nonablative devices and the most commonly encountered are herpes simplex reactivation, acne eruptions, and PIH. Knowledge of potential complications and their management is important to help ensure the best possible outcomes.

**Temporary erythema, edema, pruritus, and mild sunburn-like discomfort** after treatment are common and not considered complications. These typically last a few hours with nonfractional lasers. Erythema and edema are more prominent with fractional nonablative lasers typically lasting up to 4 days; this is often followed by darkening (referred to as bronzing) of the skin, xerosis, and desquamation for 1–2 days, which represents exfoliation of the microscopic epidermal and dermal necrotic debris. See Common Follow-ups section above for management.

**Pain** is usually only reported at the time of treatment. Pain with nonfractional lasers is minimal, typically 2–3 (on a standard pain scale of 1–10). Pain is more significant with fractional lasers, typically 5–6, and often requires cooling measures immediately after treatment such as application of ice or a cool air blower. Complaint of pain several days postprocedure is unusual and evaluation is advisable, particularly to assess for epidermal thermal injury due to overtreatment and infection.

**Prolonged erythema and edema** lasting up to 1 week most often occurs with aggressive fractional treatments. Treatments in the upper cheek at the level of the lower eyelid can result in periocular and eyelid edema. Patients with erythematous skin conditions such as telangiectasias, rosacea, and Poikiloderma of Civatte may exhibit prolonged postoperative erythema. Erythema and edema can be treated with application of wrapped ice packs applied for 15 minutes a few times per day, sleeping with the head elevated, an oral antihistamine such as cetirizine (Zyrtec®) 10 mg or diphenhydramine (Benadryl®) 12.5–25 mg daily, and a topical cortico-steroid twice daily such as a low-potency steroid (e.g., hydrocortisone 2.5%) or a medium-potency steroid (e.g., triamcinolone acetonide 0.1%) depending on the severity. Prolonged erythema and edema lasting more than 1 week is not typical and may be an indication of contact dermatitis, thermal injury due to overtreat-ment, or infection.

**Petechiae** may be seen with high fluences particularly in thin-skinned areas such as the neck (Fig. 13) and periocular areas. **Purpura** may occur with shorter wavelength lasers such as 532 nm and pulsed dye lasers, particularly when short pulse widths and/ or high fluences are used. Petechiae typically take 3–5 days to resolve and purpura can take up to 2 weeks. Utilizing larger spot sizes, lower fluences, and skin compression can reduce the incidence of purpura with lasers that are prone to purpura formation. Purpura resolves spontaneously within 3 weeks. Purpura can be distressing for patients and pointing it out to the patient if it occurs and giving an expectation for resolution are reassuring. Topical products such as arnica and vitamin K may be of limited use in preventing and treating purpura.

**Urticaria** in the treatment area may be seen immediately after treatment with nonablative lasers (Fig. 14). Once identified, patients who form urticaria in response to laser treatments may be pretreated with an oral antihistamine such as cetirizine 1 hour prior to procedure to attenuate the histamine response and a topical steroid cream postprocedure (see above for dosing).

**Contact dermatitis** is uncommon with nonablative lasers treatments but is a consideration in the setting of worsening erythema or pruritus posttreatment. Treated skin is vulnerable to irritation from various substances found in topical products such as preservatives and fragrances. Over-the-counter herbal and vitamin remedies such as vitamin E and aloe products are common causes of contact dermatitis. If contact dermatitis is suspected, postprocedure topical products are discontinued. A topical corticosteroid ointment or cream is used twice daily such as a low-potency steroid (e.g., hydrocortisone 2.5%) or a medium-potency steroid (e.g., triamcinolone acetonide 0.1%) depending on the severity for 5 days or until resolved.

**Infections** can be viral, bacterial, or fungal and although they are rare, occur more often with fractional than nonfractional laser treatments. Reactivation of **herpes**

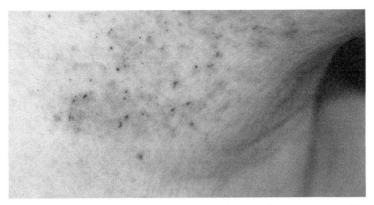

**FIGURE 13** Petechiae on the neck after nonablative skin resurfacing treatment. (Courtesy of R. Small, MD.)

**simplex virus** or herpes zoster in the treatment is one of the most frequent infectious complications and pretreatment prophylactic oral antiviral medication in patients with a known history reduces this risk (see Preprocedure Checklist section). **Acne vulgaris** is relatively common after fractional laser treatments. It typically develops within the first few weeks and resolves spontaneously. If acne persists, an oral antibiotic such as doxycycline or minocycline (e.g., 100 mg 1 tab twice daily for 2 weeks) may be used. **Impetigo** has also been reported following fractional nonablative treatments on the face and extremities. The main pathogens are *Staphylococcus aureus* (methicillin-resistant *Staphylococcus aureus* is uncommon) and group A *Streptococcus,* and impetigo occurs most often in patients who are known carriers. Consider empiric use of doxycycline 100 mg 1 tablet orally twice daily and clindamycin 300 mg 1 tablet four times per day for suspected bacterial infections, to be modified as necessary based on culture results.

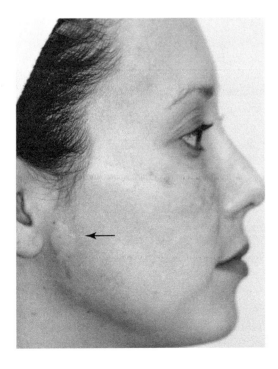

**FIGURE 14** Preauricular urticaria after nonablative skin resurfacing treatment. (Courtesy of R. Small, MD.)

Local patterns of antibiotic resistance should be taken into account when selecting antibiotics empirically.

**Milia** result from occlusion of sebaceous glands and occur more commonly with fractional nonablative lasers. Ointments used to hydrate skin can occlude sebaceous glands and contribute to milia formation. Milia do not usually resolve spontaneously and require lancing with a 20-gauge needle and extraction (i.e., gentle squeezing with cotton-tipped applicators) for removal.

**Hyperpigmentation** and **hypopigmentation** are pigmentary complications resulting from alteration to background skin color. Patients with dark Fitzpatrick skin types (IV–VI), actinic bronzing, and tanned skin have the highest risk of pigmentary changes. They occur most often with the use of fractional lasers, and with aggressive treatment parameters including short wavelengths (e.g., 532 nm), short pulse widths, and high fluences. The risk of hyperpigmentation with fractional lasers can be reduced by using lower MTZ density settings, fewer passes, and long treatment intervals; all of which may increase the number of treatments necessary to achieve desired results. In addition, overly aggressive cooling can also result in pigmentary changes. Hyperpigmentation and hypopigmentation have been reported with nonfractional lasers as a result of epidermal injury from overcooling using cryogen sprays. **Hyperpigmentation** usually resolves spontaneously over several months, although in rare instances may be permanent. Sun protection including the application of a broad-spectrum sunscreen with SPF 30 containing zinc oxide or titanium dioxide and sun avoidance are preventative measures for PIH. Topical lightening agents such as hydroquinone cream 4–8% twice daily in the PIH area, and superficial exfoliation procedures such as microdermabrasion and light chemical peels, and sun protection may be used to treat hyperpigmentation. **Hypopigmentation** is a more significant complication. Hypopigmentation is usually temporary and may resolve spontaneously with exposure to ambient light sunlight, but in some cases it is permanent. There are few treatment options for hypopigmentation but it may respond to the excimer (308 nm) laser or narrow band UVB treatment. Alternatively, skin surrounding hypopigmented areas can be lightened to reduce the demarcation between background skin and hypopigmented areas.

**Burns** are rare with nonablative resurfacing lasers but can result from aggressive treatment parameters (short pulse widths, high fluences, and inadequate epidermal cooling), particularly with devices that utilize short wavelengths (e.g., 532 nm and pulsed dye lasers). Prompt application of a wrapped ice pack to areas suspected of overtreatment at the time of treatment that are intensely erythematous and painful may reduce the area of injury. Blisters are managed with application of an occlusive ointment, like Aquaphor™ or bacitracin, and covered with a gauze dressing and tape. Patients are monitored over the next few weeks for formation of bullae, intense erythema, induration, and scarring. **Tattoos and permanent makeup** have concentrated ink pigments and treatment over these may result in lightening or a full-thickness skin burn, depending on the device used.

**Deeper than intended resurfacing** evident as skin erosions, has been reported with fractional laser treatments. Although it is a rare complication, it can occur with pulse stacking, a high number of passes, and in thin-skinned areas such as the neck and under the eyes.

**Reduced hair growth** in or adjacent to the treatment area may occur. It is advisable to emphasize this risk if dark hair is present, especially when treating over men's facial hair when using nonfractional lasers that target melanin (e.g., 532 and 585 nm).

Toxicity from topical anesthetic applied prior to fractional lasers has been reported. Complete removal of topical anesthetic prior to fractional treatments and restricting application to small areas (less than 400 cm$^2$) can reduce this risk.

Alteration to dermal fillers with nonablative lasers is controversial. While there is some evidence to suggest that nonablative lasers do not affect dermal fillers in tissue, other studies indicate that nonablative lasers can render undesired collections of dermal filler more moldable and reduce their appearance in the skin (e.g., Q-switched 1064 nm). Dermal fillers can be altered with ablative lasers, particularly in thin-skinned areas such as the tear trough.

Scarring is extremely rare with nonablative lasers, but may occur with overaggressive treatments, particularly in areas predisposed to scarring such as the sternum, or with treatments complicated by infection. See Chapter 6 for additional information and management of scars.

Ocular injury can be avoided by wearing appropriate laser safe eyewear at all times during treatment, directing the laser tip away from the eye, and treating outside of the eye orbit.

## Special Populations and Additional Considerations

- **Pregnant and nursing.** Women that are pregnant or nursing typically do not undergo elective procedures such as laser treatments. One of the potential complications from prolonged pain during a treatment might be inhibition of lactation in women who are nursing.
- **Dark Fitzpatrick skin types.** Nonfractional nonablative lasers (1064 nm, 1320 nm, 1450 nm) are safe on all skin types. Use of conservative settings with long pulse widths, low fluences, and low densities reduces the risk of complications when treating with fractional nonablative lasers (1410 nm, 1440 nm, 1540 nm, 1550 nm, 1565 nm, 1927 nm) and chromophore-dependent lasers (532 nm, 585 nm, 595 nm, intense pulsed light). Note that 1064 nm is safe on all skin types and is commonly used in skin type VI as it has deep penetration due to its long wavelength compared to the other chromophore-dependent lasers and is not highly absorbed by epidermal melanin.
- **Pediatric patients.** Pediatric patients are not generally candidates for cosmetic nonablative laser treatments.
- **Melasma.** Laser treatments of melasma are variable and the specific technology used must be taken into consideration when determining whether or not to perform nonablative resurfacing treatments in patients with melasma. For example, 1064 nm lasers improve melasma while repetitive treatments with intense pulsed light may worsen hyperpigmentation.
- **Nonfacial areas.** Nonablative resurfacing treatments are commonly performed on nonfacial areas, such as the neck and chest. While safety profiles are much improved compared to ablative lasers, these areas have delayed healing relative to the face due to fewer pilosebaceous units and have a greater risk of overtreatment and scarring. Use of conservative treatment parameters is recommended in nonfacial areas.

## Learning Techniques for Nonablative Laser Treatments for Skin Resurfacing

Consider performing treatments on the face using conservative parameters of large spot sizes, long pulse widths, and low fluences in patients with light Fitzpatrick skin types (I–III), and performing one pass only.

## Current Developments

**Combination therapy** utilizing nonablative lasers with other minimally invasive aesthetic procedures in the same visit is emerging as a popular approach to skin rejuvenation. For example, Q-switched 1064 nm laser for dermal collagen remodeling may be combined with superficial exfoliating procedures such as microdermabrasion and superficial chemical peels on the same day to enhance wrinkle reduction and reduction of melasma without increasing downtime or side effects. Combination therapy utilizing several nonablative lasers in 1 treatment is also being investigated in order to treat multiple aspects of photoaging such as textural changes and dyspigmentation (e.g., 1550 and 1927 nm lasers).

**Enhanced delivery of topical products** with fractional lasers is a under development. Treating the skin initially with a fractional laser (1550 nm) has been shown to enhance delivery of levulinic acid as part of photodynamic therapy (see Alternative Therapies section above) which shortens the incubation time and shows greater improvements in photodamaged skin. Enhancement of platelet-rich plasma (PRP) has also been shown following treatment with fractional laser (1550 nm) with improved skin elasticity along with reduced laser-induced erythema.

**Focused ultrasound** is a newer technology being used for wrinkle reduction. Ultrasound consists of high-frequency acoustic waves. Ultrasound can be focused and concentrated at select depths below the skin creating confined zones of thermal injury without damaging overlying epidermis. In this way, the dermis can be heated resulting in wrinkle reduction, and some devices heat adipose tissue for removal of focal fat. Like RF, ultrasound can be used in all skin types.

## Financial Considerations

Nonablative lasers treatments for skin resurfacing are not reimbursable by insurance companies. The charges for treatments vary and are largely determined by geographic region. Individual treatment prices range from $200–$500 per treatment for a large area such as the face or chest and $150–$250 for a small area such as the neck or hands. Several treatments are typically required to achieve maximal benefits and a series of 4 or 6 treatments may be offered to patients.

## Chapter 6

# Wrinkles—Ablative Resurfacing

Rebecca Small, M.D.

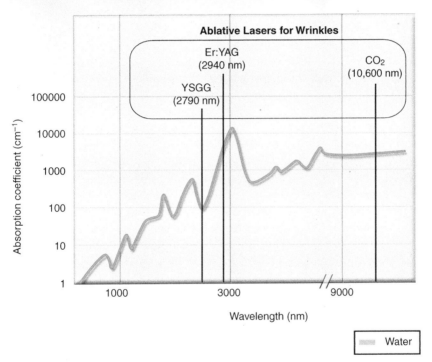

**FIGURE 1** ● Water absorption spectrum and ablative skin resurfacing lasers.

Ablative skin resurfacing is the most effective laser treatment available for wrinkle reduction. This aggressive procedure utilizes laser energy to heat and vaporize skin, creating a controlled wound in the epidermis and dermis. A healing process ensues after treatment that results in wrinkle reduction. Wrinkle reduction with ablative lasers, also referred to as ablative resurfacing or ablative laser resurfacing, is most commonly performed using carbon dioxide ($CO_2$) and erbium:yttrium aluminum garnet (Er:YAG) lasers. In the past, ablative resurfacing treatments removed all skin in a treatment area. These deep, confluent treatments were associated with prolonged recovery times as well as serious complications of infection, hypopigmentation, and scarring. More recently, ablative resurfacing treatments use a modified method of delivering laser energy whereby only a portion or "fraction" of the skin is treated, referred to as fractional resurfacing. Fractional ablative resurfacing has shorter recovery times and fewer risks compared to conventional deep laser resurfacing. It has become a primary modality used for rejuvenation of photodamaged skin particularly in patients willing to tolerate procedural discomfort and downtime.

## Anatomy

**Wrinkles** are one of the most prominent characteristics of photoaged skin. Histologically, wrinkled skin is atrophied with a thinned cellular epidermis and has reduced structural proteins in the dermal extracellular matrix (ECM) such as collagen and elastin that give skin its firmness and elastic recoil. Synthesis of ECM components slows naturally with age, and ultraviolet (UV) light stimulates degradative enzymes that weaken and accelerate protein breakdown. There is also diminished functioning of the sweat and oil glands, and fewer ECM glycosaminoglycans, which reduces skin hydration and suppleness. In certain cases of advanced photoaging, skin can have solar elastosis changes with tangled masses of damaged elastin protein in the dermis.

 **Ablative lasers used for skin resurfacing remove epidermal and dermal tissue.** A healing process ensues after treatment that stimulates synthesis of collagen and other ECM components. Immediate improvement in wrinkles is seen postprocedure due to thermally induced collagen denaturation and shrinkage, and delayed improvements subsequently occur due to fibroblast proliferation and synthesis of new collagen, referred to as dermal collagen remodeling. In addition to wrinkle reduction, collagen remodeling effects with ablative lasers also include improvement in atrophic scars, hypertrophic scars, pore size, rough skin texture, and skin laxity. Furthermore, benign epidermal pigmented lesions are also removed with ablative lasers. Pigment removal is nonspecific and results from vaporization of tissue containing epidermal pigment.

 Ablative lasers used for skin resurfacing employ either a nonfractional or fractional method of delivering laser energy to the skin. **Nonfractional ablative lasers** heat a region of skin confluently and vaporize tissue (Fig. 2A). They can penetrate superficially to the

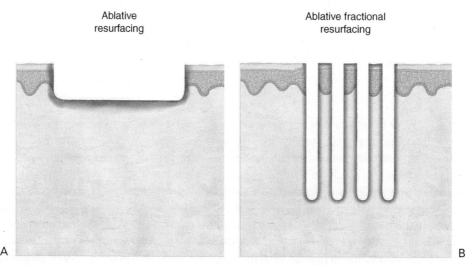

Ablative
resurfacing

Ablative fractional
resurfacing

A                               B

*FIGURE 2* ● Ablative laser patterns of injury: nonfractional **(A)** and fractional **(B)**.

epidermis, approximately 50 µm, or deeply to the papillary dermis, approximately 300 µm. Nonfractional ablative laser treatments are also referred to as "full field" or conventional resurfacing. Superficial treatments are used for reduction of fine lines and epidermal pigmented lesions, while deeper treatments have traditionally been used for severe wrinkles. Deep nonfractional ablative lasers transfer a great deal of heat to the dermis. While this has a profound effect on reducing wrinkles and skin laxity, bulk heating has significant risks of complications and as a result, deep nonfractional ablative skin resurfacing is rarely performed today.

**Fractional ablative lasers** heat and vaporize a portion of the skin in microscopic columns (Fig. 2B). These columns, referred to as microthermal treatment zones (MTZs), penetrate deeply to the reticular dermis, approximately 1500 µm. Tissue in the MTZs is ablated and untreated tissue between the MTZs serves as a reservoir for regenerative cells that migrate into the treated areas and facilitate rapid wound healing. Fractional ablative lasers are the treatment of choice today for severe wrinkles. Clinical effects are less dramatic than deep nonfractional ablative lasers, but they have fewer risks of complications.

## Laser Principles

Ablative lasers use **water as the target chromophore** to heat and vaporize tissue. The most commonly used wavelengths for ablative resurfacing are 2940 nm (erbium:yttrium aluminum garnet or Er:YAG) and 10600 nm (carbon dioxide or $CO_2$). While both wavelengths are well absorbed by water, 2940 nm takes advantage of an absorption peak and is approximately 15 times more highly absorbed by water than $CO_2$. A third, less frequently used wavelength is 2790 nm (yttrium scandium gallium garnet or YSGG). It is less well absorbed by water than 2940 nm, but better absorbed than 10600 nm.

Absorbed laser energy has two main effects on tissue: (1) **ablation**, the removal of tissue and (2) **coagulation**, heat transference to tissue. Coagulation clinically results in tissue tightening. A controlled amount of coagulation is desirable with skin resurfacing treatments, but too much thermal injury from heat transference can be associated with complications such as hypopigmentation and scarring. Due to a greater absorption by water, Er:YAG lasers ablate tissue at lower fluences (approximately 1 $J/cm^2$) compared to $CO_2$ lasers, which require higher fluences to achieve similar ablation (approximately 5 $J/cm^2$). Er:YAG lasers have less thermal transference to the surrounding tissues and therefore, have smaller zones of coagulation than $CO_2$ lasers (Fig. 3). Er:YSGG lasers are intermediate between these two lasers and ablate tissue at 3 $J/cm^2$; they have a greater zone of coagulation than Er:YAG lasers and a narrower zone of coagulation than $CO_2$ lasers. The amount of ablation and coagulation is controlled by laser fluence and pulse width. Ablation is most effectively achieved with short pulse widths and high fluences, whereas coagulation is achieved with longer pulse widths and lower fluences (Fig. 4). By varying these two parameters, ablative laser devices can independently control the amounts of ablation and coagulation achieved.

### Laser Parameters for Ablative Skin Resurfacing Treatments

Ablative laser devices have variable fluences, spot sizes, spot densities, and pulse widths all of which affect the depth of penetration, as well as the degree of ablation and coagulation achieved.

- **Wavelength.** Wavelength selection is specific for the water chromophore, which absorbs laser energy between 950–11000 nm (Fig. 6, Key References). Lasers targeting

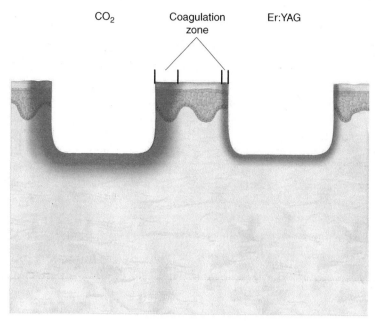

*FIGURE 3* ● Carbon dioxide ($CO_2$) and erbium: yttrium aluminum garnet (Er:YAG) pulse characteristics.

water that are used for skin resurfacing are shown in Figure 1 and include **Er:YAG (2940 nm), YSGG (2790 nm), and $CO_2$ (10600 nm).**

- **Fluence.** Laser fluence is a major determinant of the depth of penetration, where higher fluences penetrate deeper in the skin.
- **Pulse width.** The pulse width affects how much ablation versus coagulation is associated with a pulse at a given fluence. Longer pulse widths provide more coagulation than shorter pulse widths. For most ablative lasers, the pulse width is fixed and is less than 1 ms, which is the thermal relaxation time for the epidermis.
- **Spot size.** Larger spot sizes have greater absorption and deeper penetration of laser energy compared to small spot sizes.

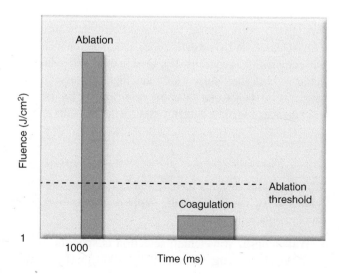

*FIGURE 4* ● Ablation and coagulation with ablative lasers.

- **Repetition rate.** Fast repetition rates allow for more rapid coverage of large treatment areas and can shorten treatment times.
- **Fractional lasers.**
  - **Spot size.** Spot sizes used with fractional devices are very small, ranging from 100–900 μm, and are not adjustable. These tiny spot sizes can penetrate very deeply (to 1.5 mm) and increasing penetration depth with increasing spot size does not hold true when considering these tiny spot sizes used with fractional lasers.
  - **Spot density.** Fractional devices also have a density setting, which determines the percentage of skin that is treated with a pulse (that range from 5–50%). High-density settings are associated with more aggressive treatments, have longer healing times, and greater improvements.
  - **Fluence.** In addition to the depth of penetration, high fluences are associated with large microthermal treatment zones (i.e., skin treatment area). Higher fluences are also associated with longer healing times.
  - **Pulse width.** The pulse width of fractional lasers determines the ratio of ablation to coagulation present at each MTZ. Very short pulse widths create ablative MTZs with very narrow surrounding thermal zones of coagulation. Longer pulse widths create MTZs with wider surrounding thermal zones of coagulation.
  - **Scanners.** Some ablative devices utilize scanners and computer software to "randomly" deliver pulses within a set pattern so that the pulses are not adjacent to one another, as opposed to stamping a pattern. Changing the energy delivery pattern from sequential to nonadjacent pulses allows for high energies to be delivered without the effects of bulk heating. This is particularly useful with $CO_2$ devices, which can cause greater thermal injury.

## Patient Selection

Ablative resurfacing has traditionally been used for patients with more **advanced signs of facial aging** including generalized static wrinkles, keratoses, severe dyschromia, sallow color, and coarse pores as seen with Glogau stage IV photoaging (see Introduction and Foundation Concepts, Glogau Classification of Photoaging section). With the advent of fractional technologies that have more rapid recovery times and fewer risks, ablative laser procedures are being performed on patients with less severe photoaging. Nonetheless, the most common indication today for fractional ablative resurfacing is still moderate to severe wrinkles and scars.

Fitzpatrick skin type is an important factor in assessing patients for laser skin resurfacing. The ideal patient has a light Fitzpatrick skin type (I-III) and patients with these skin types are the focus of this chapter. Patients with dark skin types (IV and V) have higher risks, particularly of pigmentary complications, and require more cautious treatment parameters, which can limit results.

## Patient Expectations

Ablative skin resurfacing, both conventional and fractional, has been shown to effectively reduce wrinkles and improve dyschromia such as lentigines and ephelides in photoaged skin. Although fractional ablative treatments have the advantages of reduced recovery time and reduced risks compared to conventional ablative resurfacing, results with deep conventional resurfacing are more impressive. While ablative resurfacing can improve wrinkles, significant skin laxity, and sagging jowls may be better addressed with plastic surgery. Patients must fully understand the ablative laser postoperative recovery course and agree to comply with postprocedure instructions. Re-epithelialization following fractional ablative laser treatments typically requires 5–7 days. Patients must be able to tolerate this recovery period. Anticipated professional and social obligations should be considered with patient selection and timing of the procedure.

Patients often seek laser skin resurfacing to improve wrinkles near the lower eyelids and, while significant improvements can be achieved in this area, treatment inside the orbit on the eyelids is an advanced application with risks of ectropion and there are certain contraindications to treating this area (see Contraindications section).

## Indications

- Static rhytids
- Scarring (atrophic and hypertrophic)
- Rough skin texture
- Enlarged pores
- Benign pigmented lesions (e.g., lentigines and ephelides)
- Certain epidermal lesions including actinic keratoses, seborrheic keratoses, sebaceous hyperplasia, syringomas, actinic cheilitis, dermatosis papulosa nigra, xanthelasma, and rhinophyma.

## Alternative Therapies

**Aggressive exfoliation procedures** such as dermabrasion, and deep chemical peels can achieve deep skin resurfacing with results akin to ablative laser resurfacing. **Dermabrasion** is a mechanical method of exfoliation that utilizes motorized wire bristle brushes that rotate to remove the epidermis, papillary, and upper reticular dermis. **Chemical peels** use acids to wound the epidermis and dermis. Dermabrasion and chemical peels have the advantage of being less expensive than laser resurfacing. However, due to the high risk of scarring and hypopigmentation, and need for extensive preceptored hands-on training, dermabrasion and deep chemical peels are rarely used today. Superficial and medium depth peels and microdermabrasion are commonly used to treat mild static wrinkles but results do not equate with laser skin resurfacing.

**Nitrogen plasma** (e.g., Portrait™, Rhytec) is a laser-like technology used for thermal skin resurfacing that coagulates tissue with minimal ablation and has rapid recovery. Nitrogen plasma (an ionized gas) is formed by combining high-energy radiofrequency energy with nitrogen gas. Few studies are currently available on efficacy and long-term safety, and the role of plasma resurfacing is still emerging.

While ablative lasers are indicated for treatment of **pigmentation,** patients presenting only with benign pigmented lesions, without concerns of wrinkles and textural changes, may benefit from other less aggressive options, such as pigment specific nonablative lasers and intense pulsed light, which maintain an intact epidermis and have minimal risks with little to no recovery time (see Pigmented Lesions, Chapter 2).

Other available treatments for facial lines and wrinkles include **botulinum toxin** for dynamic wrinkles and **dermal fillers** for treatment of static lines and these treatments are often performed in conjunction with laser procedures. **Plastic surgery** is an option for severe wrinkling with saggy lax skin.

# Devices Currently Available for Ablative Resurfacing

| Laser | Wavelength (nm) |
|---|---|
| Carbon dioxide (CO$_2$) | 10600 |
| Erbium:yttrium aluminum garnet (Er:YAG) | 2940 |
| Erbium:yttrium scandium gallium garnet (Er:YSGG) | 2790 |

**CO$_2$ lasers** (10600 nm) were the first ablative lasers used and are still in use today. Early devices had long pulse widths, which deposited excessive heat in tissue and commonly had complications such as prolonged erythema for many months, hyperpigmentation, hypopigmentation, infection, and scarring. There are two main types of nonfractional ablative CO$_2$ lasers used today, both of which utilize shorter pulses to reduce heat deposition in tissue such as high-energy very short pulsed systems (e.g., UltraPulse™, Lumenis) and rapidly scanning continuous lasers (e.g., Silktouch™ by Sharplan, FeatherTouch™ by Lumenis). These lasers are highly effective for reduction of deep wrinkles and acne scars due to their coagulation effects from heat deposition and also improve superficial skin lesions such as actinic keratoses, lentigines, ephelides, and fine lines. Nonfractional ablative CO$_2$ lasers are still associated with significant side effects and most CO$_2$ and other ablative lasers are performed as fractional treatments.

**Er:YAG (2940 nm)** lasers were the next generation of ablative lasers. Due to higher water absorption, these lasers penetrate less deeply and deposit less heat in tissue. As a result of decreased coagulation, these early erbium devices had inferior skin tightening effects and more bleeding relative to CO$_2$ lasers. A benefit to the erbium lasers, however, was shorter recovery times; also a function of lower coagulation as the combined depth of ablation and coagulation is the main factor that determines recovery time with ablative lasers. Subsequent advancements in erbium lasers involved lengthened and variable pulse widths, which improved coagulation effects for wrinkle reduction and hemostasis (e.g., ProFractional™, Sciton). Combination lasers of erbium and CO$_2$ (in the same pulse) were popular for a brief period as they allowed heat deposition with CO$_2$ and precise ablation with erbium (e.g., Derma-K™, Lumenis).

**Er:YSGG (2790 nm)** are a newer addition to the ablative laser family (e.g., Pearl™, Cutera). They have intermediate water absorption compared to CO$_2$ and Er:YAG lasers. Like other ablative lasers, these lasers have shown benefits for photoaged skin with reduction of wrinkles and dyspigmentation, but devices do not penetrate as deeply as Er:YAG and CO$_2$ lasers and the potential for improvements may be limited as a result.

Today, ablative lasers are most commonly used for **fractional treatments.** Fractional devices treat a portion of the skin in microscopic columns, called MTZ, with an array of customizable density and depth. Fractional ablative lasers show pigmentary and textural improvements in photoaged skin and have the advantage of shorter recovery time and lower risks of complications compared to deep nonfractional ablative lasers. One of the most notable benefits of fractional lasers is the lack of hypopigmentation (independent of scarring). Several treatments are usually required with fractional ablative lasers to achieve desired results. Regardless of the number of treatments, reduction of deep wrinkles with fractional lasers is not comparable to deep nonfractional ablative laser treatments. Nonfractional ablative treatments are still commonly performed at superficial depths (20–50 μm) in the epidermis to treat fine lines and dyspigmentation. Deep nonfractional treatments (300 μm) are rarely performed due to the associated risks.

See Supply Sources, Appendix 6 for laser manufacturers.

# Contraindications

## General Laser Contraindications

- Active infection in the treatment area (e.g., herpes simplex, pustular acne, cellulitis)
- Dermatoses in the treatment area (e.g., vitiligo, psoriasis, atopic dermatitis)
- Melanoma, or lesions suspected for melanoma in the treatment area
- Deep chemical peel, dermabrasion or radiation therapy in the treatment area within the preceding 6 months
- Keloidal scarring[‡]
- Bleeding abnormality (e.g., thrombocytopenia, anticoagulant use)
- Impaired healing (e.g., immunosuppressive medications, poorly controlled diabetes mellitus)
- Peripheral vascular disease
- Seizure disorder
- Uncontrolled systemic condition
- Cardiac pacemaker
- Skin atrophy (e.g., chronic oral steroid use, genetic syndromes such as Ehlers–Danlos syndrome)
- Livedo reticularis, a vascular disease associated with mottled skin discoloration of the arms or legs exacerbated by heat exposure
- Erythema ab igne, a rare acquired reticular erythematous or pigmented rash exacerbated by heat exposure
- Direct sun exposure within the preceding 2 weeks resulting in reddened or tanned skin
- Self-tanning product within the preceding 2 weeks
- Topical prescription retinoid within the preceding week
- Isotretinoin (Accutane™) within the preceding 6 months
- Gold therapy (e.g., used for treatment of arthritis)
- Photosensitizing medications (e.g., tetracyclines, St. John's wort, thiazides)
- Photosensitive disorder (e.g., systemic lupus erythematosus)
- Pregnant or nursing
- Unrealistic patient expectations
- Body dysmorphic disorder
- Treatment inside the eye orbit (i.e., without intraocular eye shields)

## Contraindications Specific to Ablative Laser Treatment for Skin Resurfacing

- Fitzpatrick skin types V–VI
- Aggressive skin resurfacing within 1 year (e.g., dermabrasion, deep chemical peel, deep nonfractional ablative laser treatment)
- Radiation therapy in the treatment area

---

[‡]Caution should be used in patients with hypertrophic scarring.

- Extensive electrolysis
- Unwilling to adhere to preprocedure and/or postprocedure instructions
- Resurfacing treatments near or on eyelids are contraindicated with the presence of:
  - Ectropion
  - Significant eyelid laxity (indicated by an abnormal lower eyelid "snap test")
  - Prior lower blepharoplasty

Certain procedures can reduce adnexal structures in the treatment area and impair healing such as deep chemical peels, dermabrasion, radiation therapy, deep nonfractional ablative laser treatment, and extensive electrolysis.

## Advantages of Ablative Lasers for Skin Resurfacing

- Multiple conditions treated simultaneously with high efficacy
- Ongoing improvements posttreatment with continued collagen remodeling and wrinkle reduction

## Disadvantages of Ablative Lasers for Skin Resurfacing

- Significant recovery time relative to nonablative laser treatments
- Greater potential for infection, hypopigmentation, and scarring complications compared to nonablative lasers
- Expensive

## Equipment

### Anesthesia

- Alcohol wipes
- Benzocaine/lidocaine/tetracaine (20:6:4) ointment or other topical anesthetic
- Cool air blower (optional but recommended)

### Procedure

- Ablative laser
- Smoke evacuator
- Laser-safe eyewear for patient, provider, and all personnel in the room
- Mask for provider and all personnel in the room
- Gloves nonsterile
- Gauze 4 × 4 in
- Alcohol wipes
- Nonalcohol wipes to cleanse the treatment area for removal of makeup and topical anesthetic
- Headband

### Postprocedure

- Gauze 4 × 4 in
- Normal saline 1000 mL
- Gloves nonsterile

- Large soft ice packs
- Handheld fan with soft blades (if cool air blower device not used)
- Towels (thin muslin, very soft)
- Petrolatum-based topical product (e.g., Aquaphor™)

## Preprocedure Checklist

### 4–6 Weeks Prior

- **Aesthetic consultation** is performed to review the patient's medical history including history of postinflammatory hyperpigmentation (PIH), hypertrophic or keloidal scarring, blepharoplasty, previous skin resurfacing, and date.
- **Fitzpatrick skin type** is determined (see Introduction and Foundation Concepts, Aesthetic Consultation section).
- **Examination of the treatment area** is performed. Wrinkle severity (see Introduction and Foundation Concepts, Glogau Classification of Photoaging section) and other indications for treatment are documented. Lesions suspicious for neoplasia are biopsied or referred if indicated and negative biopsy results received before proceeding with laser treatments.
- **Lower eyelid "snap test"** is performed to assess for skin elasticity for treatment on or near the lower eyelid. Resurfacing of inelastic skin in the lower eyelid area has a risk of ectropion. A snap test is performed by pulling the lower eyelid skin down and assessing skin recoil. If the lower eyelid skin does not return to its normal resting position within 3 seconds after release, avoid laser resurfacing near the lower eyelid.
- **Avoidance of direct sun exposure** and daily use of a broad-spectrum **sunscreen** with SPF 30 containing zinc oxide or titanium dioxide prior to and throughout the course of treatment is advised (see Preprocedure Skin Care Products section below).
- **Preprocedure written instructions** are reviewed (see Appendix 3f).

## Preprocedure Skin Care Products

- **Sunscreen** that is broad-spectrum with SPF 30 containing zinc oxide or titanium dioxide is recommended for all patients prior to procedure.
- **Topical lightening agents** may be used by patients prone to hyperpigmentation and dark Fitzpatrick skin types (IV and V) such as hydroquinone 4–8%, or a cosmeceutical product containing kojic acid, arbutin, niacinamide, or azelaic acid to reduce the risk of PIH. Ideally, a lightening product is begun 1 month prior to procedure and may be used twice daily.
- **Preprocedure skin care products** can be used to condition the skin and create a healthier pretreatment epidermis and dermis. A typical regimen contains a **retinoid, alpha-hydroxy acid, and antioxidant** such as vitamins C. While prescription-strength retinoids have traditionally been used as part of preprocedure regimens, these can be poorly tolerated and a less irritating retinoid such as retinol or retinaldehyde may be used instead. Topical retinoids have been shown to promote more rapid healing postprocedure and improve clinical outcomes with chemical peels, however, some studies show no benefits with laser resurfacing procedures, and the use of a preprocedure regimen is controversial. If used, a preprocedure skin care regime would be started 6 weeks prior to the laser procedure and continued for approximately 4 weeks. Active products such as retinoids and hydroxy acids such as glycolic acid are discontinued 1–2 weeks prior to a laser procedure to ensure the epidermis is intact at the time of treatment.

## 2 Weeks Prior

- **Informed consent** is obtained with a thorough review of potential adverse effects (see Introduction and Foundation Concepts, Aesthetic Consultation section). An example of a consent form is provided in Appendix 4f.
- **Photographs** are taken (see Introduction and Foundation Concepts, Aesthetic Consultation section).
- **Wound care instructions and postprocedure product use** are reviewed, and **appointments** scheduled (see Appendix 3f).
- **Medications** necessary for the procedure are prescribed, which may include the following:
  - **Antiviral** if a prior history of herpes simplex or zoster in or near the treatment area (e.g. valacyclovir 500 mg 1 tablet twice daily) for 2 days prior to the procedure and continue for 3–5 days postprocedure. There is a high incidence of latent herpes simplex virus (HSV) infection and some providers use prophylactic oral antiviral medications with all patients undergoing facial laser resurfacing.
  - **Anxiolytic** or **analgesic** (see Anesthesia section below) to be taken on the day of treatment if needed.
- **Anticoagulants are discontinued** including Aspirin, vitamin E, St. John's Wort and other dietary supplements including ginkgo biloba, evening primrose oil, garlic, feverfew, and ginseng 2 weeks prior to treatment to reduce the risk of bleeding. Other nonsteroidal anti-inflammatory medications including ibuprofen and naprosyn, and alcohol consumption, are discontinued 2 days prior to treatment.
- **Sun-protective clothing** (wide-brimmed hat and scarf) are recommended for the day of treatment.

## Anesthesia

Ablative resurfacing treatments have significant pain associated with the procedure and patients complain of a build-up of heat that is maximal at the end of the treatment. Adequate anesthesia will not only give the patient a more tolerable experience, but will also assist the provider in reaching the desirable settings for a given treatment.

Anesthesia modalities used for fractional ablative resurfacing include:

- **Topical anesthetics.** Stronger formulations such as BLT (benzocaine 20%: lidocaine 6%: tetracaine 4%) occluded with plastic wrap for 45 minutes provide good anesthesia.
- **Regional nerve block.** An infraorbital nerve block is helpful when treating the sensitive upper lip area. If using this block, topical anesthesia does not need to be applied to the upper lip area.
- **Forced air blower.** A forced air blower during the procedure can be used in addition to the other methods above.
- **Anxiolytics and analgesic medications.** In some patients, it may be helpful to give a dose 1 hour prior to the procedure. Patients taking anxiolytics or opioids require a driver to take them home after completing the procedure:
  - **Anxiolytic,** such as diazepam (Valium™) 10 mg and/or
  - **Analgesic,** such as tramadol (Ultram™) 50 mg to 100 mg, or hydrocodone with acetaminophen (Vicodin™ 5/500) 1 to 2 tablets

# Ablative Laser Resurfacing Procedure for Wrinkle Reduction

The following procedural recommendations for treatment of wrinkles including the sections on selecting initial laser parameters for treatment, general treatment technique, desirable clinical endpoints, undesirable clinical endpoints, aftercare, treatment intervals, subsequent treatments, and common follow-ups are based on treatment of the full face using a fractional ablative erbium laser 2940 nm (DermaSculpt™, Cynosure/ConBio) that is indicated for Fitzpatrick skin types (I–III). Manufacturer guidelines for the specific device used should be followed at the time of treatment.

## Selecting Initial Laser Parameters for Treatment

- **Wrinkles.** Deep wrinkles typically require more aggressive parameters with higher fluence and higher spot density. Fine lines typically require less aggressive parameters with lower fluences and lower spot density (Fig. 5).
- **Location.** Areas with thinner skin such as the periocular area require less aggressive parameters with lower fluence and lower spot density than thicker skinned areas such as the cheeks and upper lip.

## General Treatment Technique

- When treating the full face, it may be broken down into sections to help ensure complete coverage. One possible sequence for treating the face starting with section 1 and progressing to section 6 is shown in Figure 14, Introduction and Foundation Concepts.
- Fractional ablative resurfacing may be performed on a region of the face, referred to as a facial subunit. In the past, deep nonfractional ablative treatments were

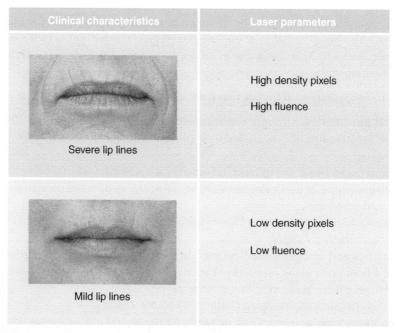

| Clinical characteristics | Laser parameters |
|---|---|
| Severe lip lines | High density pixels<br><br>High fluence |
| Mild lip lines | Low density pixels<br><br>Low fluence |

*FIGURE 5* ● Wrinkle severity and laser parameters. (Courtesy of R. Small, MD.)

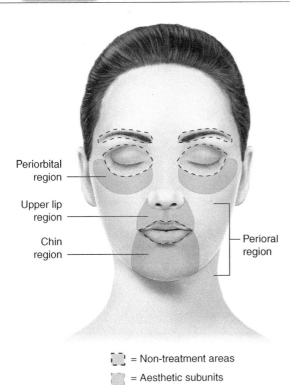

Periorbital region

Upper lip region

Chin region

Perioral region

⬚ = Non-treatment areas

▨ = Aesthetic subunits

**FIGURE 6** ● Facial aesthetic subunits commonly treated with fractional ablative skin resurfacing.

commonly associated with hypopigmentation and lines of demarcation between treated and untreated areas were obvious. However, lines of demarcation between treated and untreated areas have not proven to be a significant complication with fractional ablative lasers, and therefore, fractional ablative can be performed in discrete facial subunits. Figure 6 shows commonly treated facial aesthetic subunits. The periocular subunit is bounded inferiorly by the crest of the zygoma and superiorly by the orbital rim. The upper lip subunit extends laterally to the nasolabial folds and superiorly to the nose. The perioral subunit includes the upper lip and extends along the marionette line.

- Confluent coverage of the treatment area with laser pulses is important. This can be achieved by performing one pass and ensuring pulses are adjacent. The degree of recommended overlap and number of passes varies according to the specific device used but most device manufacturers recommend no overlap between pulses and only one pass (Fig. 7).
- Hold the laser tip perpendicular to the skin at all times
  **TIP: In the periocular area, angle the laser tip away from the eyes to reduce the risk of ocular injury and laser reflection off the patient's lead goggles.**
- The laser tip distance guide is in contact with the skin when pulsing the laser to maintain a uniform distance from the skin (Fig. 7).
- It is advisable for providers getting started with ablative lasers to restrict treatment to the area outside orbit, above the supraorbital ridge (roughly where the eyebrows sit), and below the inferior orbital rim.
  **TIP: Providers with advanced ablative laser skill may choose to treat over the eyelids with conservative settings using intraocular lead eye shields for patients.**

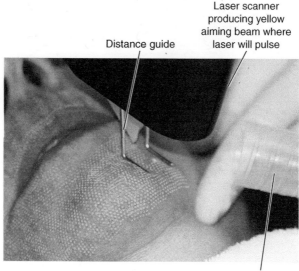

FIGURE 7 ● Clinical endpoints for fractional ablative skin resurfacing of crisp white pixels and erythema. (Courtesy of R. Small, MD.)

## Desirable Clinical Endpoints

When optimal parameters are used for fractional ablative laser treatments, one or more of the following clinical endpoints may be observed:

- **White dots** (referred to as pixels) (Fig. 7)
- **Erythema** (Figs. 7 and 8)
- **Pinpoint bleeding** (Fig. 8)

## Undesirable Clinical Endpoints

When overly aggressive laser parameters are used for treatment, one or more of the following undesirable clinical endpoints may be observed on the skin:

- **Blistering**
- **Frank bleeding**

   Frank bleeding refers to an area that drips blood and is not rapidly hemostatic by dabbing with gauze.

## Performing Ablative Laser Skin Resurfacing Procedure for Wrinkle Reduction

The following guidelines are for fractional ablative skin resurfacing on the full face to treat moderate wrinkles using a 2940 nm erbium laser. These treatment steps are specific to Cynosure/ConBio DermaSculpt™ system. Providers are advised to follow manufacturer guidelines for the specific device used at the time of treatment.

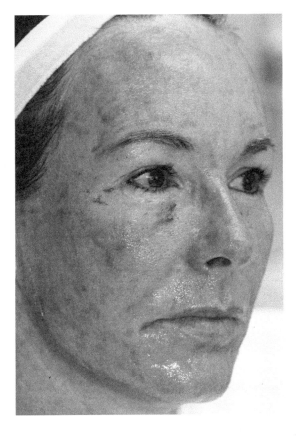

*FIGURE 8* ● Clinical endpoints for fractional ablative skin resurfacing of pinpoint bleeding and erythema. (Courtesy of R. Small, MD.)

1. Inquire about sun exposure and sunscreen use. If the patient is recently sun exposed or has tanned skin in the treatment area, consider waiting 1 month before treating to reduce the risk of pigmentary complications.
2. If the patient has not eaten prior to their procedure, provide food to help sustain blood sugar.
3. Have patients take pretreatment oral medications if indicated including an anxiolytic and/or analgesic.
4. Remove jewelry that may reflect laser light.
5. Have the patient remove contact lenses if present.
6. Pull hair away from the treatment area using a headband.
7. Wash the face and remove all makeup.
8. Cleanse the skin with an alcohol wipe prior to application of topical anesthetic to enhance penetration.
9. Apply topical anesthetic (e.g., BLT), occlude with plastic wrap and remove after 45–60 minutes using a facial wipe.
10. Position the patient supine with the treatment table flat. The physician is seated comfortably at the head of the patient.
11. Prepare the skin with an alcohol wipe and allow to fully dry.
12. Provide the patient with extraocular lead goggles and provide wavelength-specific protective eyewear to everyone in the treatment room.
13. Wear a mask to reduce particle inhalation.
14. Always operate the laser in accordance with your office's laser safety policies and the manufacturer's guidelines.

15. Have an assistant position the smoke evacuator near the area to be treated, approximately 3–4 in above the skin (Fig. 7).
    **TIP: Take care to avoid contacting the skin with the smoke evacuator as this makes a loud noise and can be startling. Also take care not to bump the laser handpiece.**

16. If using a cool air blower, have an assistant position the blower handpiece near the area to be treated, approximately 3–4 in above the skin per manufacturer guidelines.

17. Select the fluence and spot density based on the severity of wrinkles being treated and the location on the face (see Selecting Initial Laser Parameters for Treatment section).

18. Hold the handpiece at a 90-degree angle to the skin with the distance guide lightly touching the skin.

19. Perform a few pulses within the treatment area near the margin. Assess patient tolerance and observe the skin for clinical endpoints. Pain should be less than or equal to 6 on a scale of 1–10.

20. Perform one "pass" to the entire face, by covering the entire treatment area confluently with pulses, with no overlap.

21. Continually assess laser–tissue interaction and clinical endpoints throughout the treatment and adjust settings accordingly.
    - If **bleeding** occurs, discontinue treatment in that area and apply pressure until hemostatic. Pinpoint bleeding is indicative of aggressive parameters and is usually sparse, occurring in five or so locations in the treatment area, and is rapidly hemostatic. Numerous sites of pinpoint bleeding and frank bleeding that is not rapidly hemostatic are undesirable endpoints. Decrease fluence and/or spot density to make the treatment less aggressive in remaining areas.
    - If **blistering** occurs, discontinue treatment in that area and apply a wrapped ice pack for 15 minutes. Decrease fluence and/or spot density to make the treatment less aggressive in remaining areas.

22. Blend the treatment area with adjacent untreated areas by "feathering the edges" of the treatment area. This is achieved by reducing settings (i.e., using lower fluence and/or lower spot density) around the periphery of the treated area.
    **TIP: Extend treatment under the jaw line when treating near the jaw (Fig. 9).**

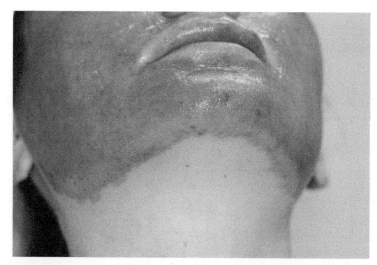

*FIGURE 9* ● Ablative laser treatments on the lower face extend under the jaw line. (Courtesy of R. Small, MD.)

23. Immediately after treatment, apply ice packs wrapped in a towel to the face and/or use a cool air blower to cool the skin for 30 minutes. Patients are often uncomfortably hot and it is important to cool them down rapidly.
24. Apply an occlusive topical ointment (e.g., Aquaphor™) after cooling.
25. Remind patient to wear sun-protective clothing (e.g., hat) upon leaving as sunscreen is not applied to the skin.

## Aftercare

Fractional ablative laser treatments have two distinct phases of healing: the open wound phase followed by the postepithelialization phase, which require different skin care. Postprocedure patient instructions are provided in Appendix 3f.

### Open Wound Phase (Days 0–7)

The open wound phase starts from the time of treatment and persists until full re-epithelialization takes place. This typically takes about 4 days with erbium lasers. Figure 10 shows the recovery process for a fractional ablative resurfacing treatment using an erbium laser on the full face of a 41-year-old woman. On the first postprocedure day the treatment area is an open wound demonstrating intense erythema, serous oozing, crusting, and pinpoint bleeding (A). By the fourth postprocedure day (B) the treatment area is almost fully re-epithelialized showing mild erythema with a few open areas. On day five this patient had fully re-epithelialized. Open wound care consists of gentle rinsing of the treatment area with dilute acetic acid (vinegar) soaks several times a day (see Appendix 3f). Figure 11 shows a patient the day after fractional ablative resurfacing prior to (A) and after (B) a vinegar wash. Note the devitalized, brown tissue and crusting

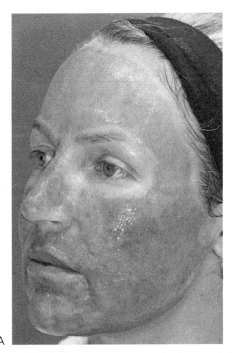 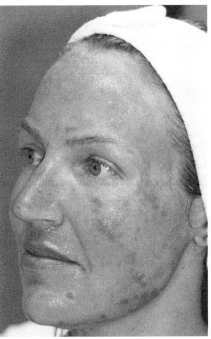

A                                                                                                   B

*FIGURE 10* ● Recovery process for fractional ablative skin resurfacing with an erbium laser on the first postprocedure day **(A)** and the fourth postprocedure day **(B)**. (Courtesy of R. Small, MD.)

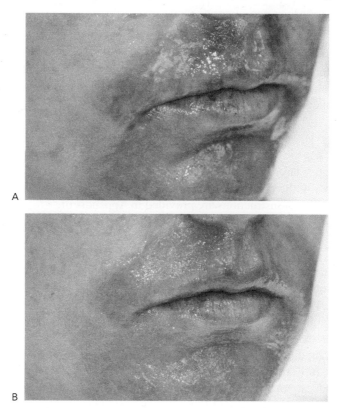

**FIGURE 11** ● Perioral fractional ablative skin resurfacing on the first postprocedure day prior to **(A)** and immediately after **(B)** cleansing with vinegar solution. (Courtesy of R. Small, MD.)

has been removed to reveal healthy pink tissue after the wash. Pinpoint bleeding may occur during the washing process, which is fine. Washing is followed by application of an occlusive ointment such as Aquaphor to promote moist wound healing. Some providers use nonocclussive products that promote wound healing (e.g., Biafine® by OrthoNeutrogena) during this phase. Excessive or prolonged use of occlusive topical products may increase the risk of milia, folliculitis, acne, bacterial and/or candidal infections, while inadequate use of hydrating products may result in crusting and delayed re-epithelialization. During the open wound phase, no sunscreen or makeup is worn and strict sun avoidance is imperative to reduce the risk of hyperpigmentation.

## Postepithelialization Phase (Days 7–30)

The postepithelialization phase commences once the open wound has healed and the epidermis is fully intact. This phase typically starts 1 week postprocedure and persists for 3 weeks. Skin is mildly erythematous and more sensitive than at baseline. Occlusive products are discontinued and products, which are soothing and hydrating (e.g., Epidermal Repair™, SkinCeuticals) may be used. Mineral makeup may be applied at this time to camouflage any remaining erythema. Direct sun exposure is avoided and a broad-spectrum sunscreen of SPF 30 containing zinc oxide or titanium dioxide is applied daily for 4 weeks after treatment to help minimize the risk of pigmentary changes. After 4 weeks, when skin is no longer sensitive, patients' preprocedural products may be resumed.

## Follow-Up Visits

Frequent follow-up is advised initially to evaluate the healing progress and monitor for early signs of complications. Visit intervals are increased once re-epithelialization has occurred. Below is one possible follow-up schedule. However, if the patient experiences any problems or complications, more frequent visits may be warranted:

- **Postprocedure day 1 or 2.** Evaluate for signs of infection and reinforce adherence to the recommended home care regimen during the open wound phase.
- **Postprocedure day 7.** Assess for full re-epithelialization. Once full re-epithelialization is observed transition to nonocclusive postcare topical products.
- **Postprocedure day 30.** Evaluate for resolution of erythema and assess clinical benefits.

## Subsequent Treatments

Fractional ablative treatments may be performed annually to maintain and enhance results, provided no complications occur with the procedure.

## Results

Ablative laser treatments can significantly improve wrinkles and dyschromias associated with photoaging such as lentigines and darkened ephelides. Wrinkle reduction is evident immediately posttreatment and benefits continue to improve for up to 6 months after treatment. Fractional ablative lasers have shown success with scar reduction such as atrophic acne scars, as well as seborrheic keratoses and actinic keratoses.

- Figure 12 shows results for facial rhytids before (A) and after (B) one deep ablative skin resurfacing treatment using an erbium laser to 120 µm depth (Contour TRL™, Sciton).

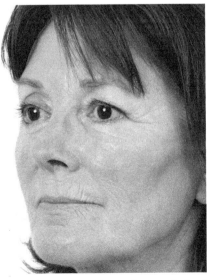 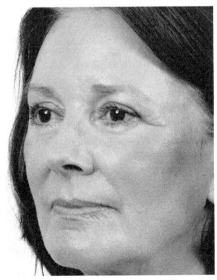

A                                                                                                    B

*FIGURE 12* ● Deep ablative skin resurfacing for facial wrinkles before **(A)** and after **(B)** one treatment to 120 µm depth using an erbium laser. (Courtesy of L. Apostolakis, MD and Sciton.)

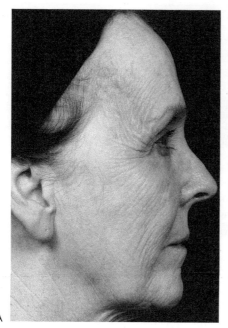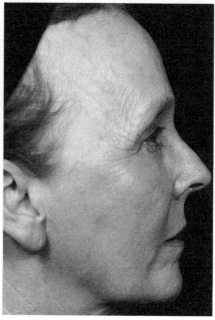

A                                                                                                      B

*FIGURE 13* ● Fractional ablative skin resurfacing for facial wrinkles before **(A)** and after **(B)** one treatment using a carbon dioxide laser. (Courtesy of Z. Rahman, MD and Solta.)

- Figure 13 shows facial rhytids before (A) and after (B) one fractional ablative skin resurfacing treatment using a carbon dioxide laser (Re:pair™, Fraxel).
- Figure 14 shows facial rhytids and mottled pigmentation before (A) and after (B) one fractional ablative skin resurfacing treatment using a carbon dioxide laser (Re:pair™, Fraxel).

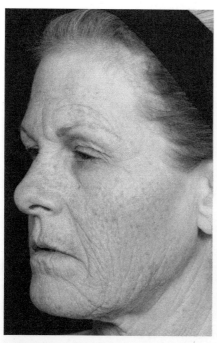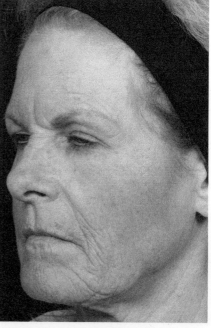

A                                                                                                      B

*FIGURE 14* ● Fractional ablative skin resurfacing for facial wrinkles and pigmentation before **(A)** and after **(B)** one treatment using a carbon dioxide laser. (Courtesy of Z. Rahman, MD and Solta.)

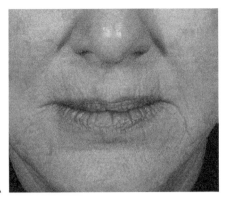 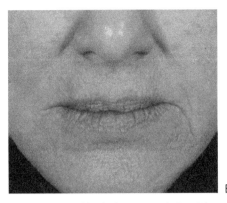

A    B

*FIGURE 15* ● Fractional ablative skin resurfacing for perioral wrinkles before **(A)** and after **(B)** one treatment using a carbon dioxide laser. (Courtesy of G. Munavalli, MD and Lumenis.)

- Figure 15 shows perioral rhytids before (A) and after (B) one fractional ablative skin resurfacing treatment using a carbon dioxide laser (TotalFX™, Lumenis).
- Figure 16 shows cheek rhytids before (A) and after (B) one fractional ablative skin resurfacing treatment with a YSGG laser (Pearl™, Cutera).
- Figure 17 shows facial wrinkles before (A) and after (B) one fractional ablative skin resurfacing treatment using an erbium laser (Profractional-XC™, Sciton).
- Figure 18 shows periocular rhytids before (A) and after (B) one fractional ablative skin resurfacing treatment using an erbium laser (Lux2940™, Cynosure/Palomar).
- Figure 19 shows acne scarring before (A) and after (B) five fractional ablative skin resurfacing treatments using an erbium laser (Profractional-XC™, Sciton).
- Figure 20 shows actinic keratoses before (A) and after (B) two fractional ablative skin resurfacing treatments using an erbium laser (Profractional™, Sciton).
- Figure 21 shows solar lentigines and ephelides before (A) and after (B) one superficial ablative skin resurfacing treatment using an erbium laser to 50 µm depth (Contour TRL™ MicroLaserPeel™, Sciton).
- Figure 22 shows seborrheic keratoses before (A) and after (B) one ablative skin resurfacing treatment using an erbium laser (Dermasculpt™ Chisel Touch™, Cynosure/ConBio).

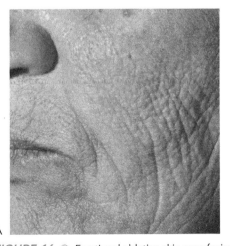 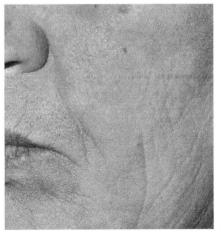

A    B

*FIGURE 16* ● Fractional ablative skin resurfacing for cheek wrinkles before **(A)** and after **(B)** one treatment using a YSGG laser. (Courtesy of B. DiBernardo, MD and Cutera.)

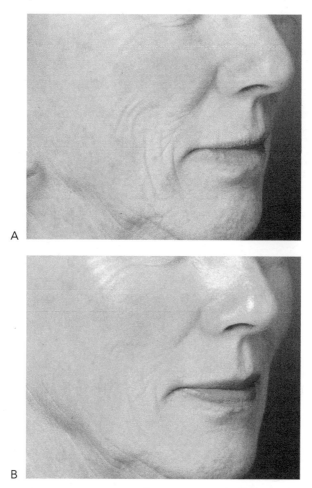

**FIGURE 17** ● Fractional ablative skin resurfacing for facial wrinkles before **(A)** and after **(B)** one treatment using an erbium laser. (Courtesy of K. Remington, MD and Sciton.)

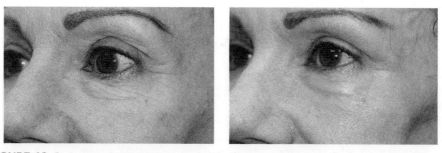

**FIGURE 18** ● Fractional ablative skin resurfacing for periocular wrinkles before **(A)** and after **(B)** one treatment using an erbium laser. (Courtesy of R. Small, MD.)

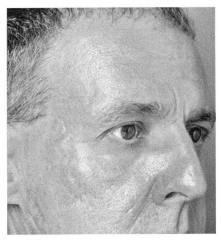 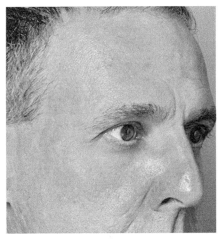

**FIGURE 19** Fractional ablative skin resurfacing for acne scarring before **(A)** and after **(B)** five treatments using an erbium laser. (Courtesy of K. Remington, MD and Sciton.)

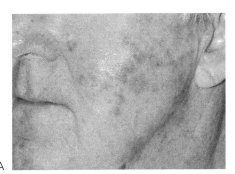 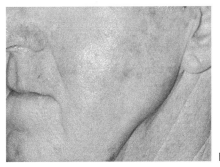

**FIGURE 20** Fractional ablative skin resurfacing for actinic keratoses before **(A)** and after **(B)** two treatments using an erbium laser. (Courtesy of R. Koch, MD and Sciton.)

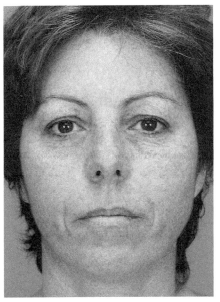 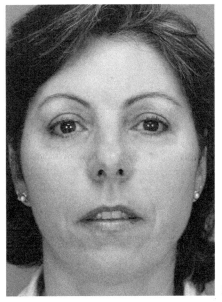

**FIGURE 21** Superficial ablative skin resurfacing for solar lentigines before **(A)** and after **(B)** one treatment to 50 μm depth using an erbium laser. (Courtesy of J. Pozner, MD and Sciton.)

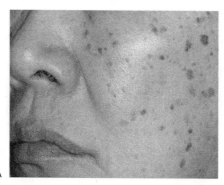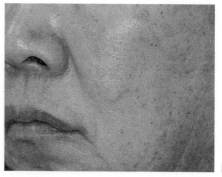

A                                                                                            B

*FIGURE 22* ● Ablative skin resurfacing for seborrheic keratoses before **(A)** and after **(B)** one treatment using an erbium laser with microtip. (Courtesy of K. Khatri, MD and Cynosure/ConBio.)

## Complications

- Pain
- Erythema
- Edema
- Contact dermatitis
- Infection (e.g., viral, fungal, and bacterial including acne vulgaris)
- Milia
- Hyperpigmentation
- Hypopigmentation
- Burn
- Bleeding
- Scarring
- Deeper than intended resurfacing
- Ectropion
- Toxicity from topical anesthetic
- Ocular injury

Complications associated with ablative laser resurfacing range from mild to severe reactions. Mild reactions include prolonged erythema, acne or milia formation, and contact dermatitis. Moderate complications include infections and PIH. More severe complications include hypertrophic scarring, delayed onset hypopigmentation, ectropion, and disseminated infection.

All ablative laser treatments create an open wound. While complications such as infection and scarring are seen most often with deep nonfractional laser treatments, they also occur with fractional ablative laser treatments despite comparatively shorter recovery times and increased safety. Early recognition of complications allows the physician to initiate appropriate treatments that can help reduce the risk of permanent damage.

**Pain** is usually reported only at the time of skin resurfacing and is typically moderate, 5–6 on a standard pain scale of 1–10, with the use of topical anesthetics and a cool air blower. Complaint of pain several days postprocedure is uncommon and evaluation is advisable, particularly to assess for infection.

**Erythema and edema** are expected after laser skin resurfacing. They are considered abnormal if they persist longer or are more intense than routinely observed. Intense erythema is expected immediately postprocedure during the open wound phase and typically lasts up to 1 week. After the first week, erythema is usually mild and can last up to 4 weeks. Postoperative erythema following $CO_2$ laser lasts longer than with erbium lasers. Treatments in the upper cheek at the level of the lower can result in periocular and eyelid edema. Patients with erythematous skin conditions such as telangiectasias, rosacea, and Poikiloderma of Civatte may be predisposed to prolonged postoperative erythema. Contact dermatitis and infection can also cause prolonged erythema. Persistent intense erythema can be an indicator of impending scar formation.

**Contact dermatitis** is a consideration in patients that have worsening erythema or pruritus after treatment. Newly resurfaced skin is vulnerable to irritation from substances found in topical products such as preservatives and fragrances. Topical antibiotics such as bacitracin, Neosporin™ (bacitracin, neomycin, and polymyxin B sulfate), and Polysporin® (bacitracin and polymyxin B) are also common causes of contact dermatitis and it is advisable to avoid these products in the immediate postoperative period. In addition, patients may self-prescribe over-the-counter herbal and vitamin remedies such as vitamin E and aloe products, which can cause contact dermatitis. If contact dermatitis is suspected, postprocedure topical products are discontinued and a topical corticosteroid ointment is used twice daily such as a low-potency steroid (e.g., hydrocortisone 2.5%) or a medium-potency steroid (e.g., triamcinolone acetonide 0.1%) depending on the severity, and cool wet compresses applied regularly. If pruritus is prominent, a nonsedating (e.g., cetirizine 10 mg) or sedating (e.g., diphenhydramine 25 mg) oral antihistamine may be taken. For severe contact dermatitis, a short course of an oral corticosteroid (prednisone 30 mg per day taper over 7–10 days) may be necessary to control inflammation and irritation.

**Infections** are not uncommon and can be viral, bacterial, or fungal. They occur most often during the first postoperative week. The appearance of infections in nonintact resurfaced skin does not always have the characteristic signs seen with intact skin. It is advisable to have a low threshold for culturing areas suspected of infection. Reactivation of **HSV** is the most frequent infectious complication following ablative resurfacing. Symptoms of HSV infection include tingling, burning, or discharge from isolated regions within the treated areas. Characteristic grouped vesicles may not be present in the early postoperative period since there is no intact epithelium. Instead, one may see small superficial erosions. If a herpetic outbreak occurs despite prophylaxis, consider switching to a different antiviral medication or increase the dosage to maximal herpes zoster doses (i.e., acyclovir 800 mg 5 times a day, or valacyclovir/famciclovir 500 mg 3 times a day).

**Bacterial** and **fungal** infections can also occur as the moist environment of resurfaced skin provides a hospitable environment for overgrowth of opportunistic pathogens. The most common **bacterial** infections are *streptococcal, staphylococcal,* and *Pseudomonas aeruginosa.* **Impetigo** has been reported following treatments on the face and extremities. The main pathogens are *Staphylococcus aureus* (methicillin-resistant *Staphylococcus aureus* is uncommon) and group A *Streptococcus,* and impetigo occurs most often in patients who are known carriers. **Fungal** infections can be difficult to diagnose as they may resemble acne or milia in nonintact skin. Pain, increased erythema, pruritus, purulent discharge, crusting, or delayed wound healing should alert one to possible bacterial or fungal infections. It is advisable to obtain wound cultures and initiate antibiotics and antifungal medications against the common pathogens prior to obtaining culture results. Consider empiric use of doxycycline 100 mg 1 tablet orally twice daily and clindamycin 300 mg 1 tablet four times per day for suspected bacterial infections, to be modified as necessary based on culture results. Local patterns of antibiotic resistance should be taken into account when selecting antibiotics empirically. Consider fluconazole 100 mg 1 tablet daily for presumed fungal and candidal infections. Infections must be treated aggressively as local spread can lead to permanent scarring and significant morbidity.

**Acne vulgaris** is a relatively common mild bacterial infection that can occur after laser skin resurfacing, usually due to prolonged application of occlusive ointments such as Aquaphor. Acne typically develops within the first few weeks. It may have a delayed onset and usually resolves spontaneously once occlusive ointments are discontinued. If acne persists despite the discontinuation of ointments, an oral antibiotic such as doxycycline or minocycline (e.g., 100 mg 1 tablet twice daily for 2 weeks) may be used.

**Milia** are tiny 1–2 mm white papules that result from occlusion of sebaceous glands. Occlusive ointments used to hydrate skin can obstruct sebaceous glands and contribute to milia formation. Milia do not usually resolve spontaneously and require lancing with a 20-gauge needle and extraction (i.e., gentle squeezing with cotton-tipped applicators) for removal.

**Postinflammatory hyperpigmentation (PIH)** commonly occurs postprocedure, particularly in the setting of prolonged erythema, unprotected sun exposure, and in patients with a predisposition to hyperpigmentation. PIH is usually observed within the first month postprocedure as erythema is fading, and spontaneously resolves during the next several months, although in rare instances may be permanent. Sun protection including the application of a broad-spectrum sunscreen with SPF 30 containing zinc oxide or titanium dioxide and sun avoidance are preventative measures for PIH. Various treatments can be initiated to speed resolution including topical lightening agents such as hydroquinone cream (4–8%) twice daily in the PIH area, superficial exfoliation procedures such as microdermabrasion and light chemical peels 1 month posttreatment, and sun protection.

**Hypopigmentation** is a serious and potentially permanent complication, which was reported more frequently with nonfractional deep ablative resurfacing, but there are reports with fractional ablative laser treatments. Figure 23 shows a patient with hypopigmentation and a distinct line of demarcation between treated and untreated skin,

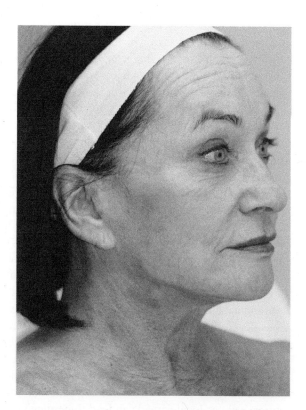

*FIGURE 23* ● Hypopigmentation twenty years after deep ablative skin resurfacing using a carbon dioxide laser. (Courtesy of R. Small, MD.)

20 years after receiving conventional deep ablative $CO_2$ skin resurfacing of the face. Hypopigmentation is usually delayed, presenting 6–12 months after ablative resurfacing. Hypopigmentation is much less common with fractional ablative lasers but is reported with coverage of 45% or greater. Hypopigmentation may be a temporary or permanent complication. There are few treatment options for hypopigmentation but it may repigment with exposure to ambient light sunlight, or respond to the excimer (308 nm) laser, or narrow band UVB treatment. One treatment strategy for hypopigmentation is to reduce the contrast between hypopigmented areas and adjacent skin by using chemical peels or nonablative lasers to decrease the surrounding skin's relative hyperpigmentation. Opaque makeup may be used for camouflage.

**Burns** with blister formation are rare with ablative resurfacing, but may result from aggressive treatment parameters. Prompt application of a wrapped ice pack to blisters may reduce the area of injury. Blisters and crusting are managed with moist wound care using an occlusive ointment such as Aquaphor™ or bacitracin until healed.

**Bleeding** is common with ablative resurfacing. Pinpoint bleeding can occur with aggressive parameters and is typically sparse, occurring in five or so pinpoint locations in the treatment area, and is rapidly hemostatic. Numerous sites of pinpoint bleeding or frank bleeding that is not rapidly hemostatic is a complication. Erbium lasers are associated with more bleeding than carbon dioxide lasers as they have less coagulation. Bleeding can almost always be managed with pressure and gauze until hemostatic. In rare instances aluminum chloride solution 35% may be necessary and can be gently applied with a cotton-tipped applicator to the bleeding sites.

**Scarring** is an uncommon but serious complication. Factors increasing the risk for scarring include aggressive laser parameters such as high fluences, pulse stacking, pulse overlapping, and high number of passes. Certain locations such as the lower eyelids, mandible, anterior neck, and chest are more susceptible to scarring and it is advisable to treat more cautiously in these areas. Sites of burns, bleeding, and postoperative infection have increased risk of scarring, especially if not treated appropriately. In addition, recent use of isotretinoin pretreatment, previous radiation therapy in the treatment area, and a history of keloid formation are also risk factors for hypertrophic scarring. Scarring is more common with nonfractional ablative resurfacing than fractional ablative resurfacing. Most of the scarring complications associated with fractional ablative lasers to date have been reported in thin skinned areas, such as under the eye, and in nonfacial areas, such as the neck and chest using skin coverage of 45% or more. Scarring is usually heralded by focal areas of intense erythema and induration and early intervention may help avoid permanent scarring. If **impending scar formation** is suspected, a very high–potency topical corticosteroid ointment may be applied (e.g., clobetasol 0.05% or betamethasone dipropionate 0.05% twice daily), topical silicone, and pulsed dye lasers (585 and 595 nm) may be used to reduce scar formation. Once formed, hypertrophic scars may be treated with the above therapies and injections of low-dose triamcinolone acetonide (Kenalog®-10, 10 mg/mL, using 1–2 mg). Injections may be repeated monthly, taking care not to overtreat, which can result in depressed atrophic scar formation. Full-thickness burns may require skin grafting.

**Ectropion**, or eversion of the eyelid, is another serious complication following laser skin resurfacing on or near the lower eyelid. Prior lower blepharoplasty increases this risk, as well as pretreatment lower lid laxity. Lower lid laxity is ruled out with a "snap test" prior to laser resurfacing (see Preprocedure Checklist section). In general, conservative laser settings and one laser pass is used when treating the lower lids due to thin skin in this area. While topical corticosteroid application, massage, and temporary taping may be tried if ectropion results, surgical correction is often required.

**Toxicity from topical anesthetic** applied prior to fractional laser skin resurfacing has been reported. Complete removal of topical anesthetic prior to fractional treatments and restricting application to small areas (less than 400 cm$^2$) can reduce this risk.

**Ocular injury** from laser light in the eye can be avoided by wearing appropriate laser-safe eyewear at all times during treatment, always directing the laser tip away from the eye, and treating outside of the eye orbit.

## Special Populations and Additional Considerations

- **Pregnant and nursing.** Women that are pregnant or nursing typically do not undergo elective procedures such as laser skin resurfacing. One of the potential complications from prolonged pain during a laser treatment is inhibition of lactation in women who are nursing.
- **Dark Fitzpatrick skin types.** Ablative lasers are typically performed in lighter skin types (I–III), but some device manufacturers include darker skin types (IV and V) as candidates. It is advisable to proceed with caution using conservative settings with low fluences and low densities if treating darker skin types to reduce the risk of complications.
- **Pediatric patients.** Pediatric patients are not generally candidates for cosmetic ablative laser treatments.
- **Melasma.** Ablative laser treatments can exacerbate melasma.
- **Nonfacial areas.** Photoaged skin of the neck, chest, and hands can be treated with the fractional ablative resurfacing. More conservative settings are advised in these areas as the skin contains fewer adnexal glands than the face and therefore, does not heal as well. These areas have a greater risk of complications and are considered advanced treatment areas, to be performed by experienced laser providers.

## Learning Techniques for Ablative Laser Treatments for Skin Resurfacing

Ablative laser treatment technique may be practiced on an eggplant initially as the white pulse pattern is clearly visible against the dark surface.

## Current Developments

Fractional ablative lasers are a relatively new class of laser and knowledge of tissue effects with specific devices and laser parameters continues to rapidly expand, improving the performance and side effect profiles of these devices.

**Combination therapy** utilizing ablative lasers and nonablative lasers sequentially in one treatment is being investigated in order to enhance results for photoaging and wrinkle reduction. For example, a nonablative 1440 nm treatment can be performed for coagulation followed by a 2940 nm fractional laser treatment for ablation to enhance collagen remodeling effects. Combination treatment can also be performed using ablative lasers to target different depths in the skin. For example, nonfractional superficial skin resurfacing with an erbium can be performed to target fine lines and skin texture, immediately followed by a deeper fractional skin resurfacing erbium treatment to target deeper wrinkles and laxity.

**Radiofrequency (RF)** has recently been used for fractional resurfacing (Matrix RF™, Syneron and Infini™, Lutronic). This is a nonlaser, nonlight-based device that uses rapidly alternating current. Radiofrequency produces thermal injury in the dermis as a result of the skin's resistance to the flow of current (impedance). Fractional RF handpieces have an array of electrode pins and the skin in contact with the pins is heated while the areas between the pins are spared. The energy is concentrated in the mid to deep dermis with limited epidermal disruption and these devices are therefore, referred to as subablative. Benefits have been demonstrated for textural improvement in facial wrinkles. These devices show promise for treatment of darker skin types due to the limited epidermal involvement, and may have lower risks of scarring.

**Focused ultrasound** is a newer technology being used for wrinkle reduction. Ultrasound consists of high-frequency acoustic. Ultrasound can be focused and concentrated at select depths below the skin creating confined zones of thermal injury without damaging overlying epidermis. In this way, the dermis can be heated resulting in wrinkle reduction, and some devices heat adipose tissue for removal of focal fat. Like radiofrequency, ultrasound can be used in all skin types.

## Financial Considerations

Ablative resurfacing is not reimbursable by insurance. The charges for treatments vary and are mainly determined by local prices. For example, fees for fractional ablative resurfacing treatments in the Northern California Bay Area range from $2700–$3500 for full face and $1000–$1200 for periocular or perioral areas.

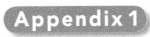

# Aesthetic Intake Form

Date:_____

Name:_____  AGE:_____ * DOB:_____
　　　Last　　　　　　　　　First
ADDRESS:_____  CITY:_____  ZIP:_____

HOME PHONE:_____  ☐ OK TO CONTACT/LEAVE MESSAGE HERE

MOBILE PHONE:_____  ☐ OK TO CONTACT/LEAVE MESSAGE HERE

WORK PHONE:_____  ☐ OK TO CONTACT/LEAVE MESSAGE HERE

E-MAIL:_____  ☐ OK TO CONTACT/LEAVE MESSAGE HERE

OCCUPATION:_____  REFERRED BY:_____

Please list in order of importance, beginning with 1, what you would like to improve about your skin:
_____ Reduction of fine lines _____ Reduction of oil/acne _____ Reduction of redness _____ Reduction of brown spots/sun damage
_____ Reduction of hair _____ Acne scars diminished _____ Tattoo_____ Other　　　　*For minors, please list guardian info.

| Medical history | Yes | No |
|---|---|---|
| Are you or is it possible that you may be pregnant? | | |
| Are you breastfeeding? | | |
| Do you form thick or raised scars from cuts or burns? | | |
| After injury to the skin (such as cuts/burns) do you have: (circle) Darkening of the skin in that area (hyperpigmentation) Lightening of the skin in that area (hypopigmentation) | | |
| Hair removal by plucking, waxing, or electrolysis in the last 4 weeks? | | |
| Tanning (tanning bed) or sun exposure in the last 4 weeks? (circle) | | |
| Tanning products or spray on tan in the last 2 weeks? | | |
| Do you have a tan now in the area to be treated? | | |
| Do you use sunscreen daily with spf 30 or higher? | | |
| History of skin cancer or unusual moles? | | |
| Have you ever had a photosensitive disorder? (E.g. lupus) | | |
| History of seizures? | | |
| Permanent make-up or tattoos? Where _____ | | |
| Have you used Accutane in last 6 months? | | |
| Are you currently taking antibiotics? Which _____ | | |
| Are you using Retin-A or Glycolic products? (circle) | | |
| Are you currently under the care of a physician? | | |
| Do you currently smoke? | | |
| Do you have an allergy or sensitivity to lidocaine, latex, sulfa medications, hydroquinone, aloe, and bee stings? (circle) | | |
| Life threatening allergy to anything? | | |
| Do you have scars on the face? | | |

| Please check all medical conditions past or present | Yes | No | |
|---|---|---|---|
| | ☐ | ☐ | Keloid scarring |
| | ☐ | ☐ | Cold sores |
| | ☐ | ☐ | Herpes (genital) |
| | ☐ | ☐ | Easy bruising or bleeding |
| | ☐ | ☐ | Active skin infection |
| | ☐ | ☐ | Moles that changed, itched, or bled |
| | ☐ | ☐ | Recent increase in amount of hair |
| | ☐ | ☐ | Asthma |
| | ☐ | ☐ | Seasonal allergies/allergic rhinitis |
| | ☐ | ☐ | Eczema |
| | ☐ | ☐ | Thyroid imbalance |
| | ☐ | ☐ | Poor healing |
| | ☐ | ☐ | Diabetes |
| | ☐ | ☐ | Heart condition |
| | ☐ | ☐ | High blood pressure |
| | ☐ | ☐ | Pacemaker |
| | ☐ | ☐ | Disease of nerves or muscles (e.g. ALS, myasthenia gravis, Lambert-Eaton or other) |
| | ☐ | ☐ | Cancer |
| | ☐ | ☐ | HIV/AIDS |
| | ☐ | ☐ | Autoimmune disease (e.g. rheumatoid arthritis, scleroderma) |
| | ☐ | ☐ | Hepatitis |
| | ☐ | ☐ | Shingles |
| | ☐ | ☐ | Migraine headaches |
| | ☐ | ☐ | Other illness, health problems, or medical conditions not listed. |

Explanation of items marked "Yes":

Explanation of items marked "Yes":
_____
_____
_____

I certify that the medical information I have given is complete and accurate. _____ Initials

**For Internal Use Only Below This Line**

*(Courtesy of Monterey Bay Laser Aesthetics.)*

# Fitzpatrick Skin Type

Name:_____     DOB: _____

| Score | 0 | 1 | 2 | 3 | 4 |
|---|---|---|---|---|---|
| What color are your eyes? | light blue, gray, green | hazel | blue | dark brown | brownish black |
| What is the natural color of your hair? | sandy red | blond | chestnut/dark blond | dark brown | black |
| What is the color of your skin (nonexposed areas)? | reddish | very pale | pale with beige tint | light brown | dark brown |
| Do you have freckles on sun-exposed areas? | many | several | few | incidental | none |

Total score for genetic disposition:

| Score | 0 | 1 | 2 | 3 | 4 |
|---|---|---|---|---|---|
| What happens when you stay too long in the sun? | Painful, redness, blistering, peeling | blistering, followed by peeling | burns sometimes followed by peeling | rare burns | never had burns |
| To what degree do you turn brown? | hardly or not at all | light color tan | reasonable tan | tan very easy | turn dark brown quickly |
| Do you turn brown within several hours of exposure? | never | seldom | sometimes | often | always |
| How does your face react to the sun? | very sensitive | sensitive | normal | very resistant | never had a problem |

Total score for reaction to sun exposure:

| Score | 0 | 1 | 2 | 3 | 4 |
|---|---|---|---|---|---|
| When did you last expose the treatment area to direct sun (or sunlamp/tanning)? | more than 3 months ago | 2–3 months ago | 1–2 months ago | less than 1 month ago | less than 2 weeks ago |
| Do you routinely expose the treatment area to sun? | never | hardly ever | sometimes | often | always |

Total score for tanning habits:

| Total Score | Score | Fitzpatirck Skin Type |
|---|---|---|
| | 0–7 | I |
| | 8–16 | II |
| | 17–25 | III |
| | 26–30 | IV |
| | Over 30 | V–VI |

*(Courtesy of Monterey Bay Laser Aesthetics.)*

Completed by:_____ Date:_____

# Hair Removal Before and After Instructions for Laser Treatments

The following instructions are for laser and intense pulsed light (collectively referred to as laser) treatments for hair removal.

## Prior to Treatment

- Avoid tanning bed, direct sun exposure, and sunless tanning products for 4 weeks prior to each treatment and the duration of treatments.
- Use a broad-spectrum sunscreen of SPF 30 containing zinc oxide or titanium dioxide daily for the duration of treatments.
- Do not use medications that cause photosensitivity (such as doxycycline and minocycline) for at least 72 hours prior to each treatment.
- If you have a history of herpes (oral cold sores, genital) or shingles in the treatment area, start your antiviral medication (valacyclovir, acyclovir) as directed for 2 days prior to treatment and continue for 3 days after treatment.
- Discontinue use of glycolic and Retin-A–containing products 1 week before treatments.
- Shave the area to be treated 1 day prior to your visit. If the hair in the treatment area is very sparse, do not shave—the provider will shave that area at the time of your treatment.
- Do not pluck, wax, undergo stringing or electrolysis, use depilatory creams or bleach for 4 weeks prior to treatments.
- At the time of treatment, the area must be free of any open sores, lesions, or skin infections (e.g., active acne).

## After Treatment

- Some skin redness and swelling along with a mild to moderate sunburn sensation in the treatment area are common. This typically resolves within a few hours but may last up to 3 days.
- Apply a wrapped cool compress or wrapped ice pack to the treated areas for 15 minutes every 1–2 hours as needed to reduce these symptoms. You may also apply hydrocortisone 1% over-the-counter cream two times per day on intact skin up to 3 days to decrease any skin irritation.
- Gently wash twice daily with mild soap, do not rub the skin vigorously and avoid hot water, as the skin will be fragile for several days.
- Avoid activities that can cause flushing for 24 hours after treatment or until any swelling resolves.

- Avoid any topical products that may cause irritation for 1 week following treatment.
- If blistering, crusting, or scabbing develops, call our office immediately. Apply a thin layer antibiotic ointment (such as bacitracin) to the area twice a day until the skin heals. Do not pick or attempt to remove scabs that form following your treatment, as this may incur infection or scarring.
- Any extruding singed hairs is normal and may occur for several weeks.

*This form is intended to serve only as an example and should be modified accordingly based on patient and provider needs. (Courtesy of Monterey Bay Laser Aesthetics.)*

# Pigmented Lesion Before and After Instructions for Laser Treatments

The following instructions are for laser and intense pulsed light (collectively referred to as laser) treatments for benign pigmented lesions.

## Prior to Treatment

- Avoid tanning bed, direct sun exposure, and sunless tanning products for 4 weeks prior to each treatment and the duration of treatments.
- Use a broad-spectrum sunscreen of SPF 30 containing zinc oxide or titanium dioxide daily for the duration of treatments.
- Do not use medications that cause photosensitivity (such as doxycycline and minocycline) for at least 72 hours prior to each treatment.
- If you have a history of herpes (oral cold sores, genital) or shingles in the treatment area, start your antiviral medication (valacyclovir, acyclovir) as directed for 2 days prior to treatment and continue for 3 days after treatment.
- Discontinue use of glycolic and Retin-A–containing products 1 week before treatments.
- At the time of treatment, the area must be free of any open sores, lesions, or skin infections (e.g., active acne).

## After Treatment

- Immediately after treatment, pigmented lesions will appear darkened. The lesions will continue to darken and flake off over 1–2 weeks.
- Some skin redness and swelling along with a mild to moderate sunburn sensation in the treatment area are common. This typically resolves within a few hours but may last up to 3 days.
- Apply a wrapped cool compress or wrapped ice pack to the treated areas for 15 minutes every 1–2 hours as needed to reduce these symptoms. You may also apply hydrocortisone 1% over-the-counter cream two times per day on intact skin up to 3 days to decrease any skin irritation.
- Gently wash twice daily with mild soap, do not rub the skin vigorously and avoid hot water, as the skin will be fragile for several days.
- Avoid activities that can cause flushing for 24 hours after treatment or until any swelling resolves.
- Avoid any topical products that may cause irritation for 1 week following treatment.

- If blistering, crusting, or scabbing develops, call our office immediately. Apply a thin layer antibiotic ointment (such as bacitracin) to the area twice a day until the skin heals. Do not pick or attempt to remove scabs that form following your treatment, as this may incur infection or scarring.

*This form is intended to serve only as an example and should be modified accordingly based on patient and provider needs. (Courtesy of Monterey Bay Laser Aesthetics.)*

# Vascular Lesion Before and After Instructions for Laser Treatments

The following instructions are for laser and intense pulsed light (collectively referred to as laser) treatments for red vascular lesions.

## Prior to Treatment

- Avoid tanning bed, direct sun exposure, and sunless tanning products for 4 weeks prior to each treatment and the duration of treatments.
- Use a broad-spectrum sunscreen of SPF 30 containing zinc oxide or titanium dioxide daily for the duration of treatments.
- Do not use medications that cause photosensitivity (such as doxycycline and minocycline) for at least 72 hours prior to each treatment.
- If you have a history of herpes (oral cold sores, genital) or shingles in the treatment area, start your antiviral medication (valacyclovir, acyclovir) as directed for 2 days prior to treatment and continue for 3 days after treatment.
- Discontinue use of glycolic and Retin-A–containing products 1 week before treatments.
- At the time of treatment, the area must be free of any open sores, lesions, or skin infections (e.g., active acne).

## After Treatment

- Immediately after treatment, vascular lesions may disappear, lighten or change color turning gray or bluish-purple. The lesions will typically lighten over the next week.
- Some skin redness and swelling along with a mild to moderate sunburn sensation in the treatment area are common. This typically resolves within a few hours but may last up to 3 days.
- Apply a wrapped cool compress or wrapped ice pack to the treated areas for 15 minutes every 1–2 hours as needed to reduce these symptoms. You may also apply hydrocortisone 1% over-the-counter cream two times per day on intact skin up to 3 days to decrease any skin irritation.
- Gently wash twice daily with mild soap, do not rub the skin vigorously and avoid hot water, as the skin will be fragile for several days.
- Avoid activities that can cause flushing for 24 hours after treatment or until any swelling resolves.
- Avoid any topical products that may cause irritation for 1 week following treatment.

- If blistering, crusting, or scabbing develops, call our office immediately. Apply a thin layer antibiotic ointment (such as bacitracin) to the area twice a day until the skin heals. Do not pick or attempt to remove scabs that form following your treatment, as this may incur infection or scarring.

*This form is intended to serve only as an example and should be modified accordingly based on patient and provider needs. (Courtesy of Monterey Bay Laser Aesthetics.)*

# Tattoo Removal Before and After Instructions for Laser Treatments

## Prior to Treatment

- Avoid tanning bed, direct sun exposure, and sunless tanning products for 4 weeks prior to each treatment and the duration of treatments.
- Use a broad-spectrum sunscreen of SPF 30 containing zinc oxide or titanium dioxide daily for the duration of treatments.
- Do not use medications that cause photosensitivity (such as doxycycline and minocycline) for at least 72 hours prior to each treatment.
- If you have a history of herpes (oral cold sores, genital) or shingles in the treatment area, start your antiviral medication (valacyclovir, acyclovir) as directed for 2 days prior to treatment and continue for 3 days after treatment.

## After Treatment

- Immediately after treatment, apply a wrapped cool compress or wrapped ice pack to the treatment area for 15 minutes every 1–2 hours or as directed. The area may feel warm, appear swollen, reddish, or bruised. Blistering or scabbing can occur particularly if ice is not applied as directed and will generally heal in 1–2 weeks.
- Discomfort typically resolves within 1 day and can be relieved with icing.
- If the skin is irritated (without scabs or bleeding), apply sunscreen SPF 30 or greater daily. A bandage of gauze and paper tape may be applied over the area if desired, but this is not needed.
- If the tattoo is in an area prone to abrasion, for example, where pants or bra strap contact skin, keep tattoo dressed (as above) until fully healed, and the skin is no longer shiny.
- Avoid activities that can cause flushing for 24 hours after treatment or until any swelling resolves.
- Avoid products that can cause irritation for 1 week following treatment.
- If blistering, crusting, or scabbing develops, contact our office immediately. Use bacitracin or Aquaphor daily to keep the area moist, place a bandage over the area (as described above) and replace every day until all scabs are fully healed to prevent infection. Do not pick any crusted or scabbed areas as it may interfere with healing and cause scarring.
- Keep the area clean with gentle cleansing. Do not rub the area with a washcloth or towel; pat dry instead.

- Avoid direct contact with hot water (e.g., hot tubs, saunas) for 1 week following treatment.
- If swimming or participating in water activites, cover tattoo with bacitracin and gauze and place a tegaderm (or other waterproof bandage) on top of the gauze with at least 1 in of adhesive around the gauze.

*This form is intended to serve only as an example and should be modified accordingly based on patient and provider needs. (Courtesy of Monterey Bay Laser Aesthetics.)*

# Wrinkles-Nonablative Resurfacing Before and After Instructions for Laser Treatments

The following instructions are for laser and intense pulsed light (collectively referred to as laser) nonablative skin resurfacing treatments.

## Prior to Treatment

- Avoid tanning bed, direct sun exposure, and sunless tanning products for 4 weeks prior to each treatment and the duration of treatments.
- Use a broad-spectrum sunscreen of SPF 30 containing zinc oxide or titanium dioxide daily for the duration of treatments.
- Do not use medications that causes photosensitivity (such as doxycycline and minocycline) for at least 72 hours prior to each treatment.
- If you have a history of herpes (oral cold sores and genital) or shingles in the treatment area, start your antiviral medication (valacyclovir and acyclovir) as directed for two days prior to treatment and continue for 3 days after treatment.
- Discontinue use of glycolic and Retin-A–containing products 1 week before treatments.
- At the time of treatment, the area must be free of any open sores, lesions, or skin infections (e.g., active acne).

## After Treatment

- Some skin redness and swelling along with a mild to moderate sunburn sensation in the treatment area are common. This typically resolves within a few hours but may last up to 3 days.
- Apply a wrapped cool compress or wrapped ice pack to the treated areas for 15 minutes every 1–2 hours as needed to reduce these symptoms. You may also apply hydrocortisone 1% over-the-counter cream two times per day on intact skin up to 3 days to decrease any skin irritation.
- Gently wash twice daily with mild soap, do not rub the skin vigorously, and avoid hot water, as the skin will be fragile for several days.
- Avoid activities that can cause flushing for 24 hours after treatment or until any swelling resolves.
- Avoid any topical products that may cause irritation for 1 week following treatment.

- If blistering, crusting, or scabbing develops, call our office immediately. Apply a thin layer of antibiotic ointment (such as bacitracin) to the area twice a day until the skin heals. Do not pick or attempt to remove scabs that form following your treatment, as this may incur infection or scarring.

*This form is intended to serve only as an example and should be modified accordingly based on patient and provider needs. (Courtesy of Monterey Bay Laser Aesthetics.)*

# Wrinkles-Ablative Resurfacing Before and After Instructions for Laser Treatments

## Prior to Treatment

- Avoid tanning bed, direct sun exposure, sunless tanning products and use a broad-spectrum sunscreen of SPF 30 containing zinc oxide or titanium dioxide daily for 4 weeks prior to treatment and 4 weeks after the treatment.
- Avoid deep facial peel procedures for 4 weeks prior to your laser treatment (e.g., aggressive chemical peels, laser resurfacing, dermabrasion).
- Avoid Ginko biloba, vitamin E, aspirin products (e.g., Excedrin) for 2 weeks prior to the laser procedure to minimize bruising risk. Avoid anti-inflammatory medications such as ibuprofen (e.g., Motrin, Advil), naproxen (e.g., Aleve), and celecoxib (e.g., Celebrex) for 1 week prior to your procedure. Tylenol (acetaminophen) is fine.
- Do not use medications that cause photosensitivity (such as doxycycline, minocycline) for at least 72 hours prior to treatment.
- If you have a history of herpes (oral cold sores, genital) or shingles in the treatment area, start your antiviral medication (valacyclovir, acyclovir) as directed for 2 days prior to treatment and continue for 3 days after treatment.
- Discontinue use of glycolic and Retin-A–containing products 1 week before treatment.
- For discomfort, you may take Ultram 50 mg 1 hour prior to your procedure. Alternatively, the doctor can prescribe stronger medications for discomfort such as Vicodin, Darvocet, and/or Valium.
- At the time of treatment, the area must be free of any open sores, lesions, or skin infections (e.g., active acne).

## Preparation for Procedure

- Meet with skincare specialist for appropriate home care products for postprocedure.
- Products for facial cleansing (vinegar soak) postprocedure
  - White vinegar
  - Nonwoven gauze 4 × 4 in
  - Plastic container in which to store vinegar-soaked gauze
  - Headbands
  - Two medium-sized soft reusable ice packs

## Day of Procedure

- Eat a solid breakfast.
- Take medications if indicated for prevention of herpes outbreak and for pain such as Ultram or Darvocet (1 hour before procedure) as prescribed.
- Bring sun-protective items for postprocedure such as wide-brimmed hat and sunglasses.

## Postprocedure

- Sleep and rest with your head and shoulders elevated postprocedure day 0–4 to help minimize the swelling that may occur around the eyes and cheeks.
- Avoid activities that can cause flushing for 2 weeks after treatment.
- Avoid aggressive facial treatments such as microdermabrasion and chemical peels for 4 weeks and any topical products that may cause irritation for 6 weeks following treatment.
- Acne lesions or milia (white-colored tiny keratin plugs) can occur up to a month after treatment.
- Contact our office if you develop acne or milia. If you have been prescribed a medicine for acne, continue to take all medication as prescribed.
- If blistering, crusting, or scabbing develops, call our office immediately. Apply a thin layer of antibiotic ointment (such as bacitracin) to the area twice a day until the skin heals. Do not pick or attempt to remove scabs that form following your treatment, as this may incur infection or scarring.

## Postprocedure Days 0–4

- Immediately after treatment, the skin will be red and feel sensitive and sunburned. There may be pinpoint bleeding. There may be some facial swelling, particularly around the eye area.
- Cleanse the treatment area only with vinegar soaks (see below) 6–8 times/day for day 0–2, then three to four times/day for day 3–4. Apply an occlusive moisturizer such as Hydra Balm generously as needed to keep the skin moist at all times.
- Apply a cool compress or wrapped ice pack 15 minutes/1–2 hours as needed.

## Vinegar Soaks

Always wash hands before touching the treated skin. Make a vinegar solution with 1 teaspoon of white vinegar in 2 cups of water. Soak the gauze in the vinegar solution and gently apply dripping wet to the treated areas allowing the gauze to remain in place for approximately 10–15 minutes. Using gentle pressure, wipe the treated area using the gauze. Do not tug or pull at skin. Serous drainage and/or tiny areas of bleeding in the treated areas may be present on day 0–1. Avoid aggressively rubbing the treated area.

## Postprocedure Days 5–7

- The skin will be less red and should not feel uncomfortable. There should not be any pinpoint bleeding. Dryness, itchiness, and skin peeling or flaking may occur. Redness typically lasts 1–2 weeks and mild redness may be prolonged.

- Gently wash twice daily with mild facial cleanser (e.g., Gentle Cleanser), do not rub the skin vigorously and avoid hot water as the skin will be fragile.
- When advised by provider, switch to using less occlusive moisturizer such as Epidermal Repair for 2 weeks, then change to Emollience. Apply a physical sunscreen (with titanium and/or zinc) after the application of the moisturizer is fully absorb. If the treated area still feels dry consult the skincare specialist.
- Mineral makeup may be applied if desired once sunscreen is being used.

*This form is intended to serve only as an example and should be modified accordingly based on patient and provider needs. (Courtesy of Monterey Bay Laser Aesthetics.)*

# Hair Removal
# Consent for Laser Treatments

This consent form provides the necessary information to make an informed decision about whether or not to undergo laser/intense pulsed light (collectively referred to as laser) treatments for the removal of unwanted hair.

The laser energy targets and destroys the pigmented hair follicles in the active growth phase while the lighter surrounding skin is typically left unaffected. As hair follicles grow in different cycles, multiple treatments are needed. Results vary and no guarantees can be made that a specific patient will benefit from treatment or achieve any level of improvement.

Possible risks, side effects, and complications of laser treatments include, but are not limited to:

1. Discomfort/pain during treatment, temporary redness, and swelling may occur.
2. Bruising, blistering, burns, scabbing, and infection may also occur, but are rare.
3. Patients with darker skin types have an increased risk of complications such as hypopigmentation, hyperpigmentation, blistering, scarring, and more variable results.
4. Laser treatments may produce visible patterns within the skin. The occurrence of this is not predictable and is typically temporary but may be permanent.
5. Very rare risk of accidental eye injury if struck by any laser beam even though laser safety precautions and eye protection are always used throughout all laser treatments.
6. Recurrent viral infections such as herpes simplex (cold sores, genital herpes) or varicella (shingles) may be activated by laser treatments.
7. Tattoos and permanent makeup in the treatment area may be altered unintentionally.

Patients with the following conditions may not receive laser treatments: history of abnormal raised scarring or keloid formation, pregnancy or lactation, history of seizures, tanned skin, tanning bed use, or active sun exposure 4 weeks prior to treatment.

My signature below certifies that I have fully read this consent form and understand the information provided to me regarding the proposed procedure.

Patient Name _____

Patient Signature _____  Date _____

Witness _____  Date _____

*This form is intended to serve only as an example and should be modified accordingly based on patient and provider needs. (Courtesy of Monterey Bay Laser Aesthetics.)*

# Pigmented Lesion
# Consent for Laser Treatments

This consent form provides the necessary information to make an informed decision about whether or not to undergo laser/intense pulsed light (collectively referred to as laser) treatments for benign pigmented lesions.

The laser energy targets and reduces pigmented lesions including sun spots, mottled pigmentation, and melasma while leaving the surrounding skin typically unaffected.

Individual results vary and no guarantees can be made that a specific patient will benefit from treatment or achieve any level of improvement. Results are cumulative and several treatments may be necessary to achieve maximum benefit.

Possible risks, side effects, and complications of laser treatments include, but are not limited to:

1. Discomfort/pain during treatment, temporary redness, and swelling may occur.
2. Bruising, blistering, burns, scabbing, and infection may also occur, but are rare.
3. Undesired skin texture changes or undesired pigment changes such as hypopigmentation (skin lightening) or hyperpigmentation (skin darkening or discoloration) may occur. These pigment changes typically resolve in 3–6 months, but in rare cases may be permanent.
4. Patients with darker skin types have an increased risk of complications such as hypopigmentation, hyperpigmentation, blistering, scarring, and more variable results.
5. Laser treatments may produce visible patterns within the skin. The occurrence of this is not predictable and is typically temporary but may be permanent.
6. Very rare risk of accidental eye injury if struck by any laser beam even though laser safety precautions and eye protection are always used throughout all laser treatments.
7. Recurrent viral infections such as herpes simplex (cold sores, genital herpes) or varicella (shingles) may be activated by laser treatments.
8. Hair follicles, tattoos, and permanent makeup in the treatment area may be altered unintentionally.

Patients with the following conditions may not receive laser treatments: history of abnormal raised scarring or keloid formation, pregnancy or lactation, history of seizures, tanned skin, tanning bed use, or active sun exposure 4 weeks prior to treatment.

My signature below certifies that I have fully read this consent form and understand the information provided to me regarding the proposed procedure.

Patient Name _____

Patient Signature _____        Date _____

Witness _____        Date _____

*This form is intended to serve only as an example and should be modified accordingly based on patient and provider needs. (Courtesy of Monterey Bay Laser Aesthetics.)*

# Vascular Lesion Consent for Laser Treatments

This consent form provides the necessary information to make an informed decision about whether or not to undergo laser/intense pulsed light (collectively referred to as laser) treatments for benign pigmented lesions.

The laser energy targets red vascular lesions including facial blood vessels and rosacea to help improve appearance while leaving the surrounding skin typically unaffected.

Individual results vary and no guarantees can be made that a specific patient will benefit from treatment or achieve any level of improvement. Several treatments may be necessary to achieve maximum benefit.

Possible risks, side effects, and complications of laser treatments include, but are not limited to:

1. Discomfort/pain during treatment, temporary redness, and swelling may occur.
2. Bruising, blistering, burns, scabbing, and infection may also occur, but are rare.
3. Undesired skin texture changes or undesired pigment changes such as hypopigmentation (skin lightening) or hyperpigmentation (skin darkening or discoloration) may occur. These pigment changes typically resolve in 3–6 months, but in rare cases may be permanent.
4. Patients with darker skin types have an increased risk of complications such as hypopigmentation, hyperpigmentation, blistering, scarring, and more variable results.
5. Laser treatments may produce visible patterns within the skin. The occurrence of this is not predictable and is typically temporary but may be permanent.
6. Very rare risk of accidental eye injury if struck by any laser beam even though laser safety precautions and eye protection are always used throughout all laser treatments.
7. Recurrent viral infections such as herpes simplex (cold sores and genital herpes) or varicella (shingles) may be activated by laser treatments.
8. Hair follicles, tattoos, and permanent makeup in the treatment area may be altered unintentionally

Patients with the following conditions may not receive laser treatments: history of abnormal raised scarring or keloid formation, pregnancy or lactation, history of seizures, tanned skin, tanning bed use, or active sun exposure 4 weeks prior to treatment.

My signature below certifies that I have fully read this consent form and understand the information provided to me regarding the proposed procedure.

Patient Name _____

Patient Signature _____     Date _____

Witness _____     Date _____

*This form is intended to serve only as an example and should be modified accordingly based on patient and provider needs. (Courtesy of Monterey Bay Laser Aesthetics.)*

# Tattoo Removal
# Consent for Laser Treatments

This consent form provides the necessary information to make an informed decision about whether or not to undergo laser tattoo removal treatments.

The purpose of this procedure is removal of the tattoo or to make the pattern as unrecognizable as possible by lightening the tattoo pigment. Anesthesia with local injectable, topical, or no anesthesia may be used. The laser energy directly targets tattoo ink in the skin, which disrupts the ink and allows the body's immune system to break it down and get rid of it.

Individual results vary and no guarantees can be made that a specific patient will benefit from treatment or achieve any level of improvement. Multiple treatments will be necessary to achieve desired results.

Possible risks, side effects, and complications of the procedure include, but are not limited to:

1. Pain during treatment, temporary redness, and swelling.
2. Bleeding, bruising, blistering, burns, scabbing, and infection may occur.
3. Undesired skin texture changes or undesired pigment changes such as hypopigmentation (skin lightening) or hyperpigmentation (skin darkening or discoloration) may occur.
4. Patients with darker skin types have an increased risk of complications such as hypopigmentation, hyperpigmentation, blistering, scarring, and more variable results.
5. Very rare risk of accidental eye injury if struck by any laser beam even though laser safety precautions and eye protection are always used throughout all laser treatments.
6. Recurrent viral infections such as herpes simplex (cold sores and genital herpes) or varicella (shingles) may be activated by laser treatments.
7. Hair follicles may be altered unintentionally.
8. Residual tattoo pigment or persistence of tattoo pattern is possible.

Patients with the following conditions may not receive laser treatments: history of abnormal raised scarring or keloid formation, pregnancy or lactation, history of seizures, tanned skin, tanning bed use, or active sun exposure 4 weeks prior to treatment.

My signature below certifies that I have fully read this consent form and understand the information provided to me regarding the proposed procedure.

Patient Name _____

Patient Signature _____    Date _____

Witness _____    Date _____

*This form is intended to serve only as an example and should be modified accordingly based on patient and provider needs. (Courtesy of Monterey Bay Laser Aesthetics.)*

# Wrinkles-Nonablative Resurfacing Consent for Laser Treatments

This consent form provides the necessary information to make an informed decision about whether or not to undergo laser/intense pulsed light (collectively referred to as laser) treatments for nonablative laser resurfacing.

The laser energy heats the dermis, the deeper layer of the skin, resulting in a process referred to as *collagen remodeling*, which can reduce wrinkles, pore size, depression scars, and improve rough skin texture.

Individual results vary and no guarantees can be made that a specific patient will benefit from treatment or achieve any level of improvement. Results are cumulative and several treatments may be necessary to achieve maximum benefit.

Possible risks, side effects, and complications of laser treatments include, but are not limited to:

1. Discomfort/pain during treatment, temporary redness, and swelling may occur.
2. Bruising, blistering, burns, scabbing, and infection may also occur, but are rare.
3. Undesired skin texture changes or undesired pigment changes such as hypopigmentation (skin lightening) or hyperpigmentation (skin darkening or discoloration) may occur. These pigment changes typically resolve in 3–6 months, but in rare cases may be permanent.
4. Patients with darker skin types have an increased risk of complications such as hypopigmentation, hyperpigmentation, blistering, scarring, and more variable results.
5. Laser treatments may produce visible patterns within the skin. The occurrence of this is not predictable and is typically temporary but may be permanent.
6. Very rare risk of accidental eye injury if struck by any laser beam even though laser safety precautions and eye protection are always used throughout all laser treatments.
7. Recurrent viral infections such as herpes simplex (cold sores, genital herpes) or varicella (shingles) may be activated by laser treatments.
8. Hair follicles, tattoos, and permanent makeup in the treatment area may be altered unintentionally.

Patients with the following conditions may not receive laser treatments: history of abnormal raised scarring or keloid formation, pregnancy or lactation, history of seizures, tanned skin, tanning bed use, or active sun exposure 4 weeks prior to treatment.

My signature below certifies that I have fully read this consent form and understand the information provided to me regarding the proposed procedure.

Patient Name _____

Patient Signature _____  Date _____

Witness _____  Date _____

*This form is intended to serve only as an example and should be modified accordingly based on patient and provider needs. (Courtesy of Monterey Bay Laser Aesthetics.)*

# Wrinkles-Ablative Resurfacing Consent for Laser Treatments

This consent form provides the necessary information to make an informed decision about whether or not to undergo ablative laser resurfacing treatments.

The laser energy heats the dermis tissue and starts a natural healing process that forms new, healthy skin, which can reduce wrinkles, pore size, depression scars, and improve rough skin texture. Individual results vary, and no guarantees can be made that a specific patient will benefit from treatment or achieve any level of improvement. In general, most people do experience improvement, which is typically seen 3–6 months after treatment, although improvements may be seen sooner.

Possible risks, side effects, and complications of laser resurfacing include, but are not limited to:

1. Discomfort or pain during and after treatment that typically resolve within 2–3 days.
2. Redness and swelling immediately after treatment and that typically resolve within 1 week.
3. Pigment changes such as hypopigmentation (skin lightening) or hyperpigmentation (skin darkening or discoloration) that usually resolve in 3–6 months but may be permanent. Patients with darker skin types have increased risks.
4. Risk of bacterial, fungal, or viral infection with broken skin barrier.
5. Blistering, scabbing, and scarring are rare but can occur.
6. Laser treatments may produce visible patterns within the skin. The occurrence of this is not predictable and is typically temporary but may be permanent.
7. Very rare risk of accidental eye injury if struck by any laser beam even though laser safety precautions, and eye protection are always used throughout all laser treatments.
8. Recurrent viral infections such as herpes simplex (cold sores and genital herpes) or varicella (shingles) may be activated by laser treatments.
9. Hair follicles, tattoos, and permanent makeup in the treatment area may be altered unintentionally.

Patients with the following conditions may not receive laser treatments: history of abnormal raised scarring or keloid formation, pregnancy or lactation, history of seizures, tanned skin, tanning bed use, or active sun exposure 4 weeks prior to treatment.

My signature below certifies that I have fully read this consent form and understand the information provided to me regarding the proposed procedure.

Patient Name _____

Patient Signature _____      Date _____

Witness _____      Date _____

*This form is intended to serve only as an example and should be modified accordingly based on patient and provider needs. (Courtesy of Monterey Bay Laser Aesthetics.)*

# Hair Removal Procedure Note for Laser Treatments

Name:_____     DOB:_____

**Fitzpatrick Skin Type:** _____

| | | Wavelength | Pulse width | Fluence | Passes |
|---|---|---|---|---|---|

**Date:_____ Tx #_____**   Area:_____   _____nm   _____ms   _____J/cm   _____

Handpiece:_____   _____nm   _____ms   _____J/cm

**Initial Visit**   |   **Pregnancy:**☐ No   ☐Yes   |   **Response from Tx:**   **Pain Score:____/10**

**Subjective:**
☐ Unwanted hair
☐ Reduce hair/folliculitis

NOTES:_____
_____

Shaved at visit:   ☐ Yes   ☐ No

**Objective:**
☐ Blond/Gray/Red/Dark hair
☐ Course/Fine hair
☐ Good/Fair/Poor candidate

**Skin prep:**
☐ cleansed
☐ other:_____
☐ gel applied

☐Singed hair smell ☐Hair extrusion ☐Erythema ____
☐Perifollicular edema (PFE) mild/moderate
☐Complication _____

**Post-Tx:**
☐Cold Compress   ☐HC 1%   ☐HC 2.5%/TAC .5%
☐Sunblock   ☐Other:_____

**Provider:**_____

---

**Date:_____ Tx #_____**   Area:_____   _____ms   _____J/cm   _____

Handpiece:_____   _____ms   _____J/cm

**Pregnancy:**☐ No   ☐Yes   |   **Response from Tx:**   **Pain Score:____/10**

**Subjective:**
Last sun exposure was _____
Hair growth reduction from initial
   ☐ Yes ____% ☐ No
☐Patchy regrowth
☐Hair is lighter/finer

Shaved at visit:   ☐ Yes   ☐ No

**Objective:**
Hair growth reduction from
initial visit
   ☐ Yes ____% ☐ No

**Skin prep:**
☐ cleansed
☐ other:_____
☐ gel applied

☐Singed hair smell ☐Hair extrusion ☐Erythema ____
☐Perifollicular edema (PFE) mild/moderate
☐Complication _____

**Post-Tx:**
☐Cold Compress   ☐HC 1%   ☐HC 2.5%/TAC .5%
☐Sunblock   ☐Other:_____

**Provider:**_____

---

**Date:_____ Tx #_____**   Area:_____   _____ms   _____J/cm   _____

Handpiece:_____   _____ms   _____J/cm

**Pregnancy:**☐ No   ☐Yes   |   **Response from Tx:**   **Pain Score:____/10**

**Subjective:**
Last sun exposure was _____
Hair growth reduction from initial
   ☐ Yes ____% ☐ No
☐Patchy regrowth
☐Hair is lighter/finer

Shaved at visit:   ☐ Yes   ☐ No

**Objective:**
Hair growth reduction from
initial visit
   ☐ Yes ____% ☐ No

**Skin prep:**
☐ cleansed
☐ other:_____
☐ gel applied

☐Singed hair smell ☐Hair extrusion ☐Erythema ____
☐Perifollicular edema (PFE) mild/moderate
☐Complication _____

**Post-Tx:**
☐Cold Compress   ☐HC 1%   ☐HC 2.5%/TAC .5%
☐Sunblock   ☐Other:_____

**Provider:**_____

*This form is intended to serve only as an example and should be modified accordingly based on patient and provider needs. (Courtesy of Monterey Bay Laser Aesthetics.)*

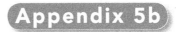

# Pigmented Lesion Procedure Note for Laser Treatments

Name:_____     DOB:_____

**Fitzpatrick Skin Type:** _____

| | | Wavelength | Pulse width | Fluence | Passes |
|---|---|---|---|---|---|

| Date:_____ Tx #_____ | Area:_____ | ____nm | ____ms | ____J/cm | ____ |
| | Handpiece:_____ | ____nm | ____ms | ____J/cm | ____ |

**Initial Visit**

**Subjective:**
☐ Uneven pigment
☐ Lentigos

**NOTES:**_____
_____

**Pregnancy:** ☐ No   ☐ Yes

**Objective:**
☐ Uneven pigment
☐ Lentigos

**Skin prep:**
☐ cleansed
☐ other:_____
☐ gel applied

**Response from Tx:**          **Pain Score:**_____/10
☐ ↑Pigmentation   ☐ Erythema:_____
☐ Complication _____

**Post-Tx:**
☐ Cold Compress   ☐ HC 1%   ☐HC 2.5%/TAC .5%
☐ Sunblock   ☐ Other:_____

**Provider:**_____

---

| Date:_____ Tx #_____ | Area:_____ | ____ms | ____J/cm | ____ |
| | Handpiece:_____ | ____ms | ____J/cm | ____ |

Any swelling/redness/purpura from last tx lasted _____ days
☐ Pigment darkened & flaked

Last sun exposure was _____

**S  &  O** (subjective/objective)
☐__ % ☐__% Improve from initial
☐         ☐Uneven pigment
☐         ☐Lentigos

**Pregnancy:** ☐ No   ☐ Yes

**Objective:**
☐ Uneven pigment
☐ Lentigos

**Skin prep:**
☐ cleansed
☐ other:_____
☐ gel applied

**Response from Tx:**          **Pain Score:**_____/10
☐ ↑Pigmentation   ☐ Erythema:_____
☐ Complication _____

**Post-Tx:**
☐ Cold Compress   ☐ HC 1%   ☐HC 2.5%/TAC .5%
☐ Sunblock   ☐ Other:_____

**Provider:**_____

---

| Date:_____ Tx #_____ | Area:_____ | ____ms | ____J/cm | ____ |
| | Handpiece:_____ | ____ms | ____J/cm | ____ |

Any swelling/redness/purpura from last tx lasted _____ days
☐ Pigment darkened & flaked

Last sun exposure was _____

**S  &  O** (subjective/objective)
☐__ % ☐__% Improve from initial
☐         ☐Uneven pigment
☐         ☐Lentigos

**Pregnancy:** ☐ No   ☐ Yes

**Objective:**
☐ Uneven pigment
☐ Lentigos

**Skin prep:**
☐ cleansed
☐ other:_____
☐ gel applied

**Response from Tx:**          **Pain Score:**_____/10
☐ ↑Pigmentation   ☐ Erythema:
☐ Complication _____

**Post-Tx:**
☐ Cold Compress   ☐ HC 1%   ☐HC 2.5%/TAC .5%
☐ Sunblock   ☐ Other:_____

**Provider:**_____

*This form is intended to serve only as an example and should be modified accordingly based on patient and provider needs. (Courtesy of Monterey Bay Laser Aesthetics.)*

# Vascular Lesion Procedure Note for Laser Treatments

Name:_____     DOB:_____

**Fitzpatrick Skin Type:** _____

| | | Wavelength | Pulse width | Fluence | Passes |
|---|---|---|---|---|---|

Date:_____ Tx #_____    Area:_____    ____nm    ____ms    ____J/cm    ____

Handpiece:_____    ____nm    ____ms    ____J/cm    ____

**Initial Visit**    **Pregnancy:**☐ No    ☐Yes    **Response from Tx:**    **Pain Score:**____/10

**Subjective:**    **Objective:**    ☐Vessel changes _____    ☐ Erythema_____
  ☐ Telangiectasias      ☐ Telangiectasias    ☐ Complication(s) _____
  ☐ Angiomas      ☐ Angiomas
    **Post-Tx:**
    **Skin prep:**    ☐ Cold Compress  ☐ HC 1%  ☐HC 2.5%/TAC .5%
NOTES:_____    ☐ cleansed    ☐ Sunblock  ☐ Other _____
_____    ☐ other _____
    ☐ gel applied    **Provider:**_____

---

Date:_____ Tx #_____    Area:_____    _____ms    _____J/cm$^2$    _____

Handpiece:_____    _____ms    _____J/cm$^2$    _____

Swelling/redness/purpura from    **Pregnancy:**☐ No    ☐Yes    **Response from Tx:**    **Pain Score:**____/10
last tx: ☐ No    ☐Yes
Lasted _____ days    **Objective:**    ☐Vessel changes _____    ☐ Erythema_____
      ☐ Telangiectasias    ☐ Complication(s) _____
Last sun exposure was _____    ☐ Angiomas
    **Post-Tx:**
**S  & O** (subjective/objective)    **Skin prep:**    ☐ Cold Compress  ☐ HC 1%  ☐HC 2.5%/TAC .5%
☐__ % ☐__% Improved from initial    ☐ cleansed    ☐ Sunblock  ☐ Other _____
☐      ☐    Vessel(s) diminishing    ☐ other _____
    ☐ gel applied    **Provider:**_____

---

Date:_____ Tx #_____    Area:_____    _____ms    _____J/cm$^2$    _____

Handpiece:_____    _____ms    _____J/cm$^2$    _____

Swelling/redness/purpura from    **Pregnancy:**☐ No    ☐Yes    **Response from Tx:**    **Pain Score:**____/10
last tx: ☐ No    ☐Yes
Lasted _____ days    **Objective:**    ☐Vessel changes    ☐ Erythema
      ☐ Telangiectasias    ☐ Complication(s) _____
Last sun exposure was _____    ☐ Angiomas
    **Post-Tx:**
**S  & O** (subjective/objective)    **Skin prep:**    ☐ Cold Compress  ☐ HC 1%  ☐HC 2.5%/TAC .5%
☐__ % ☐__% Improved from initial    ☐ cleansed    ☐ Sunblock  ☐ Other _____
☐      ☐    Vessel(s) diminishing    ☐ other _____
    ☐ gel applied    **Provider:**_____

*This form is intended to serve only as an example and should be modified accordingly based on patient and provider needs. (Courtesy of Monterey Bay Laser Aesthetics.)*

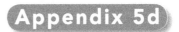

# Tattoo Removal
# Procedure Note
# for Laser Treatments

Name:_____     DOB:_____

**Fitzpatrick Skin Type:** _____

| | | Wavelength | Spot Size | Fluence | Frequency | Passes |
|---|---|---|---|---|---|---|

Date:_____ Tx #_____ | Area:_____ | _____nm _____mm _____J/cm ___HZ _____

Color(s):_____ | _____nm _____mm _____J/cm ___HZ _____

**Initial Visit** | **Pregnant:** ☐ No   ☐ Yes | **Response from Tx:**          **Pain Score:**_____/10
☐ Edema                    ☐ Whitening/yellowing

**Subjective:** | **Objective:** | ☐ Petechiae              ☐ Pinpoint bleeding
Last sun exposure was _____ | | ☐ Complication/Other _____
Tattoo placed on ___/___/_____ |
By professional artist ☐ Yes   ☐ No | **Skin prep:** | **Post-Tx:**
Cover up          ☐ Yes   ☐ No | ☐ cleansed | ☐ Cold Compress  ☐ HC 1%  ☐ HC 2.5%/TAC .5%
Color(s): _____ | ☐ other: _____ | ☐ Sunblock  ☐ Other:_____

**Provider:** _____

Date:_____ Tx #_____ | Area:_____ | _____nm _____mm _____J/cm ___HZ _____

Color(s):_____ | _____nm _____mm _____J/cm ___HZ _____

**Subjective:** | **Pregnant:** ☐ No   ☐ Yes | **Response from Tx:**          **Pain Score:**_____/10
Reduction from initial _____% | | ☐ Edema                   ☐ Whitening/yellowing
Last sun exposure _____ | **Objective:** | ☐ Petechiae             ☐ Pinpoint bleeding
Response from last treatment: | Shiny/unhealed ☐ Yes  ☐ No | ☐ Complication/Other _____
Blisters        ☐ Yes   ☐ No |
Crusting       ☐ Yes   ☐ No | | **Post-Tx:**
Abraded       ☐ Yes   ☐ No | **Skin prep:** | ☐ Cold Compress   ☐ HC 1%   ☐ HC 2.5%/TAC .5%
Hyperpigm    ☐ Yes   ☐ No | ☐ cleansed | ☐ Sunblock   ☐ Other:_____
Hypopigm    ☐ Yes   ☐ No | ☐ other: _____ |

**Provider:** _____

Date:_____ Tx #_____ | Area:_____ | _____nm _____mm _____J/cm ___HZ _____

Color(s):_____ | _____nm _____mm _____J/cm ___HZ _____

**Subjective:** | **Pregnant:** ☐ No   ☐ Yes | **Response from Tx:**          **Pain Score:**_____/10
Reduction from initial _____% | | ☐ Edema                   ☐ Whitening/yellowing
Last sun exposure _____ | **Objective:** | ☐ Petechiae             ☐ Pinpoint bleeding
Response from last treatment: | Shiny/unhealed ☐ Yes  ☐ No | ☐ Complication/Other _____
Blisters        ☐ Yes   ☐ No |
Crusting       ☐ Yes   ☐ No | | **Post-Tx:**
Abraded       ☐ Yes   ☐ No | **Skin prep:** | ☐ Cold Compress   ☐ HC 1%   ☐ HC 2.5%/TAC .5%
Hyperpigm    ☐ Yes   ☐ No | ☐ cleansed | ☐ Sunblock   ☐ Other:_____
Hypopigm    ☐ Yes   ☐ No | ☐ other: _____ |

**Provider:** _____

*This form is intended to serve only as an example and should be modified accordingly based on patient and provider needs. (Courtesy of Monterey Bay Laser Aesthetics.)*

# Wrinkles-Nonablative Resurfacing Procedure Note for Laser Treatments

Name:_____     DOB:_____

Fitzpatrick Skin Type:_____

| | | Wavelength | Spot Size | Fluence | Frequency | Passes |
|---|---|---|---|---|---|---|

| Date:_____ Tx #_____ | Area:_____ | ____nm  ____mm  ____J/cm  ____HZ  ____ |
|---|---|---|
| | | ____mm  ____nm  ____J/cm  ____HZ  ____ |

**Initial Visit**

Pregnancy:☐ No   ☐Yes

**Subjective:**
☐ Rough texture/fine lines
☐ Enlarged pore size

**Objective:**
☐ Rough texture/fine lines
☐ Enlarged pore size

**Skin prep:**
☐ cleansed
☐ other:_____

NOTES:_____
_____

**Response from Tx:**          Pain Score:_____/10

☐↑Pigmentation   ☐ Plumes   ☐ Erythema:_____
☐ Complication _____

**Post-Tx:**
☐ Cold Compress   ☐ HC 1%   ☐HC 2.5%/TAC .5%
☐ Sunblock   ☐ Other:_____

**Provider:**_____

---

| Date:_____ Tx #_____ | Area:_____ | ____mm  ____J/cm  ____HZ  _____ |
|---|---|---|
| | | ____mm  ____J/cm  ____HZ  _____ |

Any swelling/redness/purpura from last tx lasted _____ days

Last sun exposure was _____ days

**S & O** (subjective/objective)
☐__ %  ☐__% Improve from initial
☐        ☐Texture/fine lines improve
☐        ☐Pore size diminishing

Pregnancy:☐ No   ☐Yes

**Objective:**
☐ Rough texture/fine lines
☐ Enlarged pore size

**Skin prep:**
☐ cleansed
☐ other:_____

**Response from Tx:**          Pain Score:_____/10

☐↑Pigmentation   ☐ Plumes   ☐ Erythema:_____
☐ Complication _____

**Post-Tx:**
☐ Cold Compress   ☐ HC 1%   ☐HC 2.5%/TAC .5%
☐ Sunblock   ☐ Other:_____

**Provider:**_____

---

| Date:_____ Tx #_____ | Area:_____ | ____mm  ____J/cm  ____HZ  _____ |
|---|---|---|
| | | ____mm  ____J/cm  ____HZ  _____ |

Any swelling/redness/purpura from last tx lasted _____ days

Last sun exposure was _____ days

**S & O** (subjective/objective)
☐__ %  ☐__% Improve from initial
☐        ☐Texture/fine lines improve
☐        ☐Pore size diminishing

Pregnancy:☐ No   ☐Yes

**Objective:**
☐ Rough texture/fine lines
☐ Enlarged pore size

**Skin prep:**
☐ cleansed
☐ other:_____

**Response from Tx:**          Pain Score:_____/10

☐↑Pigmentation   ☐ Plumes   ☐ Erythema:_____
☐ Complication _____

**Post-Tx:**
☐ Cold Compress   ☐ HC 1%   ☐HC 2.5%/TAC .5%
☐ Sunblock   ☐ Other:_____

**Provider:**_____

*This form is intended to serve only as an example and should be modified accordingly based on patient and provider needs. (Courtesy of Monterey Bay Laser Aesthetics.)*

# Wrinkles-Ablative Resurfacing Procedure Note for Laser Treatments

Name:_____     DOB:_____

**Physical exam:**                          Date:_____
Fitzpatrick Skin Type: _____

| Medications | □ See Med list |
|---|---|
| Coumadin | Y     N |
| Aspirin | Y     N |
| Antiviral _____ | |
| Other Meds _____ | |
| Allergies _____ | |

History of:

| Vitiligo | Y | N |
|---|---|---|
| Herpes | Y | N |
| Candida | Y | N |
| Smoker | Y | N |
| Accutane past year | Y | N |

| Pre-procedure checklist performed | Y | N |
|---|---|---|
| Consent signed in the chart | Y | N |
| Pre/Post instructions reviewed | Y | N |
| Follow-up appointments made | Y | N |

Lid snap test        strong/weak lower elasticity

Vital signs:  BP _____ HR _____ Temp _____

**Indications for treatment:** _____

Medications:
        Med and dose: _____
Anesthesia:
        Topical anesthetic: _____ was applied with/without occlusion for _____ minutes
        Injectable anesthetic: ____ml of _____ with/without epinephrine was injected at_____
The laser was passed over the _____ (treatment area), and the following parameters were used:
Mode: Fractional/Nonfractional/Other _____
Spot size: _____ mm
Beam density: _____
Beam shape: _____
Frequency: _____Hz
Fluence: _____J/cm$^2$
Overlap: None/_____%
No. of passes: _____

**Procedure:**  Ablative laser skin resurfacing

Time:_____

Immediately post-procedure:
        Mild/Mod/Severe erythema: _____area of skin
        Blood loss:                □ < 1ml□ _____ml       Vital signs:  BP _____ HR _____
        Complications:             □ None                  □ _____

Post-laser Skin Care
        Patient reported ____/10 pain level immediately post treatment
        Sterile saline saturated gauze and ice pack placed over treatment area for _____ minutes
        Occlusive petrolatum topical product _____ applied

Notes: _____

Follow-up appointment(s):     Date: _____     Time: _____

                              Provider Signature:_____

*This form is intended to serve only as an example and should be modified accordingly based on patient and provider needs.*
*(Courtesy of Monterey Bay Laser Aesthetics.)*

# Supply Sources

## Laser and Intense Pulsed Light Devices

| Supplier | Hair Removal | Pigmented Lesions* | Vascular Lesions* | Tattoo Removal | Wrinkles—Nonablative Resurfacing | Wrinkles—Ablative Resurfacing |
|---|---|---|---|---|---|---|
| Aerolase | X | X | X | | X | X |
| Alma Lasers | X | X | X | X | X | X |
| Asclepion Lasers | X | | | X | | X |
| CoolTouch | X | X | | | X | |
| Cutera | X | X | X | | X | X |
| Cynosure/Deka/ Palomar/ConBio | X | X | X | X | X | X |
| Ellipse | X | X | X | | | |
| Energist Medical Group | X | X | X | | X | X |
| Focus Medical | X | X | X | X | | X |
| Fotona | X | X | X | X | | X |
| General Project | X | X | X | | | |
| Lasering USA | X | X | X | | X | X |
| Lumenis | X | X | X | X | X | X |
| Lutronic | X | X | X | X | X | X |
| Novalis Medical | X | X | X | | X | |
| Radiancy | X | X | X | | X | |
| Sciton | X | X | X | | X | X |
| SharpLight Technologies | X | X | X | | | |
| Solta Medical | | | | | X | X |
| Syneron/Candela | X | X | X | X | X | X |

*Devices for benign pigmented lesions and red vascular lesions are primarily for lesions found in photodamaged skin (i.e., not for congenital lesions such as vascular malformations and nevi).

Aerolase
914-345-8300
www.aerolase.com

Alma Lasers
866-414-2562
www.almalasers.com

Asclepion Lasers
49 (0) 3641 7700 100
www.asclepion.com

CoolTouch
877-858-2665
www.cooltouch.com

Cutera
888-428-8372
www.cutera.com

Cynosure, Cynosure/Deka, Cynosure/
  Palomar and Cynosure/ConBio
800-886-2966
www.cynosure.com

Ellipse A/S
45-4576-8808
www.ellipse.com

Energist Medical Group
44 (0)1792 798768
www.energistgroup.com

Focus Medical
866-633-5273
www.focusmedical.com

Fotona
888-550-4113
www.fotona.com

General Project
908-454-8875
www.generalproject.com

Lasering
866-471-0469
www.laseringusa.com

Lumenis
408-764-3000
www.lumenis.com

Novalis Medical
866-627-4475
www.novalismedical.com

Radiancy
888-661-2220
www.radiancy.com

Sciton
888-646-6999
www.sciton.com

SharpLight Technologies
866-512-7797
www.sharplightech.com

Solta Medical
510-782-2286
www.solta.com

Syneron/Candela
866-259-6661
www.syneron-candela.com

**Laser Eyewear**
Glendale
800-500-4739
www.glendale-laser.com

Innovative Optics
763-425-7789
www.Innovativeoptics.com

Oculo-Plastik
888-381-3292
www.oculoplastik.com

**Smoke Evacuator**
Buffalo Filter PlumeSafe Turbo™
800-343-2324
www.buffalofilter.com

**Analgesic Devices**
ArTek Air™ (forced air cooling)
ThermoTek
972-874-4949
www.thermotekusa.com

Zimmer Cryo 6™ (forced air cooling)
LaserMed, LLC
800-530-8041
www.zimmercoolers.com

Serenity Pro™ (pneumatic skin flattening)
Syneron/Candela
866-259-6661
www.syneron-candela.com

## Icing Supplies

Instant Cold Compress™ (disposable)
Cypress Medical Products
800-334-3646
www.cypressmed.com

Jact Frost™ (reusable)
Cardinal Health
614-757-5000
www.cardinal.com

Ice Roller (reusable)
Cynosure/Palomar
800-886-2966
www.cynosure.com

## Topical Anesthetics

Benzocaine:lidocaine:tetracaine (20:6:4)
  ointment
American Health Solutions Pharmacy
310-838-7422
www.AHSRx.com

EMLA® (lidocaine 2.5%:prilocaine 2.5%)
Fresenius Kabi USA/APP Pharmaceuticals
888-386-1300
www.fresenius-kabi.us

L-M-X® (lidocaine 4–5%)
PharmaDerm
973-514-4240
www.pharmaderm.com

## Topical Silicone

ScarAway® (gel sheet)
Mitchell-Vance Laboratories LLC
866-943-7225
www.MyScarAway.com
Mepitel® (gel sheet)
Molnlycke Health Care
800-882-4582
www.molnlycke.com

bioCorneum® (Quick-drying gel)
Enaltus LLC
678-684-1426
www.biocorneum.com

## Hemostasis Agents

Aluminum chloride 35% solution
Medical Chemical Corporation (MCC)
800-424-9394
www.med-chem.com

## Posttreatment Products

Aquaphor™ ointment
Biersdorf Inc.
800-227-4703
www.aquaphorhealing.com

Epidermal Repair™
SkinCeuticals
800-771-9489
www.skinceuticals.com

Emollience™
SkinCeuticals
800-771-9489
www.skinceuticals.com

Gentle Cleanser™
SkinCeuticals
800-771-9489
www.skinceuticals.com

Mineral Make-up
Jane Iredale
800-762-1132
www.janeiredale.com

## Laser Safety Training Courses

American Society for Laser Medicine and
  Surgery (ASLMS)
715-845-9283
www.aslms.org

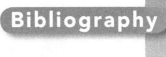

## Aesthetic Procedure Statistics and Overview

Cosmetic Surgery National Data Bank 2014 Statistics. *American Society for Aesthetic Plastic Surgery.* Accessed November 8, 2014.

Small R. Aesthetic procedures in office practice. *Am Fam Physician.* 2009;80(11):1231–1237.

## Photoaging Pathophysiology and Skin Anatomy

Antell D. How environment and lifestyle choices influence the aging process. *Ann Plast Surg.* 2009;43(Volume 6): 585–588.

Choudhary S, Tang JC, Leiva A, et al. Photodamage, Part 1: pathophysiology, Clinical Manifestations, and Photoprotection. *Cosmet Dermatol.* 2010;23:460–466.

El-Domyati M, Attia S, Saleh F, et al. Intrinsic aging vs. photoaging: a comparative histopathological, immunohistochemical, and ultrastructural study of skin. *Exp Dermatol.* 2002;11(5):398–405.

Fisher GJ, Kang S, Varani J, et al. Mechanisms of photoaging and chronological skin aging. *Arch Dermatol.* 2002;138:1462–1470.

Grunebaum LD, Heffelfinger RN. Photoaging. *Curr Probl Dermatol.* 2011;42:122–130.

Lockman AR, Lockman DW. Skin changes in the maturing woman. *Clin Fam Pract.* 2002;4(1):113–134.

Lowe NJ, Meyers DP, Wieder JM. Low doses of repetitive ultraviolet A induce morphologic changes in human skin. *J Invest Dermatol.* 1995;105:739–743.

Rabe JH, Mamelak AJ, McElgunn PJ, et al. Photoaging: mechanisms and repair. *J Am Acad Dermatol.* 2006; 55:1–19.

Yamaguchi Y, Brenner M, Hearing VJ. The regulation of skin pigmentation. *J Biol Chem.* 2007;282(38):27557–27561.

Zimbler MS, Kokoska MS, Thomas JR. Anatomy and pathophysiology of facial aging. *Facial Plast Surg Clin North Am.* 2001;9(2):179–187, vii.

## Dark Skin Types

Szabo G, Gerald AB, Pathak MA, et al. Racial differences in the fate of melanosomes in human epidermis. *Nature.* 1969;222(5198):1081–1082.

Alexis A. Photoaging in skin of color. *Cosmet Dermatol.* 2011;24(8):367.

## Consultation

Fitzpatrick TB. The validity and practicality of sun-reactive skin types I through VI. *Arch Dermatol.* 1988;124(6):869–871.

Glogau RG. Aesthetic and anatomic analysis of the aging skin. *Semin Cutan Med Surg.* 1996;15(3):134–138.

Kuhnel T, Wolf S. Mirror system for photodocumentation in plastic and aesthetic surgery. *Brit J Plast Surg.* 2005;58(6):830–832.

Small R. Aesthetic principles and consultation. In: Usatine R, Pfenninger J, Stuhlberg D, et al., eds. *Dermatologic and Cosmetic Procedures in Office Practice.* Philadelphia, PA: Elsevier; 2011:230–239.

Small R. Aesthetic procedures introduction. In: Mayeaux E, ed. 2nd ed. *The Essential Guide to Primary Care Procedures.* Philadelphia, PA: Lippincott Williams & Wilson, 2015:195–199.

## Laser Principles

Alam M, Hsu TS, Dover JS, et al. Nonablative laser and light treatments: histology and tissue effects–a review. *Lasers Surg Med.* 2003;33(1):30–39.

Anderson RR, Parrish JA. Selective photothermolysis: precise microsurgery by selective absorption of pulsed radiation. *Science*. 1983;220:524–527.

Caroll L, Humphreys TR. LASER-tissue interactions. *Clin Dermatol*. 2006;24(1):2–7.

Kennedy JC, Pottier RH, Pross DC. Photodynamic therapy with endogenous protoporphyrin IX: basic principles and present clinical experience. *J Photochem Photobiol B*. 1990;6(1–2):143–148.

Liu H, Dang Y, Wang Z, et al. Laser induced collagen remodeling: a comparative study in vivo on mouse model. *Lasers Surg Med*. 2008;40(1):13–19.

Manstein D, Herron GS, Sink RK. Fractional photothermolysis: a new concept for cutaneous remodeling using microscopic patterns of thermal injury. *Lasers Surg Med*. 2004;34:426–438.

Anderson RR, Parrish JA. The optics of human skin. *J Invest Dermatol*. 1981;77(1):13–19.

Margolis RJ, Dover JS, Polla LL, et al. Visible action spectrum for melanin-specific selective photothermolysis. *Lasers Surg Med*. 1989;9(4):389–397.

Watanabe S. Basics of laser application to dermatology. *Arch Dermatol Res*. 2008;300(suppl 1):S21–S30.

## Laser Safety

American national standard for the safe use of lasers in health care facilities (ANSI) Z136.3 2011:ISBN#:978–0–9122035–69–7.

Smalley PJ. Laser safety: Risk assessment and quality management. In: *Lasers and Energy Devices for the Skin*. Denver, CO: CRC Press; 2013:364–381.

## Anesthesia

Bernstein EF. Pneumatic skin flattening reduced pain during laser hair reduction. *Lasers Surg Med*. 2008;40:183–187.

Foley K, Pianalto D. Facial anesthesia. *Emerg Med*. 2005;37(6):30–34.

Kawesk S. Topical anesthetic creams [Safety and Efficacy Report]. *Plast Recon Surg*. 2008;121(6):2161–2165.

Latham J, Martin S. Infiltrative anesthesia in office practice. *Am Fam Physician*. 2014;89(12):956–964.

Lee MS. Topical triple-anesthetic gel compared with 3 topical anesthetics. *Cosmet Dermatol*. 2003;26(61):35–38.

Mulroy MF. *Regional Anesthesia, An Illustrated Procedural Guide*. 3rd ed. Philadelphia, PA: Lippincott Williams & Wilkins; 2002.

Salam GA. Regional anesthesia for office procedures: part 1. Head and neck surgeries. *Am Fam Physician*. 2004;69(3):585–590.

Small R. Anesthesia for cosmetic procedures. In: Usatine R, Pfenninger J, Stuhlberg D, et al., eds. *Dermatologic and Cosmetic Procedures in Office Practice*. Philadelphia, PA: Elsevier; 2011.

## Cooling and Analgesic Devices

Kelly KM, Nelson JS, Lask GP, et al. Cryogen spray cooling in combination with nonablative laser treatment of facial rhytides. *Arch Dermatol*. 1999;135(6):691–694.

Lask GP, Friedman D, Eman M, et al. Pneumatic skin flattening (PSF): a novel technology for marked pain reduction in hair removal with high energy density lasers and IPLs. *J Cosmet Laser Ther*. 2006;8(2):76–81.

Zenzie HH, Altschuler GB, Smirnov MZ, et al. Evaluation of cooling methods for laser dermatology. *Lasers Surg Med*. 2000;26(2):130–144.

## Topical Products with Laser Procedures

Darlenski R, Surber C, Fluhr JW. Topical retinoids in the management of photodamaged skin: from theory to evidence-based practical approach. *Brit J Derm*. 2010;163(6):1157–1165.

Nyriady J, Grossman R. Use of tretinoin in precosmetic and postcosmetic procedures: a review. *Cosmet Dermatol*. 2003;16:7–17.

Rendon MI, Cardona L, Benitez A. The safety and efficacy of trolamin/sodium alginate topical emulsion in postlaser resurfacing wounds. *J Drugs Dermatol*. 2008;7(5):S23–S28.

Rendon MI, Gaviria JI. Review of skin-lightening agents. *Dermatol Surg*. 2005;31:886–889.

Tanzi EL, Perez M. The effect of a mucopolysaccharide-cartilage complex healing ointment on Er:YAG laser resurfaced facial skin. *Dermatol Surg*. 2002;28:305–308.

Sachsenberg-Studer EM. Tolerance of topical retinaldehyde in humans. *Dermatology*. 1999;199(suppl 1):61–63.

## Intense Pulsed Light (IPL)

Babilas P, Schreml S, Szeimies RM, et al. Intense pulsed light (IPL): a review. *Lasers Surg Med*. 2010;42(2):93–104.

Ciocon DH, Boker A, Goldberg DJ. Intense pulsed light: what works, what's new, what's next. *Facial Plast Surg*. 2009;25(5):290–300.

Goldberg DJ. Current trends in intense pulsed light. *J Clin Aesthet Dermatol*. 2012;5(6):45–53.

Goldman MP, Weiss RA, Weiss MA. Intense pulsed light as a nonablative approach to photoaging. *Dermatol Surg*. 2005;31(9 Pt 2):1179–1187.

Kligman DE, Zhen Y. Intense pulsed light treatment of photoaged facial skin. *Dermatol Surg*. 2004;30(8):1085–1090.

Schoenewolf NL, Barysch MJ, Dummer R. Intense pulsed light. *Curr Probl Dermatol*. 2011;42:166–172.

Wat H, Wu DC, Rao J, et al. Application of intense pulsed light in the treatment of dermatologic disease: a systematic review. *Dermatol Surg*. 2014;40(4):359–377.

Weiss RA, Weiss MA, Beasly KL. Rejuvenation of photoaged skin: 5 years results with intense pulsed light of the face, neck and chest. *Dermatol Surg*. 2002;28:1115–1119.

## Light Emitting Diode (LED)

Weiss RA, McDaniel DH, Geronemus RG, et al. Clinical experience with light-emitting diode (LED) photomodulation. *Dermatol Surg*. 2005;31(9 Pt 2):1199–1205.

## Photodynamic Therapy (PDT)

Dover JS, Bhatia AC, Stewart B, et al. Topical 5-aminolevulinic acid combined with intense pulsed light in the treatment of photoaging. *Arch Dermatol*. 2005;141(10):1247–1252.

Macgregor JL, Dover JS. The Evolving Role of Photodynamic Therapy for the Treatment of Photoaged Skin. *Dermatol Surg*. 2009;36(1):49–51.

## Home-Use Lasers

Alster TS, Tanzi EL. Effect of a novel low-energy pulsed-light device for home-use hair removal. *Dermatol Surg*. 2009;35:483–489.

Brown AS. At-home laser and light-based devices. *Curr Probl Dermatol*. 2011;42:160–165.

Elm CM, Wallander ID, Walgrave SE, et al. Clinical study to determine the safety and efficacy of a low-energy, pulsed light device for home use hair removal. *Lasers Surg Med*. 2010;42:287–291.

Emerson R, Town G. Hair removal with a novel, low fluence, home-use intense pulsed light device. *J Cosmet Laser Ther*. 2009;11(2):98–105.

Garden JM, Zelickson B, Gold MH, et al. Home hair removal in all skin types with a combined radiofrequency and optical energy source device. *Dermatol Surg*. 2014;40(2):142–151.

Haedersdal M, Beerwerth F, Nash JF. Laser and intense pulsed light hair removal technologies: from professional to home use. *Br J Dermatol*. 2011;165(suppl 3):31–36.

Leyden J, Stephens TJ, Herndon JH, Jr. Multicenter clinical trial of a home-use nonablative fractional laser device for wrinkle reduction. *J Am Acad Dermatol*. 2012;67(5):975–984.

Metelitsa AI, Green JB. Home-use laser and light devices for the skin: an update. *Semin Cutan Med Surg*. 2011;30:144–147.

Mulholland RS. Silk'n–a novel device using Home Pulsed Light for hair removal at home. *J Cosmet Laser Ther*. 2009;11(2):106–109.

Sadick NS. A study to determine the efficacy of a novel handheld light-emitting diode device in the treatment of photoaged skin. *J Cosmet Dermatol*. 2008;7(4):263–267.

Spencer JM. Clinical evaluation of a handheld self-treatment device for hair removal. *J Drugs Dermatol*. 2007;6(8):788–792.

Wheeland RG. Permanent hair reduction with a home-use diode laser: safety and effectiveness 1 year after eight treatments. *Lasers Surg Med*. 2012;44(7):550–557.

Wheeland RG. Simulated consumer use of a battery-powered, hand-held, portable diode laser (810 nm) for hair removal: a safety, efficacy and ease-of-use study. *Lasers Surg Med*. 2007;39:476–493.

## Photoaging

Choudhary S, Tang J, Leiva A, et al. Photodamage, Part 2: management of photoaging. *Cosmet Dermatol*. 2010;23(11):496–509.

Dierickx CC, Anderson RR. Visible light treatment of photoaging. *Dermatol Ther*. 2005;18(3):191–208.

Northington M. Procedural options for aging. *Cosmet Dermatol*. 2011;24(09):426–430.

Papadavid F, Katsambas A. Lasers for facial rejuvenation: a review. *Int J Dermatol*. 2003;42(6):480–487.

Peterson JD, Goldman MP. Rejuvenation of the aging chest: a review and our experience. *Dermatol Surg*. 2011;37(5):555–571.

Rinaldi F. Laser: a review. *Clin Dermatol*. 2008;26(6):590–601.

Rohrer TE. Lasers and cosmetic dermatologic surgery for aging skin. *Clin Geriatr Med*. 2001;17(4):769–794, vii.

Waibel JS. Photorejuvenation. *Dermatol Clin*. 2009;27:445–457, vi.

## Hair Removal

### Overview

Gan SD, Graber EM. Laser hair removal: a review. *Dermatol Surg*. 2013;39(6):823–838.

Battle EF, Hobbs LM. Laser-assisted hair removal for darker skin types. *Dermatol Ther*. 2004;17:177–183.

Ibrahimi OA, Avram MM, Hanke CW, et al. Laser hair removal. *Dermatol Ther*. 2011;24(1):94–107.

Page G. Lasers and pulsed-light devices: hair removal. In: *Pfenninger and Fowler's Procedures for Primary Care*. 3rd ed. Pfenninger JL, Folwer GC, eds. Philadelphia, PA: Mosby/Elsevier; 2010.

Small R. Laser hair removal. In: Mayeaux E, ed. *The Essential Guide to Primary Care Procedures*. Phlidelphia, PA: Lippincott Williams & Wilson; 2009:234–248.

Small R, Chen J. Hair Reduction with Lasers. In: Usatine R, Pfenninger J, Stuhlberg D, et al., eds. *Dermatologic and Cosmetic Procedures in Office Practice*. Philadelphia, PA: Elsevier; 2012:309–321.

## Devices

Amin SP, Goldberg DJ. Clinical comparison of four hair removal lasers and light sources. *J Cosmet Laser Ther*. 2006;8(2):65–68.

Bakus AD, Garden JM, Yaghmai D, et al. Long-term fine caliber hair removal with an electro-optic Q-switched Nd:YAG Laser. *Laser Surg Med*. 2010;42:706–711.

Bouzari N, Tabatabai H, Abbasi Z, et al. Laser hair removal: comparison of long-pulsed Nd:YAG, long-pulsed alexandrite, and long-pulsed diode lasers. *Dermatol Surg*. 2004;30(4 pt 1):498–502.

Campos VB, Dierickx CC, Farinelli WA, et al. Hair removal with an 800-nm pulsed diode laser. *J Am Acad Dermatol*. 2000;43:442–447.

Dierickx CC. Hair removal by lasers and intense pulsed light sources. *Semin Cutan Med Surg*. 2000;19(4):267–275.

Eremia S, Li C, Newman N. Laser hair removal with alexandrite versus diode laser using four treatment sessions: 1-year results. *Dermatol Surg*. 2001;27(11):925–929; discussion 929–930.

Gold MH, Bell MW, Foster TD, et al. One-year follow-up using an intense pulsed light source for long-term hair removal. *J Cutan Laser Ther*. 1999;1(3):167–171.

Gorgu M, Aslan G, Akoz T, et al. Comparison of alexandrite laser and electrolysis for hair removal. *Dermatol Surg*. 2000;26:37–41.

Haedersdal M, Haak CS. Hair removal. *Curr Probl Dermatol*. 2011;42:111–121.

Handrick C, Alster TS. Comparison of long-pulsed diode and long-pulsed alexandrite lasers for hair removal: a long-term clinical and histologic study. *Dermatol Surg*. 2001;27:622–626.

Liew S, Gault D. Clinical comparison of the ruby, alexandrite, Nd:YAG in removing hair – A preliminary report. *Cosmet Dermatol*. 2000;13(5):17–19.

Lou WW, Quintana AT, Geronemus RG, et al. Prospective study of hair reduction by diode laser (800 nm) with long-term follow-up. *Dermatol Surg*. 2000;26(5):428–432.

Nanni CA, Alster TS. Laser-assisted hair removal side-effects of Q-switched Nd:YAG, long-pulsed ruby, and alexandrite lasers. *J Am Acad Dermatol*. 1999;41:165–171.

Ormiga P, Ishida CE, Boechat A, et al. Comparison of the effect of diode laser versus intense pulsed light in axillary hair removal. *Dermatol Surg*. 2014;40(10):1061–1069.

## Complications

Bernstein EF. Hair growth induced by diode laser treatment. *Dermatol Surg*. 2005;31:584–586.

Landa N, Corrons N, Zabalza I, et al. Urticaria induced by laser epilation: a clinical and histopathological study with extended follow-up in 36 patients. *Lasers Surg Med*. 2012;44(5):384–389.

Alajlan A, Shapiro J, Rivens J, et al. Paradoxical hypertrichosis after laser epilation. *J Am Acad Dermatol*. 2005;53:85–88.

Willey A, Torrontegui J, Azpiazu J, et al. Hair stimulation following laser and intense pulsed light photo-epilation: review of 543 cases and ways to manage it. *Lasers Surg Med*. 2007;39:297–301.

## Pigmented Lesions

### Overview

Bogdan Allemann I, Goldberg DJ. Benign pigmented lesions. *Curr Probl Dermatol*. 2011;42:81–96.

Gilchrest BA, Fitzpatrick TB, Anderson RR, et al. Localization of melanin pigmentation in the skin with Wood's lamp. *Brit J Dermatol*. 1977;96(3):245–248.

Kilmer SL. Laser eradication of pigmented lesions and tattoos. *Dermatol Clin*. 2002;20:37–53.

Kristel D, Polder KD, Landau JM, et al. Laser eradication of pigmented lesions: a review. *Dermatol Surg*. 2011;37(5):572–595.

Kurban AK, Morrison PR, Trainor SW, et al. Pulse duration effects on cutaneous pigment. *Lasers Surg Med*. 1992;12(3):282–287.

Lowe NJ, Kafaja S. Pigmentation of the aging face- evaluation and treatment. In: Lowe NJ, ed. *Textbook of Facial Rejuvenation: The Art of Minimally Invasive Combination Therapy*. Boca Raton, FL: Taylor and Francis; 2002:73–83.

Murphy GF, Shepard RS, Paul BS, et al. Organelle-specific injury to melanin-containing cells in human skin by pulsed laser irradiation. *Lab Invest*. 1983;49(6):680–685.

Ortonne JP, Pandya AG, Lui H, et al. Treatment of solar lentigines. *J Am Acad Dermatol*. 2006;54(5 suppl 2):S262–S271.

Polder KD, Landau JM, Vergilis-Kalner IJ, et al. Laser eradication of pigmented lesions: a review. *Dermatol Surg*. 2011;37(5):572–595.

Ross EV, Smirnov M, Pankratov M. Intense pulsed light and laser treatment of facial telangiectasias and dyspigmentation: some theoretical and practical comparisons. *Dermatol Surg.* 2005;31(9 Pt 2):1188–1198.

Sherwood KA, Murray S, Kurban AK, et al. Effect of wavelength on cutaneous pigment using pulsed irradiation. *J Invest Dermatol.* 1989;92(5):717–720.

Small R. Laser photo rejuvenation. In: Mayeaux E, ed. *The Essential Guide to Primary Care Procedures.* Philadelphia, PA: Lippincott Williams & Wilson; 2009:249–264.

Small R, Hoang D. Photorejuvenation with lasers. In: Usatine R, Pfenninger J, Stuhlberg D, et al., eds. *Dermatologic and Cosmetic Procedures in Office Practice.* Philadelphia, PA: Elsevier; 2012:322–335.

Van Aardt R. *Lasers and Pulsed-Light Devices: Photofacial Rejuvenation in Pfenninger and Fowler's Procedures for Primary Care.* 3rd ed. Philadelphia, PA: Chapter 49 Elsevier; 2010.

## Devices

Barysch MJ, Rummelein B, Kolm I, et al. Split-face study of melasma patients treated with nonablative fractionated photothermolysis (1540 nm). *J Eur Acad Dermatol Venereol.* 2012;26(4):423–430.

Bitter PH. Noninvasive rejuvenation of photodamaged skin using serial, full-face intense pulsed light treatments. *Dermatol Surg.* 2000;26:835–843.

Cho SB, Kim JS, Kim MJ. Melasma treatment in Korean women using a 1064-nm Q-switched Nd:YAG laser with low pulse energy. *Clin Exp Dermatol.* 2009;34(8):e847–e850.

Cho SB, Park SJ, Kim JS, et al. Treatment of post-inflammatory hyperpigmentation using 1064-nm Q-switched Nd:YAG laser with low fluence: report of three cases. *J Eur Dermatol Venereol.* 2009;23(10):1206–1207.

Galeckas KJ, Ross EV, Uebelhoer NS. A pulsed dye laser with a 10-mm beam diameter and a pigmented lesion window for purpura-free photorejuvenation. *Dermatol Surg.* 2008;34(3):308–313.

Ho WS, Chan HH, Ying SY, et al. Prospective study on the treatment of postburn hyperpigmentation by intense pulsed light. *Lasers Surg Med.* 2003;32(1):42–45.

Kauvar AN. The evolution of melasma therapy: targeting melanosomes using low-fluence Q-switched neodymium-doped yttrium aluminium garnet lasers. *Semin Cutan Med Surg.* 2012;31(2):126–132.

Kawada A, Shiraishi H, Asai M, et al. Clinical improvement of solar lentigines and ephelides with an intense pulsed light source. *Dermatol Surg.* 2002;28(6):504–508.

Kilmer SL. Diode laser treatment of pigmented lesions. *Lasers Surg Med.* 2000;12(suppl):23.

Kilmer SL, Wheeland RG, Goldberg DJ, et al. Treatment of epidermal pigmented lesions with the frequency-doubled Q-switched Nd:YAG laser. A controlled, single-impact, dose-response, multicenter trial. *Arch Dermatol.* 1994;130(12):1515–1519.

Kono T, Manstein D, Chan HH, et al. Q-switched ruby versus long-pulsed dye laser delivered with compression for treatment of facial lentigines in Asians. *Lasers Surg Med.* 2006;38:94–97.

Kroon MW, Wind BS, Beek JF, et al. Nonablative 1550-nm fractional laser therapy versus triple topical therapy for the treatment of melasma: a randomized controlled pilot study. *J Am Acad Dermatol.* 2011;64(3):516–523.

Lapidoth M, Yagima Odo ME, Odo LM. Novel use of erbium:YAG (2,940-nm) laser for fractional ablative photothermolysis in the treatment of photodamaged facial skin: a pilot study. *Dermatol Surg.* 2008;34(8):1048–1053.

Li YT, Yang KC. Comparison of the frequency-doubled Q-switched Nd:YAG laser and 35% trichloroacetic acid for the treatment of face lentigines. *Dermatol Surg.* 1999;25(3):202–204.

Na SY, Cho S, Lee JH. Intense Pulsed Light and Low-Fluence Q-Switched Nd:YAG Laser Treatment in Melasma Patients. *Ann Dermatol.* 2012;24(3):267–273.

Rashid T, Hussain I, Haider M, et al. Laser therapy of freckles and lentigines with quasi-continuous, frequency-doubled, Nd:YAG (532 nm) laser in Fitzpatrick skin type IV: a 24-month follow-up. *J Cosmet Laser Ther.* 2002;4(3–4):81–85.

Rosenbach A, Lee SJ, Johr RH. Treatment of medium-brown solar lentigines using an alexandrite laser designed for hair reduction. *Arch Dermatol.* 2002;138(4):547–548.

Rusciani A, Motta A, Fino P, et al. Treatment of poikiloderma of Civatte using intense pulsed light source: 7 years of experience. *Dermatol Surg.* 2008;34(3):314–319.

Scattone L, de Avelar Alchorne MM, Michalany N, et al. Histopathologic changes induced by intense pulsed light in the treatment of poikiloderma of Civatte. *Dermatol Surg.* 2012;38(7 Pt 1):1010–1016.

Todd MM, Rallis TM, Gerwels JW, et al. A comparison of 3 lasers and liquid nitrogen in the treatment of solar lentigines: a randomized, controlled, comparative trial. *Arch Dermatol.* 2000;136(7):841–846.

Trafeli JP, Kwan JM, Meehan KJ, et al. Use of a long-pulse alexandrite laser in the treatment of superficial pigmented lesions. *Dermatol Surg.* 2007;33(12):1477–1482.

Wang CC, Sue YM, Yang CH, et al. A comparison of Q-switched alexandrite laser and intense pulsed light for the treatment of freckles and lentigines in Asian persons: a randomized, physician-blinded, split-face comparative trial. *J Am Acad Dermatol.* 2006;54(5):804–810.

Wanner M, Tanzi EL, Alster TS. Fractional photothermolysis treatment of facial and non-facial cutaneous photodamage with the 1,550-nm erbium-doped fiber laser. *Dermatol Surg.* 2007;33:23–28.

Wattanakrai P, Mornchan R, Eimpunth S. Low-Fluence Q-Switched Neodymium-Doped Yttrium Aluminum Garnet (1,064 nm) Laser for the Treatment of Facial Melasma in Asians. *Dermatol Surg.* 2010;36:76–87.

Zoccali G, Piccolo D, Allegra P, et al. Melasma treated with intense pulsed light. *Aesthetic Plast Surg.* 2010;34(4):486–493.

## Vascular Lesions

### Overview

Adamic M, Troilius A, Adatto M, et al. Vascular lasers and IPLS: guidelines for care from the European Society for Laser Dermatology (ESLD). *J Cosmet Laser Ther.* 2007;9:113–124.

Astner S, Anderson RR. Treating vascular lesions. *Dermatol Ther.* 2005;18(3):267–281.

Dudelzak J, Hussain M, Goldberg DJ. Vascular-specific laser wavelength for the treatment of facial telangiectasias. *J Drugs Dermatol.* 2009;8(3):227–229.

Ross EV, Smirnov M, Pankratov M. Intense pulsed light and laser treatment of facial telangiectasias and dyspigmentation: some theoretical and practical comparisons. *Dermatol Surg.* 2005;31(9 Pt 2):1188–1198.

Small R. Laser photo rejuvenation. In: Mayeaux E, ed. *The Essential Guide to Primary Care Procedures.* Philidelphia, PA: Lippincott Williams & Wilson; 2009;249–264.

Small R, Hoang D. Photorejuvenation with Lasers. In: Usatine R, Pfenninger J, Stuhlberg D, et al., eds. *Dermatologic and Cosmetic Procedures in Office Practice.* Philadelphia, PA: Elsevier; 2012:322–335.

Srinivas CR, Kumaresan M. Lasers for vascular lesions: standard guidelines of care. *Indian J Dermatol Venereol Leprol.* 2011;77:349–368.

Ting PT, Rao J. Vascular lesions. *Curr Probl Dermatol.* 2011;42:67–80.

Travelute AC, Carniol PJ, Hruza GJ. Laser treatment of facial vascular lesions. *Facial Plast Surg.* 2001;17:193–201.

### Devices

Behroozan DS, Goldberg LH, Glaich AS, et al. Fractional photothermolysis for treatment of poikiloderma of Civatte. *Dermatol Surg.* 2006;32:298–301.

Bernstein EF, Kligman A. Rosacea treatment using the new-generation, high-energy, 595 nm, long pulse-duration pulsed-dye laser. *Lasers Surg Med.* 2008;40(4):233–239.

Bitter PH. Noninvasive rejuvenation of photodamaged skin using serial, full-face intense pulsed light treatments. *Dermatol Surg.* 2000;26:835–843.

Bitter PH. Report of a new technique for enhanced non-invasive skin rejuvenation using a dual mode, pulsed light and radiofrequency energy source: selective radio-thermolysis. *J Cosm Derm.* 2002;1:142–145.

Butler EG, McClellan SD, Ross EV. Split treatment of photodamaged skin with KTP 532 nm laser with 10 mm handpiece versus IPL: a cheek-to-cheek comparison. *Lasers Surg Med.* 2006;38:124–128.

Carniol PJ, Price J, Olive A. Treatment of telangiectasias with the 532-nm and the 532/940-nm diode laser. *Facial Plast Surg.* 2005;21:117–119.

Clark C, Cameron H, Moseley H, et al. Treatment of superficial cutaneous vascular lesions: experience with the KTP 532 nm laser. *Lasers Med Sci.* 2004;19(1):1–5. Epub 2004 Apr 14.

Clementoni MT, Gilardino P, Muti GF, et al. Facial teleangectasias: our experience in treatment with IPL. *Lasers Surg Med.* 2005;37(1):9–13.

Dai T, Diagaradjane P, Yaseen MA, et al. Laser-induced thermal injury to dermal blood vessels: analysis of wavelength (585 nm vs. 595 nm), cryogen spray cooling, and wound healing effects. *Lasers Surg Med.* 2005;37(3):210–218.

Glaich AS, Goldberg LH, Dai T, et al. Fractional photothermolysis for the treatment of telangiectatic matting: a case report. *J Cutan Laser Ther.* 2007;9:101–103.

Goodman GJ, Roberts S, Bezborodoff A. Studies in long-pulsed potassium tritanyl phosphate laser for the treatment of spider naevi and perialar telangiectasia. *Australas J Dermatol.* 2002;43(1):9–14.

McCoppin HH, Goldberg DJ. Laser treatment of facial telangiectasias: an update. *Dermatol Surg.* 2010;36(8):1221–1230.

Rose AE, Goldberg DJ. Successful Treatment of Facial Telangiectasias Using a Micropulse 1,064-nm Neodymium-Doped Yttrium Aluminum Garnet Laser. *Dermatol Surg.* 2013;39:1062–1066.

Ross EV, Uebelhoer NS, Domankevitz Y. Use of a novel pulse dye laser for rapid single-pass purpura-free treatment of telangiectasias. *Dermatol Surg.* 2007;33(12):1466–1469.

Rusciani A, Motta A, Fino P, et al. Treatment of poikiloderma of Civatte using intense pulsed light source: 7 years of experience. *Dermatol Surg.* 2008;34:314–319.

Sadick NS, Krueger N. Vascular Lesions. *Cosmet Dermatol.* 2012;25:108–109.

Schroeter CA, Haaf-von Below S, Neumann HA. Effective treatment of rosacea using intense pulsed light systems. *Dermatol Surg.* 2005;31(10):1285–1289.

Smit JM, Bauland CG, Wijnberg DS, et al. Pulsed dye laser treatment, a review of indications and outcome based on published trials. *Br J Plast Surg.* 2005;58(7):981–987.

Tanghetti E, Sherr E. Treatment of telangiectasia using the multi-pass technique with the extended pulse width, pulsed dye laser (Cynosure V-Star). *J Cosmet Laser Ther.* 2003;5(2):71–75.

Uebelhoer NS, Bogle MA, Stewart B, et al. A split-face comparison study of pulsed 532-nm KTP laser and 595-nm pulsed dye laser in the treatment of facial telangiectasias and diffuse telangiectatic facial erythema. *Dermatol Surg.* 2007;33(4):441–448.

Vidimos AT. Vascular laser an intense pulsed light treatment of rosacea-associated telangiectasia and erythema. *Cosmet Dermatol.* 2002;15:39–43.

Yaghmai D, Garden J. Treating facial vascular lesions with lasers. In: Lowe NJ, ed. *Textbook of Facial Rejuvenation: The Art of Minimally Invasive Combination Therapy.* Boca Raton, FL: Taylor and Francis; 2002;85–100.

Zelickson BD, Kilmer SL, Bernstein E, et al. Pulsed dye laser therapy for sun damaged skin. *Lasers Surg Med.* 1999;25:229–236.

## Complications

Alam M, Omura NE, Dover JS, et al. Clinically significant facial edema after extensive treatment with purpura-free pulsed-dye laser. *Dermatol Surg*. 2003;29(9):920–924.

# Tattoo Removal

## Tattoos

Bagnato G, De Pasquale R, Glacobbe O, et al. Urticaria in a tattooed patient. *Allergol Immunopathol (Madr)*. 1992;(71):70–73.
Bendsoe N, Hansson C, Sterner O. Inflammatory reactions from organic pigments in red tattoos. *Acta Derm Venereol*. 1991;71(1):70–73.
Bjornberg A. Allergic reaction to cobalt in light-blue tattoo markings. *Acta Dermatol Venereologica*. 1961;(41):259.
Bjornberg A. Allergic reactions to chrome in green tattoo markings. *Acta Derm Venereol*. 1959;39(1):23–29.
Blumental G, Okun MR, Ponitch JA. Pseudolymphomatous reaction to tattoos. Report of three cases. *J Am Acad Dermatol*. 1982;6(4 Pt 1):485–488.
Tazelaar DJ. Hypersensitivity to chromium in a light-blue tattoo. *Dermatologica*. 1970;141(4):282–287.
Winkelmann RK, Harris RB. Lichenoid delayed hypersensitivity reactions in tattoos. *J Cutan Pathol*. 1979; 6(1):59–65.

## Overview

Kent KM, Graber EM. Laser tattoo removal: a review. *Dermatol Surg*. 2012;38(1):1–13.
Adatto MA, Halachmi S, Lapidoth M. Tattoo removal. *Curr Probl Dermatol*. 2011;42:97–110.
Choudhary S, Elsaie ML, Leiva A, et al. Lasers for tattoo removal: a review. *Lasers Med Sci*. 2010;25(5):619–627.
Green JB, Metelitsa AI. Optimizing outcomes of laser tattoo removal. *Skin Therapy Lett*. 2011;16(10):1–3.
Kirby W, Kartono F, Small R. Tattoo Removal with Lasers. In: Usatine R, Pfenninger J, Stuhlberg D, et al., eds. *Dermatologic and Cosmetic Procedures in Office Practice*. Philadelphia, PA: Elsevier; 2012:377–382.
Kim KH, Geronemus RG. Tattoo Removal. *Med Lett*. 2003;45(95):96.
Luebberding S, Alexiades-Armenakas M. New tattoo approaches in dermatology. *Dermatol Clin*. 2014;32(1):91–96.
Wenzel SM. Current concepts in laser tattoo removal. *Skin Therapy Lett*. 2010;15(3):3–5.

## Devices

Agneta M. Effective treatment of traumatic tattoos with a q-switched Nd:YAG laser. *Lasers Surg Med*. 1998;(22):103–108.
Bernstein EF, Civiok JM. A continuously variable beam-diameter, high-fluence, Q-switched Nd:YAG laser for tattoo removal: comparison of the maximum beam diameter to a standard 4-mm-diameter treatment beam. *Lasers Surg Med*. 2013;45(10):621–627.
Brauer JA, Reddy KK, Anolik R, et al. Successful and rapid treatment of blue and green tattoo pigment with a novel picosecond laser. *Arch Dermatol*. 2012;148(7):820–823.
Fitzpatrick RE, Goldman MP. Tattoo removal using the alexandrite laser. *Arch Dermatol*. 1994;130:1508–1514.
Fusade T, Toubel G, Grognard C, et al. Treatment of gunpowder traumatic tattoo by Q-switched Nd:YAG laser: an unusual adverse effect. *Dermatol Surg*. 2000;26(11):1057–1059.
Gorouhi F, Davari P, Kashani MN, et al. Treatment of traumatic tattoo with the Q-switched Nd:YAG laser. *J Cosmet Laser Ther*. 2007;9(4):253–255.
Grevelink JM, Duke D, van Leeuwen RL, et al. Laser treatment of tattoos in darkly pigmented patients: efficacy and side effects. *J Am Acad Dermatol*. 1996;34(4):653–656.
Karsai S, Pfirrmann G, Hammes S, et al. Treatment of resistant tattoos using a new generation Q-switched Nd:YAG laser: influence of beam profile and spot size on clearance success. *Lasers Surg Med*. 2008;40(2):139–145.
Kilmer SL, Anderson RR. Clinical use of the Q-switched ruby and the Q-switched Nd:YAG (1064 nm and 532 nm) lasers for treatment of tattoos. *J Dermatol Surg Oncol*. 1993;19(4):330–338.
Kilmer SL, Lee MS, Grevelink JM, et al. The Q-switched Nd:YAG laser effectively treats tattoos. A controlled, dose response study. *Arch Dermatol*. 1993;129(8):971–978.
Lee CN, Bae EY, Park JG, et al. Permanent makeup removal using Q-switched Nd:YAG laser. *Clin Exp Dermatol*. 2009;34(8):e594–e596.
Mariwalla K, Dover JS. The use of lasers for decorative tattoo removal. *Skin Therapy Lett*. 2006;11:8–11.
Saedi N, Metelitsa A,. Petrell K, et al. Treatment of tattoos with a picosecond alexandrite laser. *Arch Dermatol*. 2012;148(12):1360–1363.

## Complications

Anderson RR, Geronemus RG, Kilmer SL, et al. Cosmetic tattoo ink darkening. A complication of Q-switched and pulsed-laser treatment. *Arch Dermatol*. 1993;129:1010–1014.
Ashinoff R, Levine VJ, Soter NA. Allergic reactions to tattoo pigment after laser treatment. *Dermatol Surg*. 1995;21:291–294.

England R. Immediate cutaneous hypersensitivity after treatment of tattoo with Nd:YAG laser: a case report and review of the literature. *Ann Allergy Asthma Immunol.* 2002;(89):215–217.

Kirby W, Kartono F, Desai A, et al. Treatment of Large Bulla Formation after Tattoo Removal with a Q-Switched Laser. *Clinical and Aesthetic Derm.* 2010;3(1):39–41.

Taylor CR. Laser ignition of traumatically embedded firework debris. *Lasers Surg Med.* 1998;22(3):157–158.

Wenzel S, Landthaler M, Baumler W et al. Recurring mistakes in tattoo removal. A case series. *Dermatology.* 2009;218(2):164–167.

## Skin Resurfacing

Agrawal N, Smith G, Heffelfinger R. Ablative skin resurfacing. *Facial Plast Surg.* 2014;30(1):55–61.

Aslam A, Alster TS. Evolution of laser skin resurfacing: from scanning to fractional technology. *Dermatol Surg.* 2014;40(11):1163–1172.

Alexiades-Armenakas MR, Dover JS, Arndt KA. The spectrum of laser skin resurfacing: nonablative, fractional, and ablative laser resurfacing. *J Am Acad Dermatol.* 2008;58(5):719–737.

Buford G. Lasers and Pulsed-Light Devices: skin Resurfacing. Chapter 53. In: Pfenninger JL, Folwer GC, eds. *Pfenninger and Fowler's Procedures for Primary Care.* 3rd ed. Philadelphia, PA: Mosby/Elsevier; 2010.

Chwalek J, Goldberg DJ. Ablative skin resurfacing. *Curr Probl Dermatol.* 2011;42:40–47.

Fitzpatrick RE. Resurfacing procedures: how do you choose? *Arch Dermatol.* 2000;136(6):783–784.

Freedman JR, Greene RM, Green JB. Histologic effects of resurfacing lasers. *Facial Plast Surg.* 2014;30(1): 40–48.

Preissig J, Hamilton K, Markus R. Current laser resurfacing technologies: a review that delves beneath the surface. *Semin Plast Surg.* 2012;26(3):109–116.

Yu K, Small R, Maas C. Skin Resurfacing with Ablative Lasers. In: Usatine R, Pfenninger J, Stuhlberg D, et al., eds. *Dermatologic and Cosmetic Procedures in Office Practice.* Philadelphia, PA: Elsevier; 2010.

## Wrinkles—Nonablative Skin Resurfacing

### Overview

Alam M, Dover JS. Nonablative laser and light therapy: an approach to patient and device selection. *Skin Therapy Lett.* 2003;8(4):4–7.

Goldberg DJ. Nonablative resurfacing. *Clin Plast Surg.* 2000;27(2):287–292, xi.

Small R. Wrinkle reduction with non-ablative lasers. In: Usatine R, Pfenninger J, Stuhlberg D, et al., eds. *Dermatologic and Cosmetic Procedures in Office Practice.* Philadelphia, PA: Elsevier; 2012:336–350.

### Devices

Berlin AL, Dudelzak J, Hussain M, et al. Evaluation of clinical, microscopic, and ultrastructural changes after treatment with a novel Q-switched Nd:YAG laser. *J Cosmet Laser Ther.* 2008;10(2):76–79.

Bhatia AC, Dover JS, Arndt KA, et al. Patient satisfaction and reported long-term therapeutic efficacy associated with 1,320 nm Nd:YAG laser treatment of acne scarring and photoaging. *Dermatol Surg.* 2006;32:346–352.

Carniol PJ, Farley S, Friedman A. Long-pulse 532-nm diode laser for nonablative facial skin rejuvenation. *Arch Facial Plast Surg.* 2003;5(6):511–513.

Chernoff WG. Nonexfoliating laser rejuvenation of facial rhytids. In: Keller GS, Lacombe VG, Lee PK, et al., eds. *Lasers in Aesthetic Surgery.* New York, NY: Thieme; 2001:139–148.

Ciocon DH, Doshi D, Goldberg DJ. Non-ablative lasers. *Curr Probl Dermatol.* 2011;42:48–55.

Cisneros JL, Rio R, Palou J. The Q-switched neodymium (Nd):YAG laser with quadruple frequency. Clinical histological evaluation of facial resurfacing using different wavelengths. *Dermatol Surg.* 1998;24(3): 345–350.

Dayan S, Damrose JF, Bhattacharyya TK, et al. Histological evaluations following 1,064-nm Nd:YAG laser resurfacing. *Lasers Surg Med.* 2003;33(2):126–131.

Dayan SH, Vartanian AJ, Menaker G, et al. Nonablative laser resurfacing using the long-pulse (1064-nm) Nd:YAG laser. *Arch Facial Plast Surg.* 2003;5(4):310–315.

Dierickx CC. The role of deep heating for noninvasive skin rejuvenation. *Lasers Surg Med.* 2006;38(9):799–807.

Doshi SN, Alster TS. 1,450 nm long-pulsed diode laser for nonablative skin rejuvenation. *Dermatol Surg.* 2005;31:1223–1226.

Fournier N, Dahan S, Barneon G, et al. Nonablative remodeling: a 14-month clinical ultrasound imaging and profilometric evaluation of a 1540 nm Er:Glass laser. *Dermatol Surg.* 2002;28(10):926–931.

Goldberg DJ. Full-face nonablative dermal remodeling with a 1320 nm Nd:YAG laser. *Dermatol Surg.* 2000;26(10):915–918.

Goldberg DJ. Non-ablative subsurface remodeling: clinical and histologic evaluation of a 1320-nm Nd:YAG laser. *J Cutan Laser Ther.* 1999;1(3):153–157.

Goldberg DJ. New collagen formation after dermal remodeling with an intense pulsed light source. *J Cutan Laser Ther.* 2000;2(2):59–61.

Goldberg DJ, Silapunt S. Histologic evaluation of a Q-switched Nd:YAG laser in the nonablative treatment of wrinkles. *Dermatol Surg.* 2001;27(8):744–746.

Goldberg DJ, Silapunt S. Q-switched Nd:YAG laser: rhytid improvement by nonablative dermal remodeling. *J Cutan Laser Ther.* 2000;2(3):157–160.

Goldberg DJ, Hussain M, Fazeli A, et al. Treatment of skin laxity of the lower face and neck in older individuals with a broad-spectrum infrared light device. *J Cosmet Laser Ther.* 2007;9(1):35–40.

Goldberg DJ, Rogachefsky AS, Silapunt S. Non-ablative laser treatment of facial rhytides: a comparison of 1450-nm diode laser treatment with dynamic cooling as opposed to treatment with dynamic cooling alone. *Lasers Surg Med.* 2002;30:79–81.

Goldberg DJ, Samady JA. Intense pulsed light and Nd:YAG laser non-ablative treatment of facial rhytids. *Lasers Surg Med.* 2001;28(2):141–144.

Goldberg DJ, Whitworth J. Laser skin resurfacing with the Q-switched Nd:YAG laser. *Dermatol Surg.* 1997;23(10):903–906.

Hardaway CA, Ross EV, Paithankar DY. Non-ablative cutaneous remodeling with a 1.45 microm mid-infrared diode laser: phase II. *J Cosmet Laser Ther.* 2002;4:9–14.

Hernandez-Perez E, Ibiett EV. Gross and microscopic findings in patients submitted to nonablative full-face resurfacing using intense pulsed light: a preliminary study. *Dermatol Surg.* 2002;28(8):651–655.

Kono T, Groff WF, Sakurai H, et al. Comparison study of intense pulsed light versus a long-pulse pulsed dye laser in the treatment of facial skin rejuvenation. *Ann Plast Surg.* 2007;59(5):479–483.

Lee MC, Hu S, Chen MC, et al. Skin rejuvenation with 1,064-nm Q-switched Nd:YAG laser in Asian patients. *Dermatol Surg.* 2009;35(6):929–932.

Lloyd JR. Effect of fluence on efficacy using the 1440 nm laser with CAP technology for the treatment of rhytids. *Lasers Surg Med.* 2008;40(6):387–389.

Lupton JR, Williams CM, Alster TS. Nonablative laser skin resurfacing using a 1540 nm erbium glass laser: a clinical and histologic analysis. *Dermatol Surg.* 2002;28:833–835.

Paithankar DY, Clifford JM, Saleh BA, et al. Subsurface skin renewal by treatment with a 1450-nm laser in combination with dynamic cooling. *J Biomed Opt.* 2003;8(3):545–551.

Roh M, Goo B, Jung J, et al. Treatment of enlarged pores with the quasi long-pulsed versus Q-switched 1064 nm Nd:YAG lasers: a split-face, comparative, controlled study. *Laser Ther.* 2011;20(3):175–180.

Ross EV, Sajben FP, Hsia J, et al. Nonablative skin remodeling: selective dermal heating with a mid-infrared laser and contact cooling combination. *Lasers Surg Med.* 2000;26(2):186–195.

Sadick NS. Update on non-ablative light therapy for rejuvenation: a review. *Lasers Surg Med.* 2003;32(2):120–128.

Sherling M, Friedman PM, Adrian R, et al. Consensus recommendations on the use of an erbium-doped 1,550-nm fractionated laser and its applications in dermatologic laser surgery. *Dermatol Surg.* 2010;36:461–469.

Shin MK, Lee JH, Lee SJ, et al. Platelet-rich plasma combined with fractional laser therapy for skin rejuvenation. *Dermatol Surg.* 2012;38(4):623–630.

Tanaka Y, Matsuo K, Yuzuriha S. Objective assessment of skin rejuvenation using near-infrared 1064-nm neodymium: YAG laser in Asians. *Clin Cosmet Investig Dermatol.* 2011;4:123–130.

Zelickson BD, Kilmer SL, Bernstein E, et al. Pulsed dye laser therapy for sun damaged skin. *Lasers Surg Med.* 1999;25(3):229–236.

## Complications

Handley JM. Adverse events associated with nonablative cutaneous visible and infrared laser treatment. *J Am Acad Dermatol.* 2006;55(3):482–489.

# Wrinkles—Ablative Skin Resurfacing

## Overview

Alster TS. Cutaneous resurfacing with CO2 and erbium: YAG lasers: preoperative, intraoperative, and postoperative considerations. *Plast Reconstr Surg.* 1999;103(2):619–632.

Lane JE. $CO_2$ laser therapy in dermatology and dermatologic surgery. *Cosmet Dermatol.* 2011;24:412–418.

## Devices

Bentkover SH. Plasma skin resurfacing: personal experience and long-term results. *Facial Plast Surg Clin North Am.* 2012;20(2):145–162.

Fitzpatrick RE, Rostan EF, Marchell N. Collagen tightening induced by carbon dioxide laser versus erbium: YAG laser. *Lasers Surg Med.* 2000;27(5):395–403.

Hantash BM, De CE, Liu H, et al. Split-face comparison of the erbium micropeel with intense pulsed light. *Dermatol Surg.* 2008;34(6):763–772.

Khatri KA, Ross V, Grevelink JM, et al. Comparison of erbium:YAG and carbon dioxide lasers in resurfacing of facial rhytides. *Arch Dermatol.* 1999;135(4):391–397.

Kilmer S, Semchyshyn N, Shah G, et al. A pilot study on the use of a plasma skin regeneration device (Portrait PSR3) in full facial rejuvenation procedures. *Lasers Med Sci.* 2007;22(2):101–109.

Krupashankar DS; IADVL Dermatosurgery Task Force. Standard guidelines of care: CO2 laser for removal of benign skin lesions and resurfacing. *Indian J Dermatol Venereol Leprol.* 2008;74 suppl:S61–S67.

Pozner JM, Goldberg DJ. Histologic effect of a variable pulsed Er:YAG laser. *Dermatol Surg*. 2000;26(8):733–736.
Pozner JN, Goldberg DJ. Superficial erbium:YAG laser resurfacing of photodamaged skin. *J Cosmet Laser Ther*. 2006;8(2):89–91.

## Complications

Alster TS, Lupton JR. Prevention and treatment of side effects and complications of cutaneous laser resurfacing. *Plast Reconstr Surg*. 2002;109(1):308–316.
Alster TS, Nanni CA. Famciclovir prophylaxis of herpes simplex virus reactivation after laser skin resurfacing. *Dermatol Surg*. 1999;25(3):242–246.
Sullivan SA, Dailey RA. Complications of laser resurfacing and their management. *Ophthal Plast Reconstr Surg*. 2000;16(6):417–426.
Winnington P. Conquer hyperpigmentation after laser resurfacing. *Skin Aging*. 2000;8:43–58.

# Fractional Skin Resurfacing

## Overview

Bogdan AI, Kaufman J. Fractional photothermolysis. *Curr Probl Dermatol*. 2011;42:56–66.
Christian-Reed M. Commentary: fractional resurfacing: a step in progress. *Dermatol Surg*. 2010;36(10):1509.
Geronemus RG. Fractional photothermolysis: current and future applications. *Lasers Surg Med*. 2006;38(3):169–176.
Jih MH, Goldberg LH, Kimyai-Asadi A. Fractional photothermolysis for photoaging hands. *Dermatol Surg*. 2008; 34:73–78.
Laubach HJ, Tannous Z, Anderson RR, et al. Skin responses to fractional photothermolysis. *Lasers Surg Med*. 2006; 38(2):142–149.
Tannous Z. Fractional resurfacing. *Clin Dermatol*. 2007;25(5):480–486.
Tierney EP, Kouba DJ, Hanke CW. Review of fractional photothermolysis: treatment indications and efficacy. *Dermatol Surg*. 2009;35(10):1445–1461.

## Devices

Chapas AM, Brightman L, Sukal S, et al. Successful treatment of acneiform scarring with CO2 ablative fractional resurfacing. *Lasers Surg Med*. 2008;40(6):381–386.
Clementoni MT, Gilardino P, Muti GF, et al. Non-sequential fractional ultrapulsed CO2 resurfacing of photoaged facial skin: preliminary clinical report. *J Cosmet Laser Ther*. 2007;9(4):218–225.
Hunzeker CM, Weiss ET, Geronemus RG. Fractionated CO2 laser resurfacing: our experience with more than 2000 treatments. *Aesthet Surg J*. 2009;29(4):317–322.
Jung JY, Cho SB, Chung HJ, et al. Treatment of periorbital wrinkles with 1550- and 1565-nm Er:glass fractional photothermolysis lasers: a simultaneous split-face trial. *J Eur Acad Dermatol Venereol*. 2011;25:811–818.
Karsai S, Czarnecka A, Junger M, et al. Ablative fractional lasers (CO2 and Er:YAG): a randomized controlled double-blind split-face trial of the treatment of peri-orbital rhytides. *Lasers Surg Med*. 2010;42(2):160–167.
Lapidoth M, Yagima Odo ME, Odo LM. Novel use of erbium:YAG (2,940-nm) laser for fractional ablative photothermolysis in the treatment of photodamaged facial skin: a pilot study. *Dermatol Surg*. 2008;34(8): 1048–1053.
Latowsky BC, Abbasi N, Dover JS, et al. A randomized, controlled trial of four ablative fractionated lasers for photoaging: a quadrant study. *Dermatol Surg*. 2012;38(9):1477–1489.
Pozner JN, Glanz S, Goldberg DJ. Fractional erbium resurfacing: histologic and early clinical experience. *Lasers Surg Med*. 2007;39:S19–S73.
Smith KC, Schachter GD. YSGG 2790-nm superficial ablative and fractional ablative laser treatment. *Facial Plast Surg Clin North Am*. 2011;19:253–260.
Tierney EP, Hanke CW, Petersen J. Ablative fractionated CO2 laser treatment of photoaging: a clinical and histologic study. *Dermatol Surg*. 2012;38(11):1777–1789.
Tierney EP, Hanke CW, Petersen J, et al. Clinical and echographic analysis of ablative fractionated carbon dioxide laser in the treatment of photodamaged facial skin. *Dermatol Surg*. 2010;36(12):2009–2021.
Trelles MA, Mordon S, Velez M, et al. Results of fractional ablative facial skin resurfacing with the erbium:yttrium-aluminium-garnet laser 1 week and 2 months after one single treatment in 30 patients. *Lasers Med Sci*. 2009; 24(2):186–194.
Trelles MA, Velez M, Mordon S. Correlation of histological findings of single session Er:YAG skin fractional resurfacing with various passes and energies and the possible clinical implications. *Lasers Surg Med*. 2008;40(3):171–177.

## Complications

Avram MM, Tope WD, Yu T, et al. Hypertrophic scarring of the neck following ablative fractional carbon dioxide laser resurfacing. *Lasers Surg Med*. 2009;41(3):185–188.
Fife DJ, Fitzpatrick RE, Zachary CB. Complications of fractional CO2 laser resurfacing: four cases. *Lasers Surg Med*. 2009;41(3):179–184.

Graber EM, Tanzi EL, Alster TS. Side effects and complications of fractional laser photothermolysis: experience with 961 treatments. *Dermatol Surg*. 2008;34(3):301–305.

Marra DE, Yip D, Fincher EF, et al. Systemic toxicity from topically applied lidocaine in conjunction with fractional photothermolysis. *Arch Dermatol*. 2006;142:1024–1026.

Metelitsa AI, Alster TS. Fractionated laser skin resurfacing treatment complications: a review. *Dermatol Surg*. 2010;36(3):299–306.

## Combining Aesthetic Treatments

Beer K, Waibel J. Botulinum toxin type A enhances the outcome of fractional resurfacing of the cheek. *J Drugs Dermatol*. 2007;6:1151–1152.

Bass LS, DelGuzzo M, Dougherty S, et al. Combined ablative and nonablative fractional treatment for facial skin rejuvenation. *Lasers Surg Med*. 2009;15(suppl):29.

Carruthers J, Carruthers A. The effect of full-face broadband light treatments alone and in combination with bilateral crow's feet Botulinum toxin type A chemodenervation. *Dermatol Surg*. 2004;30:355–366.

Cohen J, Ross V. Combined fractional ablative and nonablative laser resurfacing treatment: a split-face comparative study. *J Drugs Dermatol*. 2013;12(2):175–178.

de Maio M. The minimal approach: an innovation in facial cosmetic procedures. *Aesthetic Plast Surg*. 2004; 28:295–300.

Effron C, Briden ME, Green BA. Enhancing cosmetic outcomes by combining superficial glycolic acid (alpha-hydroxy acid) peels with nonablative lasers, intense pulsed light, and trichloroacetic acid peels. *Cutis*. 2007;79 (1 Suppl Combining):4–8.

Farkas JP, Richardson JA, Brown S, et al. Effects of common laser treatments on hyaluronic acid fillers in a porcine model. *Aesthet Surg J*. 2008;28(5):503–511.

Goldman MP, Alster TS, Weiss R. A randomized trial to determine the influence of laser therapy, monopolar radiofrequency treatment, and intense pulsed light therapy administered immediately after hyaluronic acid gel implantation. *Dermatol Surg*. 2007;33:535–542.

Khoury JG, Saluja R, Goldman MP. The effect of botulinum toxin type A on full-face intense pulsed light treatment: a randomized, double-blind, split-face study. *Dermatol Surg*. 2008;34:1062–1069.

Small R, Hoang D. Introduction and foundation concepts. In: Small R, Hoang D, eds. *A Practical Guide to Botulinum Toxin Procedures*. Philadelphia, PA: Lippincott Williams & Wilkins; 2012;9–22.

Lee MW. Combination visible and infrared lasers for skin rejuvenation. *Semin Cutan Med Surg*. 2002;21(4):288–300.

Small R, Hoang D. Introduction and Foundation Concepts. In: Small R, Hoang D, eds. *A Practical Guide to Dermal Filler Procedures*. Philadelphia, PA: Lippincott Williams & Wilkins; 2012:5–28.

Small R, Hoang D, Linder J. Introduction and foundation concepts. In: A Practical Guide to Chemical peels, Microdermabrasion & Topical Products. Philadephia, PA: Lippincott Williams & Wilkins; 2013:5–34

Small R, Hoang D. Combination cosmetic treatments. In: Usatine R, Pfenninger J, Stuhlberg D, et al., eds. *Dermatologic and Cosmetic Procedures in Office Practice*. Philadelphia, PA: Elsevier; 2012:377–382.

Tierney EP, Hanke CW. Recent advances in combination treatments for photoaging: review of the literature. *Dermatol Surg*. 2010;36:829–840.

Wattanakrai P, Pootongkam S, Rojhirunsakool S. Periorbital Rejuvenation with Fractional 1,550-nm Ytterbium/Erbium Fiber Laser and Variable Square Pulse 2,940-nm Erbium:YAG laser in Asians: a Comparison Study. *Dermatol Surg*. 2012;38(4):610–622.

West TB, Alster TS. Effect of botulinum toxin type A on movement-associated rhytides following $CO_2$ laser resurfacing. *Dermatol Surg*. 1999;25:259–261.

Yamauchi PS, Lask G, Lowe NJ. Botulinum toxin type A gives adjunctive benefit to periorbital laser resurfacing. *J Cosmet Laser Ther*. 2004;6:145–148.

Zimbler MS, Holds JB, Kokoska MS, et al. Effect of botulinum toxin pretreatment on laser resurfacing results: a prospective, randomized, blinded trial. *Arch Facial Plast Surg*. 2001;3(3):165–169.

## General Laser Complications

Alexiades-Armenakas M, Bernstein LJ, Friedman PM, et al. The safety and efficacy of the 308-nm excimer laser for pigment correction of hypopigmented scars and striae alba. *Arch Dermatol*. 2004;140:955–960.

Alam M, Chaudhry NA, Goldberg LH. Vitreous floaters following use of dermatologic lasers. *Dermatol Surg*. 2002; 28:1088–1091.

Alam M, Warycha M. Complications of lasers and light treatments. *Dermatol Ther*. 2011;24(6):571–580.

Almoallim H, Klinkhoff AV, Arthur AB, et al. Laser induced chrysiasis: disfiguring hyperpigmentation following Q-switched laser therapy in a woman previously treated with gold. *J Rheumatol*. 2006;33(3):620–621.

Alster TS, Wanitphakdeedecha R. Improvement of postfractional laser erythema with light-emitting diode photo modulation. *Dermatol Surg*. 2009;35(5):813–815.

Bernestein LJ, Geronemus RG. Keloid formation with the 585-nm pulsed dye laser during isotretinoin treatment. *Arch Dermatol*. 1997;133(1):111–112.

Cohen JL, Bhatia AC. The role of topical vitamin K oxide gel in the resolution of postprocedural purpura. *J Drugs Dermatol*. 2009;8:1020–1024.

Fisher GH, Geronemus RG. Short-term side effects of fractional photothermolysis. *Dermatol Surg*. 2005;31(9 Pt 2): 1245–1249.

Friedman PM, Geronemus RG. Use of the 308-nm excimer laser for postresurfacing leukoderma. *Arch Dermatol.* 2001;137:824–825.

Gan SD, Bae-Harboe YS, Graber EM. Nonablative fractional resurfacing for the treatment of iatrogenic hypopigmentation. *Dermatol Surg.* 2014;40(1):87–89.

Gaston DA, Clark DP. Facial hypertrophic scarring from pulsed dye laser. *Dermatol Surg.* 1998;24:523–525.

Katz BE, Mac Farlane DF. Atypical facial scarring after isotretinoin therapy in a patient with previous dermabrasion. *J Am Acad Dermatol.* 1994;30(5 Pt 2):852–853.

Hammes S, Augustin A, Raulin C, et al. Pupil damage after periorbital laser treatment of a port-wine stain. *Arch Dermatol.* 2007;143(3):392–394.

Handley JM. Adverse events associated with nonablative cutaneous visible and infrared laser treatment. *J Am Acad Dermatol.* 2006;55(3):482–489.

Hirsch R, Stier M. Complications and their management in cosmetic dermatology. *Dermatol Clin.* 2009;27(4): 507–520, vii.

Khatri KA. Diode laser hair removal in patients undergoing isotretinoin therapy. *Dermatol Surg.* 2004;30(9):1205–1207.

Khatri KA. The safety of long-pulsed Nd:YAG laser hair removal in skin types III-V patients during concomitant isotretinoin therapy. *J Cosmet Laser Ther.* 2009;11(1):56–60.

Kontoes PP, Vlachos SP. Intense pulsed light is effective in treating pigmentary and vascular complications of CO(2) laser resurfacing. *Aesth Surg J.* 2002;22(5):489–491.

Lee SJ, Park SG, Kang JM, et al. Cryogen-induced arcuate shaped hyperpigmentation by dynamic cooling device. *J Eur Dermatol Venereol.* 2008;22(7):883–884.

Leu S, Havey J, White LE, et al. Accelerated resolution of laser-induced bruising with topical 20% arnica: a rater blinded randomized controlled trial. *Br J Dermatol.* 2010;163:557–563.

Marra DE, Yip D, Fincher EF, et al. Systemic toxicity from topically applied lidocaine in conjunction with fractional photothermolysis. *Arch Dermatol.* 2006;142:1024–1026.

Nanni C. Handling complications of laser treatment. *Dermatol Ther.* 2000;13:127–139.

Monheit GD. Facial resurfacing may trigger the herpes simplex virus. *Cosmet Dermatol.* 1995;8:9–16.

Oh IY, Kim BJ, Kim MN, et al. Efficacy of light-emitting diode photomodulation in reducing erythema after fractional carbon dioxide laser resurfacing: a pilot study. *Dermatol Surg.* 2013;39(8):1171–1176.

Park DH, Kim IT. A case of accidental macular injury by Nd:YAG laser and subsequent 6 year follow-up. *Korean J Ophthalmol.* 2009;23:207–209.

Raulin C, Greve B, Warncke SH, Gundogan C. Excimer laser. Treatment of iatrogenic hypopigmentation following skin resurfacing. *Hautarzt.* 2004;55:746–748.

Reszko A, Sukal SA, Geronemus RG. Reversal of laser-induced hypopigmentation with a narrow-band UV-B light source in a patient with skin type VI. *Dermatol Surg.* 2008;34(10):1423–1426.

Tierney EP, Hanke CW. Treatment of CO2 laser induced hypopigmentation with ablative fractionated laser resurfacing: case report and review of the literature. *J Drugs Dermatol.* 2010;9:1420–1426.

To D, Kossintseva I, de GG. Lidocaine contact allergy is becoming more prevalent. *Dermatol Surg.* 2014;40(12):1367–1372.

Trotter MJ, Tron VA, Hollingdale J, et al. Localized chrysiasis induced by laser therapy. *Arch Dermatol.* 1995; 131(12):1411–1414.

Walia S, Alster TS. Laser resurfacing infection rate with and without prophylactic antibiotics. *Dermatol Surg.* 1999;25:857–861.

West T, Alster TS. Effect of pretreatment on the incidence of hyperpigmentation following cutaneous $CO_2$ laser resurfacing. *Dermatol Surg.* 1999;25:15–17.

Willey A, Anderson RR, Azpiazu JL, et al. Complications of laser dermatologic surgery. *Lasers Surg Med.* 2006; 38(1):1–15.

Zelickson Z, Schram S, Zelickson B. Complications in cosmetic laser surgery: a review of 494 food and drug administration manufacturer and user facility device experience reports. *Dermatol Surg.* 2014;40(4):378–382.

# Index

Note: Page number followed by f and t indicates figure and table respectively.